Principles of Treatments in Multiple Sclerosis

Commissioning editor: Melanie Tait
Editorial assistant: Myriam Brearley
Production controller: Chris Jarvis
Desk editor: Angela Davies
Cover designer: Fred Rose

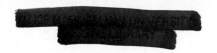

Principles of Treatments in Multiple Sclerosis

Edited by

Clive P. Hawkins, DM, FRCP
*Senior Lecturer in Neurology, Postgraduate Medical School, Keele University;
Consultant Neurologist, Royal Infirmary, Stoke on Trent, UK*

Jerry S. Wolinsky, MD
*Bartels Family Professor, Department of Neurology, University of Texas –
Houston, Health Science Center, Houston, Texas, USA*

Foreword by Ian McDonald, PhD, FRCP
*Professor Emeritus of Neurology, Institute of Neurology, University College,
London, UK*

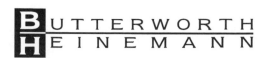

OXFORD AUCKLAND BOSTON JOHANNESBURG MELBOURNE NEW DELHI

Butterworth-Heinemann
Linacre House, Jordan Hill, Oxford OX2 8DP
225 Wildwood Avenue, Woburn, MA 01801-2041
A division of Reed Educational and Professional Publishing Ltd

ℜ A member of the Reed Elsevier plc group

First published 2000

**WL
360
P957
2000**

British Library Cataloguing in Publication Data
A catalogue record for this book is available from the British Library

Library of Congress Cataloguing in Publication Data
A catalogue record for this book is available from the Library of Congress

ISBN 0 7506 4270 X

Typeset by Avocet Typeset, Brill, Aylesbury, Bucks
Printed and bound in Great Britain by Anthony Rowe Ltd,
Reading and Chippenham

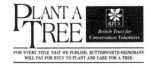

Contents

Foreword   vii

List of contributors   ix

Introduction   1

1 Pathogenesis and clinical subtypes of multiple sclerosis   2
   Clive Hawkins

Acute relapses   13

2 Treatment of acute relapses   14
   David Barnes

Disease modifying drugs – relapsing disease   23

3 Interferon beta-1b   24
   Donald Paty
4 Interferon beta-1a   38
   Lance Blumhardt
5 Glatiramer acetate   71
   Jerry Wolinsky
6 Immunoglobulins   95
   *Franz Fazekas, Ralf Gold, Hans-Peter Hartung and
   Siegrid Strasser-Fuchs*
7 Azathioprine   114
   Jacqueline Palace
8 Mitoxantrone   131
   Gilles Edan and Sean Morrissey

Disease modifying drugs – progressive disease   147

9 Treatments for progressive forms of MS   148
   Mariko Kita and Donald Goodkin

Disease modifying drugs – emerging therapies   163

10 Emerging therapies   164
   Charles Davie and David Miller

Disease modifying drugs – overview   **177**

11 Overview of treatment strategies for relapsing and progressive disease   178
     Clive Hawkins and Jerry Wolinsky

Symptomatic management   **183**

12 Management of spasticity – pharmacological agents   184
     Michael Barnes
13 Management of spasticity – botulinum toxin   201
     Anthony Ward
14 Symptomatic management: ataxia, tremor and fatigue   228
     Carolyn Young
15 The cause and management of bladder, sexual and bowel symptoms   258
     Iqbal Hussain and Clare Fowler
16 Neurobehavioural abnormalities   282
     Anthony Feinstein
17 Multidisciplinary approach   299
     Alan Thompson

Drug synonyms   **316**

Index   **318**

Foreword

A major change has taken place in the way in which patients and doctors alike view Multiple Sclerosis. It is now treatable: several agents have been approved which can modify the course of the disease and symptomatic treatment is much improved.

The course of Multiple Sclerosis is highly variable and clinical trials have been done in a variety of different ways. As a result the indications for treatment with particular agents may vary among the different forms of the disease and at different stages of it. The neurologist needs a readily accessible source which provides information for a whole range of treatments, about the mode of action, their indications, their use, their side effects, and their effectiveness. This the present volume provides in abundant measure. It is written by authors with wide experience of the disease and of the conduct of clinical trials in which the safety and efficacy of the treatments have been determined.

The treatment of Multiple Sclerosis involves much more than the use of drugs for specific manifestations of the disease such as acute relapse, tremor, spasticity or neuro-psychiatric impairment. A valuable aspect of the present book is the way in which it sets the contribution that individual treatments can make in the context of the comprehensive care and support of the patient.

Although much progress has been made in the last decade, it is unfortunately the case that present treatments are only partially effective. As the mechanism of the disease is understood better, new strategies are developed to deal with it. These issues are discussed and an indication is given where advances are likely to be made. The book provides an excellent account of the present position in relation to the treatment of Multiple Sclerosis and of the prospects for the future.

Professor Ian McDonald PhD, FRCP
Professor Emeritus of Neurology, Institute of
Neurology, University College, London, UK

List of contributors

David Barnes MD FRCP
Consultant Neurologist, Senior Lecturer, Atkinson Morley's
Hospital, Wimbledon, London, UK

Michael Barnes, MD FRCP
Professor of Neurological Rehabilitation, University of Newcastle-
upon-Tyne, UK

Lance D. Blumhardt, BSc MD FRACP FRCP
Professor of Clinical Neurology, University of Nottingham, UK

Charles Davie, MRCP MD (Hons)
Senior Lecturer, Royal Free & University College Medical School,
Royal Free Hospital, London, UK

Gilles Edan MD
Professor of Clinical Neurology, Head of the Neurological
Department, Centre Hospitalier Regional et Universitaire
De Rennes, France

Franz Fazekas, MD
Professor of Neurology, Department of Neurology and MRI
Center, Karl-Franzens University, Graz, Austria

Anthony Feinstein, MPhil PhD MRCPsych FRCPC
Associate Professor, Department of Psychiatry,
Sunnybrook Hospital, University of Toronto, Toronto, Ontario,
Canada

Clare J. Fowler, MBBS MSc FRCP
Reader and Consultant in Uro-Neurology, National Hospital for
Neurology and Neurosurgery, London, UK

Ralf Gold, MD
Associate Professor of Neurology, Department of Neurology,
Julius–Maximilians University, Würzburg, Germany

Donald E. Goodkin, MD
Associate Professor of Neurology, University of California,
San Francisco, USA

Hans-Peter Hartung, MD
Professor and Head, Department of Neurology, Karl-Franzens
University, Graz, Austria

Clive P. Hawkins, DM FRCP
Senior Lecturer in Neurology, Postgraduate Medical School, Keele
University
Consultant Neurologist, Royal Infirmary, Stoke on Trent, UK

Iqbal F. Hussain, BSc FRCS
Research Fellow in Uro-Neurology, National Hospital for
Neurology and Neurosurgery, and HST in Urology, Whittington
Hospital, London, UK

Mariko Kita, MD
Clinical Instructor, University of California, San Francisco, Mount
Zion Multiple Sclerosis Center, California, USA

David Miller, MBChB MD FRCP FRACP
Professor of Clinical Neurology, NMR Research Unit, Institute of
Neurology, The National Hospital, UK

Sean Morrissey, MD
Neurologist, Bezirksklinikum Regensburg, Universitats Str-84,
Germany

Jacqueline Palace, BM DM MRCP
Consultant Neurologist, Radcliffe Infirmary, Oxford, UK

Donald W. Paty, MD FRCPC
Professor, Division of Neurology, University of British Columbia,
Vancouver, Canada

Siegrid Strasser-Fuchs, MD
Assistant Professor of Neurology, Department of Neurology, Karl-
Franzens University, Graz, Austria

Alan J. Thompson, MD FRCP FRCPI
Garfield Weston Professor of Clinical Neurology and
Neurorehabilitation, Institute of Neurology, University College,
London, UK

Anthony Ward, BSc MB ChB FRCPE FRCP
Consultant in Rehabilitation Medicine, North Staffordshire
Rehabilitation Centre, Stoke on Trent, UK

Jerry S. Wolinsky, MD
Bartels Family Professor of Neurology, The University of Texas –
Houston, Health Science Center, Houston, Texas, USA

Carolyn Young, BSc MD FRCP
Consultant Neurologist, Walton Centre of Neurology and
Neurosurgery, Liverpool, UK

Introduction

Pathogenesis and clinical subtypes of multiple sclerosis

Introduction

There have been important recent developments in our understanding of the disease process in multiple sclerosis, which have led to a more rational approach to new treatments for the condition. In particular, the advent of magnetic resonance imaging (MRI) has allowed a more objective assessment of putative treatments and has helped to elucidate the pathological changes that occur with and without treatment. Previously there were a number of treatments that were of suggested benefit, although it was not until the last decade that major investment from the pharmaceutical industry resulted in clinical trials of drugs that have been shown to be of proven benefit in relapsing and progressive disease.

Multiple sclerosis

The definitive clinical and pathological description of multiple sclerosis (MS) was established in 1868 by Charcot. It usually follows a relapsing and remitting course, with progression of disability leading to visual loss, spastic weakness and ataxia (McDonald, 1986). The hallmarks of the condition are demyelination, inflammatory change and gliosis histologically (Charcot, 1868; Dawson, 1916; Perier and Gregoire, 1965; Allen, 1984; Prineas *et al.*, 1984; Adams *et al.*, 1985), progressing to a multifocal disorder of the central nervous system.

Aetiology

There is evidence for both genetic and environmental factors in the aetiology of the disease. Support for the former comes from family studies. The risk of developing MS in a monozygotic twin if the other twin is affected ranges from 21–50 per cent, whereas for a dizygotic twin the risk is lower at 0 17 per cent (Sawcer *et al.*, 1997). Thus the genetic contribution to the disease is thought to be in the region of 35 per cent. There is an association between MS and certain HLA groups, particularly DR2, DR4 and DQW1 (Batchelor *et al.*, 1978; Compston, 1986; Francis *et al.*, 1987a). Genome screens in MS have confirmed linkage with the major histocompatibility group on chromosome 6p21, and have also suggested linkage to chromosome 19q (Ebers *et al.*, 1996; Haines *et al.*, 1996; Sawcer *et al.*, 1996). Evidence for an environmental factor comes from migration studies; children migrating from a region of high risk to one of low risk have a lower incidence of the condition than migrating adults, suggesting that the disease may be conditioned by viral infection in childhood (Sawcer *et al.*, 1997). Further support for an environmental factor is provided by the 'epidemic' of MS that occurred in the Faroe Islands between 1943 and 1960, which was attributed to the influx of British troops during the Second World War (Kurtzke *et al.*, 1985).

Disease process

Considering the mechanism of the disease process, there are several lines of evidence to conclude that MS is an immune-mediated condition resulting from an abnormality of systemic immunity (Lisak, 1986; Hafler and Weiner, 1989; Waxman, 1998) or more localized central nervous system pathology (Esiri, 1980; Calder *et al.*, 1989). The nature of the immune antigen(s) is uncertain, although it is presumed to be a myelin antigen, and it is noticeable that a clinically similar condition involving the spinal cord and optic nerves (previously known as Jamaican myelopathy or tropical spastic paraparesis) was shown to be associated with slow virus infection (HTLV1) (Gessain *et al.*, 1985; Cruickshank *et al.*, 1990). Animal models of demyelination can be induced, as a result of viral infection, in which the chronic phase of demyelination is mediated by activated immune cells (Watanabe *et al.*, 1987).

In addition, there are parallels in the morphological (and probably the pathogenetic) characteristics between MS and the model of immune-mediated demyelination, experimental allergic encephalomyelitis (EAE) (Lassmann, 1983). In both conditions there is inflammatory demyelination and blood–brain barrier breakdown, with, in the chronic form of EAE, a relapsing remitting or progressive course. Genetic restriction operates in both, and there may be similar immune mechanisms; EAE is T-lymphocyte (CD4) mediated, and changes in peripheral blood lymphocyte subsets (for example, the CD4/CD8 ratio) are seen in MS (Lisak, 1986; Lassmann *et al.*, 1998). There is evidence for abnormal antibody production in EAE lesions, and oligoclonal IgG bands are a frequent finding in the cerebrospinal fluid in MS (Lassmann, 1983; Lisak, 1986). A breach of the blood–brain barrier in both conditions allows immune cells, particularly T-lymphocytes and monocytes, access to the relatively forbidden ground of the central nervous system (Wekerle *et al.*, 1986), with the potential for antigen presentation by locally resident cells including macrophages, microglia and astroglia.

Inflammation and barrier breakdown

Blood–brain barrier breakdown was observed in multiple sclerosis as long ago as the 1940s, when Broman showed leakage of Trypan blue into active plaques (and less so into chronic ones) after supravital injection (Broman, 1949, 1964). Other evidence for a central role of vascular changes in the evolution of the MS plaque came from Dawson (1916), who described finger-like projections of plaque along draining venules and veins, and Fog (1965), who established that virtually all lesions in the cerebral hemispheres are perivenular in distribution. Allen found changes of perivascular inflammation in the normal-appearing white matter of patients with mild or spinal MS (Allen *et al.*, 1981; Allen, 1984).

Vascular damage in MS and evidence for past blood–brain barrier breakdown was observed in many vessels in and around plaques by haemosiderin deposition, indicating past extravasation of red blood cells (Adams *et al.*, 1985; Adams, 1988). Adams indeed considered MS as a form of central nervous system venulitis or vasculitis (plasmatic vasculosis – Lendrum, 1963). The most convincing evidence that inflammatory and vascular changes can occur in the absence of myelin breakdown products in MS, and that demyelination is not a necessary precursor, comes from the observation that retinal periphlebitis with leakage of injected fluorescein (in an area generally devoid of myelin) is a frequent finding in patients with optic neuritis (Lightman *et al.*, 1987), which is often the presenting feature of MS (Compston *et al.*, 1978; McDonald, 1986; Francis *et al.*, 1987b).

With the advent of CT scanning and, later, magnetic resonance imaging (MRI), it was possible to visualize the MS lesion *in vivo* for the first time. Vascular changes were observed by MRI using the contrast agent gadolinium-DTPA (Gd-DTPA). Gd-enhancement was seen in patients with active disease (Grossman *et al.*, 1986; Kappos *et al.*, 1988; Miller *et al.*, 1988; Kermode *et al.*, 1990), and shown to be of relatively short duration – in general 2 weeks to 2 months (Miller *et al.*, 1988). In chronic relapsing EAE Gd-enhancement was similarly short-lived, and histological studies showed that areas of enhancement corresponded to blood–brain barrier breakdown and accompanying inflammatory change (perivascular inflammation) in the spinal cord (Hawkins *et al.*, 1990, 1991). Barrier breakdown in the chronic MS plaque may be due to vesicular transport of solute across the vascular endothelial cells, as appears to be the case in chronic relapsing EAE (Hawkins *et al.*, 1992).

Cytokines thought to be associated with breach of the blood–brain barrier include interleukin 1, tumour necrosis factor alpha and, possibly, interleukin 6, with sensitization of endothelial cells by interferon gamma (Brosnan *et al.*, 1992). Indeed, interferon beta has been shown to downregulate interferon gamma-induced MHC class II expression in cultures of human brain microvessels (Huynh *et al.*, 1995). Cell surface adhesion molecules, in particular the integrin receptor VLA-4 ($\alpha 4\beta 1$) on lymphocytes and monocytes which combines with VCAM on endothelial cells, are thought to be important in the trafficking of inflammatory cells across the blood–brain barrier (Cannella and Raine, 1995).

Demyelinating disease and MRI

Multiple sclerosis is therefore an inflammatory condition associated with demyelination, although whether or not inflammation and blood–brain barrier breakdown always lead to demyelination is uncertain. However, combined studies of Gd-enhancement with magnetic resonance spectroscopy to detect lipid peaks from myelin breakdown showed inflammation to be associated with active demyelination in most acute MS plaques, although lipid peaks were also seen independently of Gd-enhancement (Wolinsky *et al.*, 1990; Davie *et al.*, 1994; Narayana *et al.*, 1998). The mechanism of demyelination is generally thought to be macrophage-mediated (Prineas *et al.*, 1984), although in many plaques demyelination may be antibody-mediated (Linnington *et al.*, 1988; Lassmann *et al.*, 1998; Gemin *et al.*, 1999) and complement attack may be a contributory factor (Compston *et al.*, 1989). Lassmann (1998) has observed signs of oligo-dendrocyte dystrophy. Remyelination has been observed in MS plaques (Prineas and Connell, 1979; Lassmann *et al.*, 1997), and astrogliosis can be a prominent feature (Barnes *et al.*, 1991); it is unclear whether the latter is an active or passive response to tissue injury.

Internationally agreed Poser criteria require two episodes of inflammatory demyelination, affecting different sites of the central nervous system and sepa-rated by 1 month, to establish a diagnosis of clinically definite MS (Poser *et al.*, 1983). Brain MRI is abnormal in 95 per cent of patients with clinically definite MS (Ormerod *et al.*, 1987), having a characteristic appearance of multiple lesions in the periventricular and subcortical white matter of the brain (Paty *et al.*, 1988; Offenbacher *et al.*, 1993), and MRI can be used as a means of laboratory-supported diagnosis (including spinal cord images).

With isolated optic neuritis, brain stem disturbance or incomplete transverse myelitis of the type seen in MS, an MRI brain scan at the time of presentation will reveal white-matter lesions of variable extent in 60–70 per cent of cases. If patients are followed up for a period of 5 years, 60–70 per cent of those with an abnormal MRI brain scan at presentation will develop clinically definite MS, compared to less than 10 per cent with normal brain MRI (Morrissey *et al.*, 1993). This relationship is sustained at 10 years, with over 80 per cent of patients with an abnormal initial brain scan developing definite MS (O'Riordan *et al.*, 1998). Thus MRI is not only valuable in confirming a diagnosis of MS, but also a useful prognostic indicator; indeed, MRI is considered to be of value in moni-toring the evolution of pathological changes in MS in treatment trials (Paty and McFarland, 1998).

Different types of multiple sclerosis

In the majority of patients (up to 60 per cent or more), an initial relapsing and remitting course is followed by the development of progressive disability – sec-ondary progressive disease (SP). In a small group (up to 10–15 per cent), the con-dition is progressive from the onset (usually of the spinal type, progressive spastic paraparesis), without clinical relapses or remissions – primary progressive disease (PP). There is some evidence for immunogenetic differences between the two types of progressive MS (Olerup *et al.*, 1989). MRI has demonstrated differ-ences between the two groups (Thompson *et al.*, 1990); in a serial study with Gd-enhanced brain MRI scans, new lesions were frequent in the SP group and the majority showed Gd-enhancement. By contrast, there were fewer new lesions in the PP group and enhancement was unusual (Thompson *et al.*, 1991). These findings suggest that there may be a less marked inflammatory component in the evolution of new lesions in patients with PP as compared to SP disease, and this is supported by pathological findings (Revesz *et al.*, 1994). Thus it is important to study patients with primary and secondary progressive disease separately in treatment trials, as the pathogenetic mechanisms may be different. A proportion of patients, perhaps up to 20–30 per cent, have relatively benign MS and are minimally affected (Kurtzke EDSS 3 or less) 10 and 15 years or more after diagnosis (Lublin and Reingold, 1996). Putative treatments may be less important or the balance of risk and side effects of therapy outweigh potential benefits in this group of patients. The understanding of the natural course of multiple sclerosis has been interpreted and modified in the light of recent results from MRI studies (see Figure 1.1).

Progression of disability

Although multiple sclerosis has generally been considered to be a predominantly inflammatory demyelinating disease (Allen, 1984; Adams *et al.*, 1985; Miller *et al.*, 1988; Hawkins *et al.*, 1990), there is increasing evidence that axonal loss con-

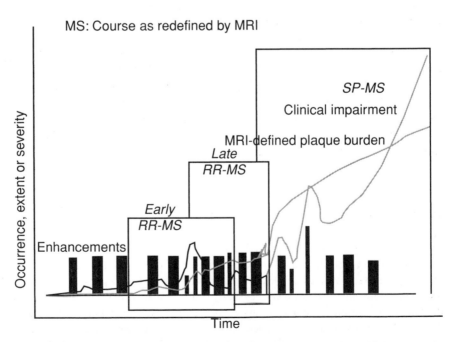

Figure 1.1 Multiple sclerosis: Course as redefined by MRI (by kind permission of J. Wolinsky).

tributes to the progression of disability in the condition. Spinal cord atrophy correlates with the degree of disability as measured by the Kurtzke EDSS, and magnetic resonance spectroscopy has shown a reduction in N-acetyl aspartate consistent with axonal loss and the expanded extracellular space seen at postmortem (Barnes *et al.*, 1991; Arnold *et al.*, 1992; Losseff *et al.*, 1996a; Edwards *et al.*, 1999). Axonal transection and damage has been a frequent finding in active inflammatory MS lesions (Ferguson *et al.*, 1997; Trapp *et al.*, 1998); indeed atrophy with axonal loss appears to be a relatively early finding in the condition (Losseff *et al.*, 1996b; Matthews *et al.*, 1998; Liu *et al.*, 1999). Whether axonal loss is conditioned by previous inflammatory episodes or is the result of continuing inflammation and demyelination is not clear. It is interesting to review the long-term progress of patients in the pivotal North American trial of interferon beta-1b in relapsing–remitting disease. Although there was suppression of disease activity by 80 per cent on MRI, and a favourable trend was evident, overall there was no major change in the progression of neurological disability after 5 years in the extended follow-up study (Paty *et al.*, 1993; IFNB MS Study Group, 1995). This raises the question of whether alternative mechanisms are responsible for disability. One potential mechanism would be damage to myelin and axons caused by products of oxidative stress, for example nitric oxide or more complex free radicals that are protected against by glutathione (Brosnan *et al.*, 1995; Smith *et al.*, 1999; Mann *et al.*, 2000). The continuing inflammatory process may be driven by the balance of cytokines in the plaque, for example Th1 cytokines (proinflammatory – TNF, IFN gamma and IL-2) compared to Th2 (anti-inflammatory – IL-4, IL-10 and TGF beta) (Hartung and Kieseier, 1996; Hohlfeld, 1997). TNF alpha is thought to contribute to the demyelinating process (Brosnan *et al.*, 1995). Interferon gamma, induced by interleukin 12, has been implicated in the chronic MS plaque (Hafler and Weiner, 1995). There is evidence from studies of genetic polymorphisms in MS to suggest that interleukin 1 beta is associated with a more severe disease course, and interleukin 1 receptor antagonist may protect against this (Mann *et al.*, 1997, 1998; Sciacca *et al.*, 1998).

Much of our current understanding of the pathogenesis of MS, the progression of disability and its treatment is dependent on the question of axonal loss, its causes and potential limitation. These important issues will be reviewed and expanded upon in several chapters of this book.

References

Adams, C. W. M. (1988). Perivascular iron deposition and other vascular damage in multiple sclerosis. *J. Neurol. Neurosurg. Psychiatr.*, **51**, 260–65.

Adams, C. W. M., Poston, R. N., Buk, S. J. *et al.* (1985). Inflammatory vasculitis in multiple sclerosis. *J. Neurol. Sci.*, **69**, 269–83.

Allen, I. V. (1984). Demyelinating diseases. In: *Greenfield's Neuropathology*, 4th edn (J. H. Adams, J. Corsellis and L. W. Duchen, eds), pp. 338–84. Edward Arnold.

Allen, I. V., Glover, G. and Anderson, R. (1981). Abnormalities in the macroscopically normal white matter in cases of mild or spinal multiple sclerosis. *Acta Neuropathol.* (**Suppl. VII**), 176–8.

Arnold, D. L., Mathews, P. M. and Francis, G. (1992). Proton magnetic resonance spectroscopic imaging for metabolic characterization of demyelinating plaques. *Ann. Neurol.*, **31**, 235–41.

Barnes, D., Munro, P. M. G. and Youl, B. D. (1991). The longstanding lesion in multiple sclerosis. *Brain*, **114**, 1271–80.

Batchelor, J. R., Compston, D. A. S. and McDonald, W. I. (1978). HLA and multiple sclerosis. The HLA system. *Br. Med. Bull.*, **34**, 279–84.

Broman, T. (1949). *The Permeability of the Cerebrospinal Vessels in Normal and Pathological Conditions*. Munksgaard.

Broman, T. (1964). Blood–brain barrier damage in multiple sclerosis: supravital test observations. *Acta Neurol. Scand.*, **40(Suppl. 10)**, 21–4.

Brosnan, C. F., Claudio, L. and Martiney, J. A. (1992). The blood–brain barrier during immune responses. *Semin. Neurosci.*, **4**, 193–200.

Brosnan, C. F., Cannella, B., Battistini, L. and Raine, C. S. (1995). Cytokine localization in multiple sclerosis lesions: correlation with adhesion molecule expression and reactive nitrogen species. *Neurology*, **45**, S16–21.

Calder, V., Owen, S., Watson, C. *et al.* (1989). MS: a localised immune disease of the central nervous system. *Immunol. Today*, **10**, 99–103.

Cannella, B. and Raine, C. S. (1995). The adhesion molecule profile and cytokine profile of multiple sclerosis lesions. *Ann. Neurol.*, **37**, 424–35.

Charcot, J.-M. (1868). Histologie de la sclerose en plaques. *Gazette Hôpital, Paris*, **41**, 554–5, 557–8, 566.

Compston, A. (1986). Genetic factors in the aetiology of multiple sclerosis. In: *Multiple Sclerosis* (W. I. McDonald and W. H. Silberberg, eds), pp. 56–73. Butterworths.

Compston, D. A. S., Batchelor, J. R., Earl, C. J. and McDonald, W. I. (1978). Factors influencing the risk of multiple sclerosis developing in uncomplicated optic neuritis. *Brain*, **101**, 495–511.

Compston, D. A., Morgan, B. P., Campbell, A. K. *et al.* (1989) Immunocytochemical localization of the terminal complement complex in multiple sclerosis. *Neuropathol. Appl. Neurobiol.*, **1b5**, 307–16.

Cruickshank, J. K., Richardson, J. H. and Morgan, O. St C. (1990). Screening for prolonged incubation of HTLV-I infection in British and Jamaican relatives of British patients with tropical spastic paraparesis. *Br. Med. J.*, **300**, 300–304.

Davie, C. A., Hawkins, C. P., Barker, G. J. *et al.* (1994). Serial proton magnetic resonance in acute multiple sclerosis lesions. *Brain*, **117**, 49–58.

Dawson, J. W. (1916). The histology of disseminated sclerosis. *Trans. R. Soc. Edinburgh*, **50**, 517–740.

Ebers, G. C., Kukay, K., Bulman, D. E. *et al.* (1996). A full genome search in multiple sclerosis. *Nat. Genet.*, **13**, 472–6.

Edwards, S. G., Gong, Q. Y., Liu, C. *et al.* (1999). Infratentorial atrophy on magnetic resonance imaging and disability in multiple sclerosis. *Brain*, **122(2)**, 291–301.

Esiri, M. M. (1980). Multiple sclerosis: a qualitative and quantitative study of immunoglobulin-containing cells in the central nervous system. *Neuropathol. Appl. Neurobiol.*, **6**, 9–21.

Ferguson, B., Matyszak, M. K., Esiri, M. M. and Perry, V. H. (1997). Axonal damage in acute multiple sclerosis lesions. *Brain*, **120**, 393–9.

Fog, T. (1965). The topography of plaques in multiple sclerosis. *Acta Neurol. Scand.*, **41(Suppl. 15)**, 7–16.

Francis, D. A., Batchelor, J. R., McDonald, W. I. *et al.* (1987a). Multiple sclerosis in north-east Scotland. An association with HLA–DQW1. *Brain*, **110**, 181–96.

Francis, D. A., Compston, D. A. S., Batchelor, J. R. and McDonald, W. (1987b). A reassessment of the risk of multiple sclerosis developing in patients with optic neuritis after extended follow-up. *J. Neurol. Neurosurg. Psychiatr.*, **50**, 758–65.

Gemin, C. P., Canella, B., Hauser, S. L. and Raine, C. S. (1999). Identification of autoantibodies associated with myelin damage in multiple sclerosis. *Nat. Med.*, **5**, 170–75.

Gessain, A., Barin, F. and Vernant, J. (1985). Antibodies to HTLV-I in patients with tropical spastic paraparesis. *Lancet*, **ii**, 407–9.

Grossman, R. I., Gonzalez-Scarano, F., Atlas, S. W. *et al.* (1986). Multiple sclerosis: gadolinium enhancement in MR imaging. *Radiology*, **161**, 721–5.

Hafler, D. A. and Weiner, H. L. (1989). MS: a CNS and systemic autoimmune disease. *Immunol. Today*, **10**, 104–7.

Hafler, D. A. and Weiner, H. L. (1995). Immunological mechanisms and therapy in multiple sclerosis (review). *Immunol. Rev.*, **144**, 75–107.

Haines, J. L., Ter-Minassian, M., Bazyk, A. *et al.* (1996). A complete genomic screen for multiple sclerosis underscores a role for the major histocompatibility complex. *Nat. Genet.*, **13**, 469–71.

Hartung, H. P. and Kieseier, B. C. (1996). Targets for the therapeutic action of interferon-beta in multiple sclerosis. *Ann. Neurol.*, **40**, 825–26.

Hawkins, C. P., Munro, P. M. G., Mackenzie, F. *et al.* (1990). Duration and selectivity of blood–brain barrier breakdown in chronic relapsing experimental allergic encephalomyelitis studied by gadolinium-DTPA and protein markers. *Brain*, **113**, 365–78.

Hawkins, C. P., MacKenzie, F., Tofts, P. *et al.* (1991). Patterns of blood–brain barrier breakdown in inflammatory demyelination. *Brain*, **114**, 801–10.

Hawkins, C. P., Munro, P. G. M., Landon, D. N. and McDonald, W. I. (1992). Metabolically dependent blood–brain barrier breakdown in chronic relapsing experimental allergic encephalomyelitis. *Acta Neuropathol.*, **83**, 630–35.

Hohlfeld, R. (1997). Biotechnical agents for the immunotherapy of multiple sclerosis. Principles, problems and perspectives. *Brain*, **120**, 865–916.

Huynh, H. K., Oger, J. and Dorovini-Zis, K. (1995). Interferon-b downregulates interferon-induced class II MHC molecule expression and morphological changes in primary cultures of human brain microvessel endothelial cells. *J. Neuroimmunol.*, **60**, 63–73.

IFNB Multiple Sclerosis Study Group and the University of British Colombia MS/MRI Analysis Group (1995). Interferon beta-1b in the treatment of multiple sclerosis: final outcome of the randomized, controlled trial. *Neurology*, **45**, 1277–85.

Kappos, L., Stadt, D., Roharbach, E. and Keil, W. (1988). Gadolinium-DTPA enhanced magnetic resonance imaging in the evaluation of different disease courses and disease activity in MS. *Neurology*, **38(Suppl. 1)**, 255.

Kermode, A. G., Tofts, P. S., Thompson, A. J. *et al.* (1990). Heterogeneity of blood–brain barrier changes in multiple sclerosis. *Neurology*, **40**, 229–36.

Kurtzke, J. F., Beebe, G. W. and Norman, J. E. (1985). Epidemiology of multiple sclerosis in United States veterans. III. Migration and the risk of MS. *Neurology*, **35**, 672–8.

Lassmann, H. (1983). *Comparative Neuropathology of Chronic Experimental Allergic Encephalomyelitis and Multiple Sclerosis*. Springer-Verlag.

Lassmann, H. (1998). Neuropathology in multiple sclerosis: new concepts. *Multiple Sclerosis*, **4(3)**, 93–8.

Lassmann, H., Bruck, W., Lucchinetti, C. and Rodriguez, M. (1997). Remyelination in multiple sclerosis. *Multiple Sclerosis*, **3(2)**, 133–6.

Lassmann, H., Raine, C. S., Antel, J. and Prineas, J. W. (1998). Immunopathology of multiple sclerosis. *J. Neuroimmunol.*, **96**, 213–17.

Lendrum, A. C. (1963). The hypertensive diabetic kidney as a model of the so-called collagen diseases. *J. Can. Med. Assoc.*, **88**, 442–52.

Lightman, S., McDonald, W. I., Bird, A. C. *et al.* (1987). Retinal venous sheathing in optic neuritis: its significance for the pathogenesis of multiple sclerosis. *Brain*, **110**, 405–14.

Linnington, C., Bradl, M. and Lassmann, H. (1988). Augmentation of demyelination in rat acute allergic encephalomyelitis by circulating mouse monoclonal antibodies directed against a myelin/oligodendrocyte glycoprotein. *Am. J. Pathol.*, **130**, 443–54.

Lisak, R. P. (1986). Immunological abnormalities. In: *Multiple Sclerosis* (W. I. McDonald and D. H. Silberberg, eds), pp. 74–98. Butterworths.

Liu, C., Edwards, S., Gong, Q. *et al.* (1999). Three-dimensional MRI estimates of brain and spinal cord atrophy in multiple sclerosis. *J. Neurol. Neurosurg. Psychiatr.*, **66(3)**, 323–30.

Losseff, N. A., Webb, S. L., O'Riordan, J. I. *et al.* (1996a). Spinal cord atrophy and disability in multiple sclerosis. A new reproducible and sensitive MRI method with potential to monitor disease progression. *Brain*, **119**, 701–8.

Losseff, N. A., Wang, L., Lai, H. M. *et al.* (1996b). Progressive cerebral atrophy in multiple sclerosis. A serial MRI study. *Brain*, **119(6)**, 2009–19.

Lublin, F. D. and Reingold, S. C. (1996). Defining the clinical course of multiple sclerosis: results of an international survey. *Neurology*, **46**, 907–10.

Mann, C. L. A., Hutchinson, J., Davies, M. B. *et al.* (1997). Polymorphisms in the interleukin-1 receptor antagonist gene related to disability in multiple sclerosis. *J. Neurol.*, **244**, S40.

Mann, C. L. A., Davies, M. B., Boggild, M. D. *et al.* (1998). The association of 5 polymorphisms at the IL-1 gene cluster with prognosis in a cohort of 400 multiple sclerosis patients. *Multiple Sclerosis*, **4**, 355.

Mann, C. L. A., Davies, M. B., Boggild, M. D. *et al.* (2000). Glutathione-S-

Transferase gene polymorphisms and their relationship to disability in multiple sclerosis. *Neurology*, **54**, 552–57.

Matthews, P. M., De Stefano, N., Naratanan, S. *et al.* (1998). Magnetic resonance spectroscopy studies in context: axonal damage and disability in multiple sclerosis. *Sem. Neurol.*, **18**, 327–36.

McDonald, W. I. (1986). Gowers Lecture. The mystery of the origin of multiple sclerosis. *J. Neurol. Neurosurg. Psychiatr.*, **49(2)**, 113–23.

Miller, D. H., Rudge, P., Johnson, G. *et al.* (1988). Serial gadolinium-enhanced magnetic resonance imaging in multiple sclerosis. *Brain*, **111**, 927–39.

Morrissey, S. P., Miller, D. H., Kendall, B. E. *et al.* (1993). The significance of brain magnetic resonance imaging abnormalities at presentation with clinically isolated syndromes suggestive of multiple sclerosis. *Brain*, **116**, 135–46.

Narayana, P. A., Doyle, T. J., Lai, D. *et al.* (1998). Serial proton magnetic resonance spectroscopic imaging, contrast-enhanced magnetic resonance imaging, and quantitative lesion volumetry in multiple sclerosis. *Ann. Neurol.*, **43(1)**, 56–71.

Offenbacher, H., Fazekas, F., Schmidt, R. *et al.* (1993). Assessment of MRI criteria for diagnosis of MS. *Neurology*, **43**, 905–9.

Olerup, O., Hillert, J., Fredrikson, S. *et al.* (1989). Primarily chronic progressive and relapsing/remitting multiple sclerosis: Two immunogenetically distinct disease entities. *Proc. Natl. Acad. Sci. USA*, **86**, 7113–17.

O'Riordan, J. I., Thompson, A. J., Kingsley, D. P. E. *et al.* (1998). The more prognostic value of brain MRI in clinically isolated syndromes of the CNS. A 10-year follow-up. *Brain*, **121**, 495–503.

Ormerod, I. E. C., Miller, D. H., McDonald, W. I. *et al.* (1987). The role of NMR imaging in the assessment of multiple sclerosis and isolated neurological lesions. *Brain*, **110**, 1570–1616.

Paty, D. W. and McFarland, H. (1998). Magnetic resonance techniques to monitor the long-term evolution of multiple sclerosis pathology and to monitor definitive clinical trials. *J. Neurol. Neurosurg. Psychiatr.*, **64**, S47–S51.

Paty, D. W., Oger, J. J. F., Kastrukoff, L. F. *et al.* (1988). MRI in the diagnosis of MS: a prospective study with comparison of clinical evaluation, evoked potentials, oligoclonal banding and CT. *Neurology*, **38**, 180–85.

Paty, D. W., Li, D. K. B., UBC MS/MRI Study Group and IFNB Multiple Sclerosis Study Group (1993). Interferon beta-1b is effective in relapsing-remitting multiple sclerosis. II. MRI analysis results of a multi-centre, randomised, double-blind, placebo-controlled trial. *Neurology*, **43**, 662–7.

Perier, O. and Gregoire, A. (1965). Electron microscope features of multiple sclerosis lesions. *Brain*, **88**, 937–52.

Poser, C. M., Paty, D. W., Scheinburg, L. *et al.* (1983). New diagnostic criteria for multiple sclerosis: guidelines for research protocols. *Ann. Neurol.*, **13**, 227–31.

Prineas, J. W. and Connell, F. (1979). Remyelination in multiple sclerosis. *Ann. Neurol.*, **5**, 22–31.

Prineas, J. W., Kwon, E. E., Cho, E.-S. and Scharer, L. R. (1984). Continual breakdown and regeneration of myelin in progressive multiple sclerosis plaques. *Ann. NY Acad. Sci.*, **436**, 11–32.

Revesz, T., Kidd, D. and Thompson, A. J. (1994). A comparison of the pathology of primary and secondary progressive multiple sclerosis. *Brain*, **117**, 756–65.

Sawcer, S. J., Jones, H. B., Feakes, R. *et al.* (1996). A genome screen in multiple sclerosis reveals susceptibility loci on chromosomes 6p21 and 17q22. *Nat. Genet.*, **13**, 464–8.

Sawcer, S. J., Robertson, N. and Compston, A. (1997). Genetic epidemiology of multiple sclerosis. In: *Multiple Sclerosis; Clinical Challenges and Controversies* (A. J. Thompson, C. Polman and R. Hohlfeld, eds), pp. 13–34. Martin Dunitz.

Sciacca, F. L., Ferri, C., Gobbi, C. *et al.* (1998). Soluble interleukin-1 receptor antagonist intron 2 polymorphism is associated with occurrence and clinical disability in patients with multiple sclerosis. *J. Neurol.*, **245**, 355.

Smith, K. J., Kapoor, R. and Felts, P. A. (1999). Demyelination: the role of reactive oxygen and nitrogen species. *Brain Pathol.*, **9**, 69–92.

Thompson, A. J., Kermode, A. G., MacManus, D. G. *et al.* (1990). Patterns of disease activity in multiple sclerosis: clinical and magnetic resonance imaging study. *Br. Med. J.*, **300**, 631–4.

Thompson, A. J., Kermode, A. G., Wicks, D. *et al.* (1991). Major differences in the dynamics of primary and secondary progressive multiple sclerosis. *Ann. Neurol.*, **29**, 53–62.

Trapp, B. D., Peterson, J., Ransohoff, R. M. *et al.* (1998). Axonal transection in the lesions of multiple sclerosis. *N. Engl. J. Med.*, **338(5)**, 278–85.

Watanabe, R., Wege, H. and Ter Meulen, V. (1987). Comparative analysis of corona virus JHM-induced demyelinating encephalomyelitis in Lewis and Brown Norway rats. *Lab. Invest.*, **37**, 375–84.

Waxman, S. (1998). Demyelinating diseases: new pathological insights, new therapeutic targets. *N. Engl. J. Med.*, **338**, 323–5.

Wekerle, H., Linington, C., Lassman, H. and Meyermann, H. (1986). Cellular immune reactivity within the CNS. *Trends Neurosci*, **9**, 271–7..

Wolinsky, J. S., Narayana, P. A. and Fenstermacher, M. J. (1990). Proton magnetic resonance spectroscopy in multiple sclerosis. *Neurology*, **40**, 1764–79.

Acute relapses

2

Treatment of acute relapses

Introduction

In clinical practice, the management of relapses in MS has two components; that of the relapse itself, with glucocorticoid (steroid) preparations, and that of the resulting symptoms. The former will be discussed in this chapter. Despite the ubiquitous prescription of steroids by doctors involved in the management of patients with MS in relapse, there are several important areas of uncertainty in the medical literature concerning this practice. As a result, there is relatively little concordance amongst doctors with respect to when and to whom steroids should be given, and which regimen to use. This chapter summarizes the available information concerning the probable mechanisms of action of steroids in MS relapse, the efficacy data in different disease types, and current prescribing habits amongst UK neurologists. Finally, some practical guidelines for the use of steroids in MS are proposed.

Possible modes of action of steroids in MS

Steroids were first heralded as being of therapeutic value in human diseases when Hench postulated the existence of 'substance X' in 1925, and reported cortin's ability to cure rheumatoid arthritis in 1949. In those days Nobel prizes were awarded on the basis of the previous year's events, and it was only over the next couple of years that Hench, having received his, found the effect was not sustained and that side effects were significant. The Nobel committee thereafter extended the period of its deliberations!

It is known from various lines of evidence, and as described elsewhere in this book, that relapses in MS are associated with immunologically-mediated damage to the blood–brain barrier at an early stage in the evolution of lesions. Further events, centred on activated T-cells, involve the upregulation and expression of adhesion molecule and cytokine systems and the recruitment of non-specific T-cells and macrophages.

Experimental and human studies have shown that glucocorticoids have wide-ranging effects on the immune system, mediated by the type II glucocorticoid receptor (Pitzalis *et al.*, 1997). These effects include:

1. Demarginating neutrophils, raising the peripheral white cell count and inducing eosinophil apoptosis (programmed cell death)
2. Decreasing class II antigen expression in macrophages and suppressing cytokine, leukotriene and prostaglandin production
3. Causing redistribution of T-lymphocytes, inducing apoptosis in mature T-cells, and decreasing their activation, helper capacity, cytotoxicity and suppression
4. Inhibiting the production and activity of pro-inflammatory cytokines, including some interferons (IL-1, IL-2 and IL-6)
5. Inhibiting endothelial cell activity, particularly in relation to adhesion molecule expression (including ICAM-1, VCAM-1 and ELAM-1) and adhesion molecule receptor expression on T-cells.

Some of these actions (such as T-cell adhesion molecule expression) may not be reflected in serum levels of these substances in human disease, and they are therefore difficult to implicate with certainty in MS relapses. Nevertheless, it is possible to summarize by stating that: steroids display potent immunosuppressant activity, which, by a variety of possible (but largely unproven) mechanisms, may ameliorate the disease process in MS when in relapse.

Perhaps one of their most important effects in MS is that of stabilization of the damaged blood–brain barrier. There is considerable MRI evidence to indicate that this effect of steroids on the blood–brain barrier is at least partly responsible for their beneficial effects in MS relapses (Miller *et al.*, 1988; Gasperini *et al.*, 1998). Gd-enhanced images show an almost complete disappearance of the enhancement within hours of the first dose, which indicates reversal of the blood–brain barrier leakage associated with acute lesions. However, this effect is lost within hours of stopping the steroid treatment, and cannot therefore be the sole mechanism whereby steroids accelerate clinical recovery from relapses. This is also indicated by the observation that longer steroid courses (for example, 3 weeks) are not significantly more effective than shorter ones (3 days).

The clinical efficacy of steroids in MS relapses

The simpest way of summarizing the usefulness of steroids in the context of MS is to say that they have been shown to shorten the recovery time of relapses, but they do not generally appear to influence the ultimate degree of recovery or to have any influence on the longer-term natural history of the disease.

The first form of steroid therapy to enjoy widespread use in MS was adrenocorticotrophic hormone (ACTH). The problem with the ACTH form of steroid therapy was that it caused unselected release of steroids from the adrenal glands in unpredictable quantities. Unfortunately, there were no good data at the time regarding the efficacy of ACTH to justify its use or to allow comparison with other forms of steroids.

Gradually, however, studies were published that first suggested and then proved the efficacy of steroids in hastening recovery from relapse, and by the 1970s steroids were an accepted form of treatment in MS. Over the next 20 years, clinical and then MRI data emerged that confirmed their efficacy and suggested that at least some of the possible mechanisms of action already discussed may be important.

Several studies have demonstrated the superiority of steroids over placebo in shortening recovery from relapses, though the best regimens remain unclear. One of the first controlled trials of ACTH for the treatment of relapses showed significant improvement in 11 of 22 patients by the end of the 3-week trial period, compared with 4 of 18 in the control group (Miller *et al.*, 1961). This result was reproduced in a similar study of 197 MS patients (Rose *et al.*, 1970). In the latter trial the proportion of treated patients improved significantly at each time interval; the largest differences were observed at 2 weeks, when 57 per cent of treated and 38 per cent of control patients improved, and at 4 weeks (65 per cent and 48 per cent respectively).

By the mid-1980s, the general perception of steroids in MS was that ACTH was less predictable and no more effective than other regimens, and it was therefore dropped from general usage. Intravenous methylprednisolone (IVMP) was shown in trials to be at least as effective as ACTH, and took its place. One trial directly compared the efficacy of ACTH and IVMP, and was unable to demonstrate a difference between the two treatment groups (Thompson *et al.*, 1989).

More recently, various low- and high-dose oral steroid regimens have been the subject of numerous reports that suggest that, as well as being less expensive and more convenient, they are probably safer in terms of side effects than IVMP. The most recent, from Denmark, described a randomized study of 25 patients in relapse treated with placebo and 26 treated with oral methylprednisolone, 500 mg for 5 days followed by a 10-day oral taper. Their results strongly favoured the treated group over an 8-week period (Sellebjerg *et al.*, 1998). How oral MP and IVMP compare with regard to efficacy is still not fully established. Alam *et al.* (1993) compared identical doses (500 mg a day for 5 consecutive days) of oral MP and IVMP in small groups of patients, and was unable to show any differences between them. Nevertheless, there is still an intuitive impression amongst neurologists that the IVMP regimens are somehow better.

In a attempt to test this hypothesis, Barnes *et al.* (1997) devised and reported a study of 80 patients treated with either IVMP (1 g for 5 days) or oral MP (48 mg for 7 days, 24 mg for 7 days and 12 mg for 7 days). Several outcome measures were used, none of which showed any significant benefit of either regimen, at any time interval.

Although many of these studies, especially the earlier ones, are open to criticism, the fact remains that none of them have been able to demonstrate any long-term implications for the use of steroids in MS relapses, either in terms of improving the outcome of relapses or of long-term disability. However the same cannot be said for the studies of optic neuritis.

With the publication of the optic neuritis treatment trial in 1992 came the suggestion that, even allowing for pre-study differences in brain MRI appearances, patients treated with low-dose oral prednisone seemed to have a greater likelihood of developing clinically definite MS at 6 months (Beck *et al.*, 1993). This observation, though not an original endpoint of the study, did carry conviction, and many clinicians – particularly in Canada and the USA – significantly modified their steroid prescribing for MS. However, when the 3-year follow-up data were published any observed difference seemed to have disappeared (Beck, 1995), and the concern about the use of low-dose steroids in MS has diminished although not completely disappeared.

Other studies of optic neuritis have suggested that in some subgroups steroids may beneficially affect recovery of vision. Those patients with longer lesions of the optic nerve on MRI and those with intra-canalicular disease evident on MRI seem to do worse, and steroids probably improve their eventual visual outcome. However, these patients are difficult to distinguish clinically, and a more recent study has suggested that is not the case (Kapoor *et al.*, 1998).

To summarize the evidence concerning the use of steroids in relapses of MS; they are effective in hastening recovery from clinical relapse but do not usually benefit eventual outcome, either in terms of degree of recovery or subsequent disease activity. In certain patients with optic neuritis, however, recovery may be improved by steroids. The best regimen remains undecided, but there is good evidence to show that both oral and IV treatments are effective; there are no controlled data showing superiority of one over the other at any dosage in MS. It does appear, however, that optic neuritis, when isolated, seems more responsive to higher than to lower dose regimens.

Clinical efficacy of steroids for progressive MS

It is now common practice to use steroids for MS relapses, but the situation in other types of MS is not well documented. Trials are needed, as there are no proper data for the treatment of progressive MS with continuous steroid therapy over a number of years. Long-term steroids are therefore not currently indicated for either primary or secondary progressive MS, as they are of no proven benefit and are potentially harmful in the long term. Any consideration of longer-term steroid use in MS is inappropriate with the current state of knowledge – in other words, the potential risks outweigh the potential benefits.

The only exception to this rule is the very rare patient with true steroid-dependency, in whom withdrawal leads to an objective neurological deterioration rather than just a feeling of malaise. Such patients are uncommon, and it may be difficult to be sure that some other process such as sarcoidosis or a vasculitis is not responsible.

Having stated that long-term steroids currently have no place in the management of MS, many clinicians feel that no patient with progressive neurological disability due to MS should be allowed to worsen without being given a course of steroids at least once; the response is sometimes worthwhile and the risk is minimal. It is not always easy to make a judgement regarding the pattern of the disease, and some patients who appear to be progressing are in fact having relapses. It is cases such as these that lend justification to the policy – not universally held – of giving steroids to every MS sufferer at least once.

A few studies have suggested that some patients with secondary progressive MS do seem to benefit from a 3- or 4-monthly course of oral prednisolone, even though steroids are not generally used in progressive MS unless there is a super-imposed relapse of sufficient severity to justify their prescription. This policy is supported by the sparse literature available on the subject, which suggests that there may be benefit in the short or medium term, particularly in pyramidal function from regular steroid courses.

Current practice amongst UK neurologists

It is clear that the majority of relapses in MS patients never come to the attention of the specialist. Many patients either do not mention less severe attacks or they contact their GPs, who may give them an oral course of steroids without reference to the local neurologist. It is therefore unknown to whom, in what form, and how frequently steroids are actually given in MS. However, in these days of evidence-based medicine it is important to understand the current situation among specialists in a field. This knowledge allows determination of the extent to which the evidence that does exist is incorporated into clinical practice, and identification of those areas where more evidence is clearly needed.

To this end, two recent surveys of UK neurologists have been carried out, the first by a group in Cardiff and the second in London (Tremlett *et al.*, 1998; Barnes, unpublished data). The results of these surveys can be summarized as follows:

1. Nearly all respondents agreed that steroids are effective in shortening recovery from relapses, but the majority disagreed with the suggestion that they may improve the eventual outcome of a relapse. About 80 per cent said they prescribed steroids in more than a quarter of all relapses, and less than 5 per cent never used steroids. More than 50 per cent always, and 99 per cent sometimes, used IVMP as the steroid of first choice. Conversely, only 5 per cent used oral steroids routinely as their first choice, and 70 per cent rarely if ever used oral steroids in MS. Curiously, there was an even split over the question of whether IVMP was superior to oral MP; presumably the continued preference for IVMP indicated a feeling that IV should be better, a lack of conviction concerning the available comparative data, and habit. It was interesting to note that despite the publication in 1997 of the paper indicating no significant difference between oral and IV steroid efficacy (Barnes *et al.*, 1997), there was no notable change in the proportion of each prescribed between 1996 and 1998.
2. There was little evidence of fixed policies where steroid prescribing is concerned; only 20 per cent of neurologists admitted always to following one. The regimens of IVMP used varied considerably from 250 mg to 1000 mg daily for anything from 2–5 days, the most common being 1 g daily for 3 days or 0.5 g daily for 5 days. Very few UK neurologists, however, used an oral taper after the IV course. It appears that few patients refuse the offer of steroids, and that admission to hospital solely for IVMP is becoming less popular, although about a third of neurologists arranged this at least some of the time.

Conversely, the majority of IVMP courses are administered to inpatients, so presumably these patients have the worst attacks, justifying admission. When oral steroids were used prednisolone was the preferred agent, although some routinely used oral dexamethasone or methylprednisolone. The latter probably has the best claim to usage, if the recently published report of its very clear superiority (in high dose) over placebo is correct. In this study the actively treated patients did significantly better at 1, 3 and 8 weeks after initiation of treatment, according to a number of measures including the EDSS and Scripps neurological rating scale (Sellebjerg *et al.*, 1998).

3. The majority of neurologists indicated that they try to limit the number of courses any one patient receives in a given 12-month period. This policy presumably reflects a concern over the cumulative side effects of steroids. The majority of neurologists disagreed with the routine prescription of steroids for relapses in MS by GPs, although a significant minority had no such objection. Most were in the habit of reviewing the outcome of a course of steroids given for MS relapse.

4. Respondents were almost unanimous that, with the current state of knowledge, there is no place for long-term steroid use in MS. Nearly a quarter, however, felt that there is a place for steroids in MS other than for relapses. A separate question asked whether every patient with MS should have at least one course of steroids to assess responsiveness, a suggestion with which just over half disagreed. Response was mixed regarding truly steroid-dependent patients with MS, with only a small majority favouring their existence.

Practical guidelines for the use of steroids for MS relapse

When considering which relapses should be treated with steroids (with the patient's approval), it is not particularly important to consider how often they have been given in the past. In general, however, it is sensible to limit the number of courses to three a year if possible, though there are no good data indicating that more are harmful in the long term. There is also no clear association between IVMP courses and a reduction in bone density. Some patients may require more to be optimally treated, but it is not good practice to prescribe steroids indiscriminately for MS relapses. The decision should be dictated, at least in part, by the severity of the attack and the amount of disability and handicap it produces. What will be disabling for one individual may only be an inconvenience for another, and non-disabling attacks almost always recover satisfactorily without treatment.

The type of attack should also be considered; whilst it is generally thought that steroids do not influence outcome, some attacks may do better with them. For example, severe optic neuritis with complete visual loss is sometimes caused by an unusually long lesion on the optic nerve or involvement of the nerve in the bony canal. In these cases, steroids may improve the outcome and should be considered. Another example is an attack affecting cerebellar function. Ataxia and dysmetria are among the most disabling manifestations of MS, and fixed disability of this type carries a very poor long-term prognosis. Steroids should be considered for any attack that causes significant cerebellar involvement. These considerations are to some extent based on personal experience and preference, but in the absence of hard data, decisions must be taken in the best interests of the patient.

Regarding the type of steroid and its dosage, surveys indicate that in the UK the two most popular regimens for IV and oral steroids are:

1. IVMP 1 g daily for 3 days, or 0.5 g for 5 days
2. Oral prednisolone tapering from 60 mg over about 3 weeks, for example 60, 45, 30, 15 and 5 mg each for 5 days.

However, there is both clinical and experimental evidence from at least two controlled trials justifying consideration of the routine prescription of high-dose oral methylprednisolone (for example 500 mg for 5 days), as used by Sellebjerg *et al.* (1998).

Some but not all trials have suggested that an oral taper after a high-dose IV course of steroids may reduce disease progression and the recurrence of relapse. As yet, however, the use of an oral taper remains a matter of personal preference – it is more popular in the USA and less so in Europe – and higher doses and longer courses of both IV and oral steroids are not uncommonly prescribed.

At present, therefore, the listed regimens (or minor modifications of them) remain standard in most parts of the world, and significant changes to routine practice should only be introduced on the basis of proper controlled, blinded and randomized trials demonstrating a significant benefit of higher total doses, longer courses, or both.

Summary

In summary, there is clear evidence to support the use of steroids in relapses of MS; they hasten recovery, but do not, in general, improve the eventual outcome. There are no universally agreed protocols concerning which type of steroid or the dosage to use, but most clinicians use high-dose IVMP as first choice. A minority use oral prednisolone, although recent evidence supports the prescription of higher-dose methylprednisolone as the oral steroid of first choice.

Relapses should be treated on their merits, with a decision being taken on the basis of relapse severity and type, and the amount of disability and handicap it produces in that individual. There is no place for the indiscriminate use of steroids for all relapses; indeed, probably no more than 10–20 per cent of all relapses merit their use.

Regarding progressive MS, there is no evidence to support the use of steroids in these groups of patients. However, if there is any doubt about the pattern of disease in a deteriorating patient it is reasonable to recommend that steroids be tried at least once, as the risk is small. There is also a lack of evidence concerning the long-term use of steroids in MS, and they should not be used in this way except in the rare patient with true steroid dependency. Some evidence exists to suggest that oral pulses of steroid may be of benefit in secondary progressive MS in the medium term.

There is much further work that could be done in this field, but it is unlikely that many individuals will be enthusiastic, particularly with the emergence of more compounds with the potential to affect the natural history of the disease. Nevertheless, steroids have underpinned the management of MS attacks for over three decades, and should still be considered a useful weapon in the fight against the condition.

References

Alam, S. M., Kyriakides, T., Lowden, M. and Newman, P. K. (1993). Methylprednisolone in multiple sclerosis: a comparison of oral with intravenous therapy at equivalent high dose. *J. Neurol. Neurosurg. Psychiatr.*, **56**, 1219–20.

Barnes, D., Hughes, R. A. C., Morris, R. W. *et al.* (1997). Randomised trial of oral and intravenous methylprednisolone in acute relapses of multiple sclerosis. *Lancet*, **349**, 902–6.

Beck, R. W. (1995). The Optic Neuritis Treatment Trial: three-year follow-up results. *Arch. Ophthalmol.*, **113**, 136–7.

Beck, R. W., Cleary, P. A., Trobe, J. D. *et al.* (1993). The effect of corticosteroids in acute optic neuritis on the subsequent development of multiple sclerosis. *N. Engl. J. Med.*, **329**, 1764–9.

Gasperini, C., Pozzilli, C., Bastianello, S. *et al.* (1998). Effect of steroids on Gd-enhancing lesions before and during recombinant interferon beta-1a treatment in relapsing remitting multiple sclerosis. *Neurology*, **50**, 403–6.

Kapoor, R., Miller, D. H., Jones, S. J. *et al.* (1998). Effects of intravenous methylprednisolone on outcome in MRI-based prognostic subgroups in acute optic neuritis. *Neurology*, **50(1)**, 230–37.

Miller, H., Newell, D. J. and Ridley, A. (1961). Multiple sclerosis: treatment of acute exacerbations with corticotropin (ACTH). *Lancet*, **2**, 1120–22.

Miller, D. H., Rudge, P., Johnson, G. *et al.* (1988). Serial gadolinium-enhanced magnetic resonance imaging in multiple sclerosis. *Brain*, **111**, 927–39.

Pitzalis, C., Sharrack, B., Gray, I. A. *et al.* (1997). Comparison of the effects of oral versus intravenous methylprednisolone regimens on peripheral T lymphocyte adhesion molecule expression, T-cell subsets distribution and TNF alpha concentrations in multiple sclerosis. *J. Neuroimmunol.*, **74**, 62–8.

Rose, A. S., Kuzma, J. W., Kurtzke, J. F. *et al.* (1970). Cooperative study in the evaluation of therapy in multiple sclerosis: ACTH versus placebo: final report. *Neurology*, **20(Suppl. 1)**, 1–59.

Sellebjerg, F., Frederiksen, J. L., Nielsen, P. M. and Olesen, J. (1998). Double-blind randomized, placebo-controlled study of oral high-dose methylprednisolone in attacks of MS. *Neurology*, **51**, 529–34.

Thompson, A. J., Kennard, C., Swash, M. *et al.* (1989). Relative efficacy of intravenous methylprednisolone and ACTH in the treatment of acute relapses in MS. *Neurology*, **39**, 969–71.

Tremlett, H. L., Luscombe, D. K. and Wiles, C. M. (1998). Use of corticosteroids in multiple sclerosis by consultant neurologists in the United Kingdom. *J. Neurol. Neurosurg. Psychiatr.*, **65(3),** 362–5.

Disease modifying drugs – relapsing disease

3

Interferon beta-1b

History of interferon beta therapy in multiple sclerosis

In the late 1970s and early 1980s, Larry Jacobs began to perform MS studies using interferon beta (Jacobs *et al.*, 1986). At first, a small dose was administered intrathecally, and there were several uncontrolled studies followed by a controlled study using natural human interferon beta. The results were very interesting, and the Chiron Company therefore developed a recombinant interferon beta molecule that could be given systemically and safely to humans, and this drug was tried in MS. The generic name of the molecule was interferon beta-1b, known as Betaseron® in North America and Betaferon® in the rest of the world.

The molecule

The interferons are one group in a large network of intercellular messengers known as cytokines. They have overlapping but distinct biological qualities/activities. In general, the interferons have antiviral, antiproliferative, anti-tumour, and immunomodulatory properties (Reder, 1997).

There are two types of interferon:

1. Type I, which includes interferons alpha and beta
2. Type II, which is interferon gamma.

Interferon beta-1b was genetically engineered from normal human interferon beta. It contains 165 amino acids and has a molecular weight of 18 500 daltons. The differences between interferon beta-1b and natural interferon beta are as follows:

1. Interferon beta-1b has a serine residue placed at position 17 in place of the normally found cysteine
2. Interferon beta-1b is not glycosylated, whereas natural human interferon is glycosylated
3. Interferon beta-1b lacks the terminal methionine residue that occurs at position 1 in the native molecule.

The genetic engineering feat noted in (1) above was performed in order to stabilize the molecule. The changes did not affect interferon beta-1b's performance in classical tests of interferon function (Chen and Sondel, 1985).

The recombinant DNA technology was performed by extracting the human interferon beta gene from human fibroblast cells and modifying it biochemically to provide a more stable molecule. The modified gene was then inserted into an *E. coli* plasmid, and the recombinant DNA molecule was added to an *E. coli* bacterial culture. The DNA was taken up into the *E. coli*, and large numbers of interferon beta-1-producing organisms were then created. Interferon beta-1b was then harvested from the ferment and purified. Dextrose and human albumin stabilizers were added. The drug is supplied in a highly purified, sterilized, lyophilized (freeze-dried) powder for administration to humans.

Mechanism of action

The mechanism of action of interferon beta-1b is not clearly known. However, there have been a number of studies showing that interferon beta blocks the effects of interferon gamma (IFNB Multiple Sclerosis Study Group, 1993). Interferon gamma acts as an immune enhancer in both the animal model for MS (EAE) and the human (Panitch *et al.*, 1987; Huynh and Dorovini-Zis, 1993), and therefore aggravates the autoimmune process. Interferon beta seems to block immune reactions within the central nervous system (CNS), particularly those immune reactions moderated by interferon gamma. Other gamma effects include direct inhibition of the activation of T-lymphocytes, and inhibition of HLA antigen expression on the surface of T-lymphocytes. Studies have shown a reduction of interferon gamma production (Bever *et al.*, 1991) and a decrease in tumour necrosis factor alpha production (Yoshida *et al.*, 1988; Johnson and Pober, 1994). There is also evidence of an increase in transforming growth factor beta (TGFβ) production (Twardzik *et al.*, 1990). TGFβ suppresses experimental allergic encephalomyelitis (EAE) in experimental animals, and is currently being tested for its ability to suppress the exacerbations of MS (Karpus and Swanborg, 1991).

The original description of interferon beta was for its antiviral effect (Isaacs and Lindenmann, 1957). The various interferons inhibit viral replication, and it may be that interferon beta prevents the mild virus infections that enhance the autoimmune process in multiple sclerosis (Isaacs and Lindenmann, 1957; Faulds and Benfield, 1994; Panitch *et al.*, 1994).

The betaseron pilot trial

In 1986, a pilot study of interferon beta-1b was begun in 30 patients with clinically definite relapsing and remitting MS (Knobler *et al.*, 1993).

All patients were ambulatory, and they were allocated in a double-blind fashion to five treatment groups. Patients received placebo or interferon beta-1b in a dosage of 0.8, 4.0, 8.0 or 16.0 million international units (Miu) subcutaneously every other day. The dosage was based on biological activity marker studies, which suggested that the drug should be given more frequently than once every 72 hours (Goldstein *et al.*, 1989).

The goals of the pilot study were to consider interferon beta-1b's tolerability, route of injection and therapeutic potential, and the most appropriate dose. The study outcomes were counts of the number of exacerbations, and assessment on the EDSS (Kurtzke, 1983) and the neurological rating scale, NRS (Sipe *et al.*, 1984). Patients tolerated the drug well, but flu-like reactions were common, especially at the highest dose (16.0 Miu). It was decided that subcutaneous administration at 8 Miu every other day was not only tolerated but was also possibly effective in suppressing relapses.

First publication (1993) of the pivotal trial in relapsing/remitting patients

In 1988, the IFNB Multiple Sclerosis Study Group organized a full-scale multi-centre, randomized, double-blind, placebo-controlled trial of interferon beta-1b (IFNB Multiple Sclerosis Study Group, 1993). The drug was given in two doses; a low dose of 1.6 Miu subcutaneously every other day or a high dose of 8.0 Miu subcutaneously every other day.

The primary endpoints were:

• the annual exacerbation rate
• the proportion of patients remaining exacerbation-free.

The secondary endpoints were:

• the time to the first exacerbation
• the duration and severity of the exacerbation
• the change in EDSS and NRS scores from baseline (changes in the EDSS scores were confirmed at 3-month follow-up in order to be considered significant – i.e. not due to relapses)
• the MRI burden of disease (BOD) on annual scans
• MRI lesion activity determined by systematically performed unenhanced scans once every 6 weeks in a sub-population of 50 patients from Vancouver.

Entry criteria were:

1. Clinically definite or laboratory supported relapsing and remitting multiple sclerosis
2. Mild to moderate disease severity (EDSS ≤ 5.5)
3. At least two exacerbations in the 2 years prior to enrolment
4. Remission for at least 1 month prior to enrolment
5. Aged 18–50 years.

The exclusion criteria included any prior treatment with immunosuppressives, or recent treatment with corticosteroids. During the trial, courses of corticosteroids were allowed for treatment of exacerbations.

The MRI portion of the study involved 327 patients, who had annual MRI scans (Paty *et al.*, 1993). These scans were analysed in order to determine the MRI burden of disease. The results were expressed in the total area of brain involved by lesions, slice by slice, in square millimetres.

A pre-determined sub-cohort of patients in Vancouver (50 patients) were scanned at 0.15 tesla every 6 weeks for 2 years. Gadolinium enhancement was not available at the time of this study. MRI activity on the proton density/T2 weighted scan was detected using the following criteria:

1. New lesions – lesions never seen before
2. Enlarging lesions – lesions that had enlarged significantly from previously seen stable lesions
3. Reappearing lesions – lesions that disappeared after a period of activity only to reappear later (this phenomenon may be a function of the lack of spatial resolution at low field strengths).

The code was broken for investigators in December 1992, the FDA held an open hearing on the results of the drug in March, 1993, and the results were published for the first time in April 1993 in *Neurology* (IFNB Multiple Sclerosis Study Group, 1993; Paty *et al.*, 1993). The results of the study at 1, 2 and 3 years are shown in Tables 3.1 and 3.2.

Table 3.1 Interferon beta-1b in RRMS: 2- and 3-year data

	Time (years)	Placebo	1.6 Miu	8 Miu	*P* value*
Number of patients	2	112	111	115	–
	3	123	125	124	–
Mean exacerbation rate	2	1.27	1.17	0.84	0.0001
	3	1.21	1.05	0.84	0.0004
Median time to first exacerbation (days)	3	147	199	264	0.028
Mean moderate and severe exacerbation rate	2	0.45	0.32	0.23	0.002
MRI BOD, median per cent change	1	10.9	3.0	–6.2	<0.001
from baseline	2	16.5	11.4	0.8	<0.001
	3	15.0	0.2	9.3	0.002

P values are for comparison of placebo to 8 Miu.

Table 3.2 Interferon beta-1b study in RRMS: MRI activity rate

	Placebo	1.6 Miu	8 Miu	P value
Entire study ($n = 327$)				
Number of patients	115	116	111	–
Mean new lesion rate (yearly)	3.57	2.01	1.80	0.001
Percentage of MRI active patients	83.5	70.7	64.9	0.011
Frequent scanning cohort ($n = 50$)				
Number of patients	17	18	17	–
Median per cent of scans with activity	29.4	11.8	5.9	0.0062
Mean per cent of scans with activity	34.6	17.0	15.4	0.0062
Mean number of new lesions/year	3.2	1.1	1.2	0.0026

Results

Primary endpoints

The annual exacerbation rate as defined by the Schumacher Committee (Schumacher *et al.*, 1965) was reduced by approximately one-third ($P = 0.001$). The proportion of patients remaining exacerbation free during the first 2 years was 16 per cent in the placebo group and 31 per cent in the high-dose treated group ($P = 0.007$).

Secondary endpoints

The time to the first exacerbation was doubled ($P = 0.015$), and the time to subsequent exacerbations was also significantly prolonged.

The severity of the exacerbations was assessed by the maximum change in the NRS score during an exacerbation, a change of up to 7 points was defined as mild, 8–14 as moderate, and more than 15 as severe. There was a 50 per cent reduction in the number of moderate and severe exacerbations in the high-dose treated group as compared to the placebo group ($P = 0.002$).

With regard to changes in EDSS and NRS scores, the treated patients had a lower treatment failure rate (27 per cent) than did the placebo group (39 per cent) ($P = 0.08$). This change due to therapy was not statistically significant, but it showed a trend that has been shown to be significant in subsequent studies with interferon beta. Re-analysis of the EDSS data by longitudinal methods (D'Yachkova, 1997) showed a significant treatment effect. In patients with a high EDSS level at entry (≥ 4.0), the drug was shown to have a significant treatment effect on the time to EDSS change (confirmed at 6 months) (Lisa Bidel, personal communication, 1998).

Other measures that were significantly favourably affected by the treatment included:

• the number of patients hospitalized for multiple sclerosis and its complications ($P = 0.046$)

- the total number of days spent in hospital as a result of multiple sclerosis ($P = 0.023$)
- the number of patients treated with corticosteroids.

An interesting observation in this study was that the annual exacerbation rate in the placebo group declined significantly year by year over the 3 years of follow-up. The reduction in the exacerbation rate due to the administration of interferon beta-1b was in addition to this natural decline in exacerbation rates seen in the placebo group. The decline in the exacerbation rate in the placebo group was probably due to regression to the mean, since the patients selected to enter the study had a higher than average pre-study relapse rate.

MRI results

The MRI detected BOD stabilized over 3 years in the high-dose treated group. The increase in BOD in the placebo group over the first 2 years was 16.5 per cent, and –0.8 per cent in the high-dose treated group ($P = 0.001$). These differences continued to be highly significant in the third year of double-blind therapy. In addition, the percentage of patients in each group with a > 10 per cent increase or decrease or a stable disease burden at 3 years showed a highly statistically significant treatment effect of the drug at the 8 Miu dosage ($P = 0.001$).

In the Vancouver sub-cohort, 52 patients were entered into a systematic serial study with unenhanced scans repeated once every 6 weeks over 2 years. Fifty patients completed the study. Eight hundred and eighty-one scans were performed on these patients with an average of 17 scans per patient. There was a significant therapeutic effect from interferon beta-1b at both dosages. The median percentage of active scans for placebo was 29.4 per cent, for low-dose 11.8 per cent, and for high-dose 5.9 per cent ($P = 0.062$ for high-dose vs. placebo). This change represented an 80 per cent reduction in disease activity at the high-dose level. There was also a dose-dependent reduction in the median number of active lesions per patient per year, from 3.0 for placebo, 1.0 for the low dose, and 0.5 for the high dose ($P = 0.04–0.0089$).

Perhaps the most significant change was a reduction in the number of new lesions appearing per year. The median number of new lesions per year for the placebo group was 2.0, and this rate was reduced to 0.5 lesions per year in both treated groups, which represents a 75 per cent reduction in the new lesion rate.

Second publication (1995) of the pivotal trial in relapsing/remitting patients

The randomized study was extended to a median of 45 months (3.75 years) double-blind follow-up (IFNB Multiple Sclerosis Study Group, 1995). The exacerbation rate for each year continued to be reduced by one-third in the 8 Miu arm compared to placebo. MRI data continued to show significant reductions in extent and activity due to the drug throughout the study. A number of patients ($n = 154$) dropped out prior to completion, mostly due to investigator-determined treatment failure or a personal sense of completion of contract with the investigators. As might be expected, the patients who dropped out from the placebo group were worse than the dropouts from the treatment groups with a higher on-study exacerbation rates and higher on-study accumulation of MRI BOD.

Adverse events and blinding

Flu-like symptoms and local skin reactions were common in the treated groups. Blinding was maintained in the relapsing/remitting study by having a treating neurologist, who dealt with the medical and side-effect issues, and an evaluating neurologist, whose only role was to examine the patients to determine relapses, relapse severity and the EDSS score. An additional masking factor was that two doses of drug were used, each having similar side-effect profiles. However, only one dose was found to have a significant clinical therapeutic effect, even though both doses had a significant treatment effect on the MRI outcome measures.

Other adverse events included liver enzyme elevations (rarely clinically significant) and leucopenia. Depression and suicide attempts were the same in all treatment groups.

Neutralizing antibodies

The production of neutralizing antibodies against an injected protein with biological activity is a predictable event. Experience with other interferons in different disease states has shown that the development of neutralizing antibodies is associated with loss of efficacy of the drug. Using insulin as an example, the dosage may have to be increased if neutralizing antibodies occur.

The original interferon beta-1b study showed that 45 per cent of patients produced neutralizing antibodies within the first 18 months (IFNB MS Study Group). The original cross-sectional analysis of the effect of neutralizing antibodies on the drug showed reduced efficacy, presumably due to the presence of the antibodies. However, long-term follow-up of these patients with neutralizing antibodies showed that the majority of them lost their neutralizing antibodies over an extended period of time (Rice et. al., 1999). The consensus conclusions of an international meeting concerning neutralizing antibodies (Arnason and Dianzani, 1997) were as follows:

1. All endogenous and exogenous class I interferons are capable of eliciting an antibody response.
2. The appearance of anti-interferon antibodies is often transient; even at high titres, antibody levels sporadically fall and/or disappear.
3. Although anti-interferon alpha and anti-interferon beta antibodies may be associated with loss of efficacy under certain circumstances and in some patients, there is no clear indication or consistent correlation between the appearance of these antibodies and the clinical course of MS in individual

patients. A longitudinal analysis of neutralizing antibody data showed that change from antibody-negative to antibody-positive status was associated with a significant increase in exacerbation rate in a few patients (Arnason and Dianzani, 1997), but this finding was not consistent (Petkau et al., unpublished).

4. There may be a group of non-responder patients with persistently high titres of neutralizing antibodies. These treatment non-responders may be identifiable by the level of their peripheral blood lymphocyte (PBL) secretion of immunoglobulin-G (IgG) in vitro at baseline (Oger et al., 1997). In addition, longitudinal analysis of patients who became neutralizing antibody-positive showed that some of these patients had more active disease than neutralizing antibody-negative patients during the first (pre-antibody) phase of treatment with the drug (Petkau et al., unpublished).

In summary, consistent neutralizing antibody production in response to interferon beta-1b is seen in a small proportion (up to 24 per cent) of patients who also have more than average aggressive disease. They have a high relapse rate, and tend to have high levels of in vitro IgG secretion (Oger et al., 1997). This sub group of patients can be seen as resistant to therapy. Further information is necessary in order to identify such patients clearly and make therapeutic decisions based on objective clinical endpoints. In addition, long-term follow-up of a sub group of neutralizing antibody-positive patients from the original trial showed that the majority of them eventually lost the antibodies (Rice et al., 1999). It is clear that the neutralizing antibodies issue is complicated, and further work needs to be done. An interesting comparison is with interferon beta-1a (Rebif®) (PRISMS Study Group, 1998). In this study, in which two doses of drug were used, the high dose was associated with a lower neutralizing-antibody rate than the low dose.

Effect in secondary progressive multiple sclerosis

The therapeutic effects of this drug (interferon beta-1b, Betaferon®) have now been seen in a trial undertaken in secondary progressive MS (SPMS) (European Study Group on Interferon beta-1b, 1998). This trial involved 718 patients in 32 centres, who were studied using a double-blind, randomized, placebo-controlled design. The treatment was 8 Miu given subcutaneously on alternate days. When all the patients had been treated for at least 24 months, the independent advisory board recommended termination of the study because of the highly significant treatment effect on the primary outcome variable, the time to confirmed neurological deterioration ($P = 0.0008$).

Patients selected for the study were in the secondary progressive phase of MS, with disability not thought to be related to incomplete recovery from relapses. EDSS at entry was between 3.0 and 6.5. Patients had also suffered either two or more clearly identified relapses in the previous 2 years or a worsening of at least one EDSS point (or 0.5 points between EDSS scores of 6.0 and 7.0) over the preceding 24 months.

The primary outcome measure was the time to confirmed neurological deterioration (defined as progression of 1 point on the EDSS scale or 0.5 point for EDSS ≥ 6.0 at entry, present for at least 3 months).

The secondary outcome measures were:

1. The time to becoming wheelchair-bound (EDSS 7.0)
2. The annual relapse rate
3. The MRI lesion volume (lesion load or BOD) with annual MRI scans in all patients
4. The number of newly active MRI lesions in a frequent MRI scanning sub-group ($n = 124$).

Only 57 patients were lost to follow-up. An intent-to-treat analysis showed that there were significant treatment effects in all primary and secondary outcome measures. Those outcomes were as follows:

- time to EDSS progression ($P = 0.008$)
- proportion of patients progressing ($P = 0.0048$)
- time to becoming wheelchair-bound ($P = 0.0133$)
- proportion of patients becoming wheelchair-bound ($P = 0.0277$)
- relapse rate (reduced by 31 per cent) ($P = 0.0002$)
- severity of relapses ($P = 0.0083$).

The moderate and severe relapse rate was also reduced ($P = 0.001$).

As in the relapsing/remitting study, the number of hospitalizations due to MS was significantly reduced, as was the number of courses of corticosteroids required.

The MRI endpoints all were highly significant for a treatment effect. In the entire cohort, the lesion load (BOD measure) increased by 8 per cent in 2 years in the placebo group with a decrease of 5 per cent in the treated group ($P = 0.0001$). In the frequent MRI sub group, there was a marked and significant reduction of the number of new lesions at 1–6 months and 19–24 months ($P = 0.0001$). The cumulative number of new lesions in the frequent MRI sub group was reduced at 6 months, and there was also a significant reduction in MRI activity identifiable at the first scanning interval following therapy, which was at 1 month.

The safety and tolerability of interferon beta-1b in SPMS patients was similar to that in the RRMS study. Again, there was no increased incidence of depression or suicide attempts in the treated group.

Summary and discussion

Interferon beta-1b has been shown to have therapeutic benefit by reducing the relapse rate in both RR and SPMS. It has also been shown to have a significant impact on prevention of disability in the more severe RR patients and in SPMS patients.

The therapeutic impact upon MRI measures has been most impressive, with all MRI outcome measures showing a sustained treatment effect even up to 5 years of double-blind follow-up. Perhaps the most significant impact seen on MRI has been upon the new lesion formation rate (a 75 per cent reduction). The number of new lesions seen on the proton density scan is very important because the number of lesions present at the onset of clinical symptoms and the rate of formation of lesions at 5 years predicts the clinical severity of MS at 5- and 10-year follow-up (O'Riordan *et al.*, 1998). In a simple calculation, if the new lesion accumulation rate is four per year, and the average number of lesions at onset is about five, an average untreated patient will go from 5–25 lesions over 5 years. At the same time, a treated patient will go from 5–10 MRI lesions. This calculation shows an impressive impact of interferon beta-1b on the accumulating pathology of the disease. Interferon beta-1b has been proven to have a modest clinical therapeutic impact and a major MRI therapeutic impact. There is now compelling evidence that all patients with relapsing disease should be treated as early as possible in order to obtain the greatest benefit.

Clinical usage

Interferon beta-1b has been in clinical usage for 5 years and in clinical trial usage for over 10 years. It is safe and partially effective as a preventive therapy for relapsing and remitting patients, and more recently has been shown to be partially effective in secondary progressive disease as well. Systematic MRI studies show a dramatic effect on the prevention of all measures of MRI activity and the MRI detected extent of disease, including the prevention of new lesions.

Theoretically, then, the use of this drug will have the greatest long-term effect if used early in the disease. The problem with early use is that some patients who would naturally run a relatively benign course might be treated unnecessarily. However, the proposed long-term benefit from the early use of therapy, from a societal view, is to delay the time of onset of clinically important disability and unemployment, and reduction in quality of life.

From an MRI point of view, the ability to prevent the formation of new lesions seen on the PD/T2 scans may be the most important predictor of its long-term therapeutic impact (see Table 3.3). Since the new lesion formation is probably the major factor impacting on the overall extent of the disease, the reduction in new lesion formation would have a major effect on the extent of MRI lesions detectable after 5 years of therapy.

The treatment of patients with interferons is not easy. Patients have unrealistic expectations, and the initial symptomatic side effects may also be quite marked. A system for patient education and counselling must be put into place prior to starting therapy, and should include the following points.

1. Education must emphasize realistic expectations:
   - this treatment is not a cure;
   - it is a partially effective preventive treatment;
   - current symptoms are not likely to get better.
2. Side effects:
   - flu-like symptoms can usually be managed by the use of anti-inflammatory drugs such as acetaminophen and ibuprofen;
   - side effects such as skin reactions are likely to occur and can be minimized (see product monograph).
3. Monitoring for blood cell count reduction and liver function abnormalities is necessary.
4. Monitoring for the formation of neutralizing antibodies is suggested after 1 year of treatment; however, the data on neutralizing antibodies are not consistent, and even the development of high titres of neutralizing antibodies is not necessarily associated with abrogation of effectiveness of the drug. High titres can also disappear in follow-up for some unexplained reason.

Table 3.3 Impact of interferon beta-1b therapy on new MRI lesions

	Number
Average number of lesions at clinical onset of MS	5
Annual rate of formation of new lesions	4
Percentage reduction of new lesion rate in interferon beta-treated patients	75
Average number of lesions after 5 years in untreated patients	25
Average number of lesions after 5 years in a patient treated at clinical onset	10

Nobody knows how to adopt 'stopping rules' with a partially effective preventive treatment. Treatment failure can be defined as in the clinical trial, but does reaching the definition of clinical failure definition mean that the drug is not working? It is not known how to interpret clinical worsening under these circumstances. However, there are a few (10 per cent or so) patients who cannot tolerate the drug and wish to stop treatment. Other patients who continue to have relapses, in spite of therapy, might have been worse without treatment.

The onset of secondary progressive disease was previously a stopping point but now, with the secondary progressive study results, this endpoint is probably not appropriate.

Therefore the best strategy may be to treat patients as early as possible with the maximum tolerated dosage of the drug in order to have the best long-term impact for the greatest number of patients.

References

Arnason, B. G. and Dianzani, F. (1997). *International Workshop on Interferon Antibodies*. Catalyst Communications.

Bever, C. T. Jr, Panitch, H. S., Levy, H. B. *et al.* (1991). Gamma-interferon induction in patients with chronic progressive MS. *Neurology*, **41**, 1124–7.

Chen, B. P. P. and Sondel, P. M. (1985). Recombinant DNA-derived interferons alpha and beta modulate the alloactivated proliferative response of bulk and cloned human lymphocytes. *J. Biol. Response Mod.*, **4**, 287–97.

D'Yachkova, Y. (1997). Analysis of longitudinal data from the Betaseron MS Clinical Trial. MSc Thesis, Dept. of Statistics.

European Study Group (1998) on Interferon beta-1b in Secondary Progressive MS: placebo-controlled multicentre randomised trial of interferon b-1b in treatment of secondary progressive multiple sclerosis. *Lancet*, **352**, 1491–7.

Faulds, D. and Benfield, P. (1994). Interferon beta-1b in multiple sclerosis: an initial review of its rationale for use and therapeutic potential. *Clin. Immunother.*, **1**, 79–87.

Goldstein, D., Sielaff, K. M., Storer, B. E. *et al.* (1989). Human biologic response modification by interferon in the absence of measurable serum concentrations: A comparative trial of subcutaneous and intravenous interferon-b serine. *J. Natl. Cancer Inst.*, **81**, 1061–8.

Huynh, H. K. and Dorovini-Zis, K. A. (1993). Effects of interferon-g on primary cultures of human brain microvessel endothelial cells. *Am. J. Pathol.*, **142**, 1265–78.

IFNB Multiple Sclerosis Study Group (1993). Interferon beta-1b is effective in relapsing–remitting multiple sclerosis, I. Clinical results of a multi-center, randomized, double-blind, placebo-controlled trial. *Neurology*, **43**, 655–61.

IFNB Multiple Sclerosis Study Group and the University of British Columbia MS/MRI Analysis Group (1995). Interferon beta-1b in the treatment of multiple sclerosis: final outcome of the randomized controlled trial. *Neurology*, **45**, 1277–85.

IFNB Multiple Sclerosis Study Group and the University of British Columbia MS/MRI Analysis Group (1996). Neutralizing antibodies during treatment of multiple sclerosis with interferon beta-1b: Experience during the first three years. *Neurology*, **47**, 889–94.

Isaacs, A. and Lindenmann, J. (1957). Virus interference I: the interferon. *Proc. R. Soc. Lond.*, **147**, 258–67.

Jacobs, L., Herndon, R., Freeman, A. *et al.* (1986). Multi-centre double-blind study of effect of intrathecally administered natural human fibroblast interferon on exacerbations of multiple sclerosis. *Lancet*, **2**, 1411–13.

Johnson, J. R. and Pober, J. S. (1994). HLA class I heavy chain gene promoter elements mediating synergy between tumor necrosis factor and interferons. *Mol. Cell Biol.*, **14**, 1322–32.

Karpus, W. J. and Swanborg, R. H. (1991). CD4+ suppressor cells inhibit the function of effector cells of experimental autoimmune encephalomyelitis through a mechanism involving transforming growth factor-beta. *J. Immunol.*, **146**, 1163–8.

Knobler, R. I., Greenstein, J. I., Johnson, K. P. *et al.* Systemic recombinant human interferon-beta treatment of relapsing-remitting multiple sclerosis: Pilot study analysis and six-year follow-up. *J. Interferon Res.*, **13**, 333–40.

Kurtzke, J. F. (1983). The Disability Status Scale for multiple sclerosis: an expanded disability status scale (EDSS). *Neurology*, **33**, 1444–52.

Oger, J. J. F., Vorobeychik, G., Al-Fahim, A. *et al.* (1997). Neutralizing antibodies in betaseron-treated MS patients and *in vitro* immune function before treatment. *Neurology*, **48**, A80.

O'Riordan, J. I., Thompson, A. J., Kingsley, D. P. E. *et al.* (1998). The prognostic value of brain MRI in clinically isolated syndromes of the CNS. A 10-year follow-up. *Brain*, **121**, 495–503.

Panitch, H. S., Haley, A. S., Hirsch, R. L. and Jonson, K. P. (1987). Exacerbations of multiple sclerosis in patients treated with gamma interferon. *Lancet*, 893–4, Volume 1.

Panitch, H. S., Katz, E. and Johnson, K. P. (1994). Effects of beta interferon treatment on viral infections and relapses of multiple sclerosis: *Neurology*, **44(Suppl. 2),** A358.

Paty, D. W., Li, D. K. B., UBC MS/MRI Study Group and the IFNB Multiple Sclerosis Study Group (1993). Interferon beta-1b is effective in relapsing-remitting multiple sclerosis. II. MRI analysis results of a multicenter, randomized, double-blind, placebo-controlled trial. *Neurology*, **43**, 662–7.

Petkau, A. J., White, R., Ebers, G. C. *et al.* Longitudinal analyses of the effects of neutralizing antibodies in relapsing-remitting multiple sclerosis patients treated with interferon beta-1b (unpublished).

PRISMS (Prevention of Relapses and Disability by Interferon beta-1a Subcutaneously in Multiple Sclerosis) Study Group (1998). Randomized double-blind placebo-controlled study of interferon beta-1a in relapsing/ remitting multiple sclerosis. *Lancet*, **352**, 1498–1504.

Reder, A. T. (1997). *Interferon Therapy of Multiple Sclerosis*. Marcel Dekker Inc.

Rice, G. P. A., Paszner, B., Oger, J. *et al.* (1999). The evolution of neutralizing antibodies in multiple sclerosis patients treated with interferon beta-1b. The London MS Clinic, London, Ontario, Canada and The UBC MS Clinic, Vancouver, BC, Canada. *Neurology*, **52**, 1277–79.

Schumacher, G. A., Beebe, G., Kibler, R. F. *et al.* (1965). Problems of experimental trials of therapy in multiple sclerosis: report by the panel on the evaluation of experimental trials of therapy in multiple sclerosis. *Ann. NY Acad. Sci.*, **122**, 552–68.

Sipe, J. C., Knobler, R. L., Braheny, S. L. *et al.* (1984). A neurologic rating scale (NRS) for use in multiple sclerosis. *Neurology*, **34**, 1368–72.

Twardzik, D. R., Mikovitis, J. A., Ranchalis, J. E. *et al.* (1990). gamma-interferon-induced activation of latent transforming growth factor-beta by human monocytes. *Ann. NY Acad. Sci.*, **593,** 276–84.

Yoshida, R., Murray, H. W. and Nathan, C. F. (1988). Agonist and antagonist effects of interferon-alpha and beta on activation of human macrophages. *J. Exp. Med.*, **167,** 1171–85.

4

Interferon beta-1a

Naturally occurring interferon beta (nIFNB) is one of the class I interferons (IFNs) produced by almost all appropriately stimulated mammalian cells, particularly fibroblasts, macrophages and epithelial cells. It is encoded by a gene on chromosome 9 and, unlike interferon alpha or the mutant IFNB-1b discussed in the previous chapter, exists only in a single, glycosylated form (about 20 per cent carbohydrate) comprised of 166 amino acids. It shares actions with interferon alpha by binding to the same receptors, despite differing by 70 per cent of its amino acid sequence.

The recombinant form of interferon beta-1a (rIFNB-1a) is produced by mass tissue culture technology using a Chinese hamster ovarian cell line. It has the same molecular weight and glycosylated amino acid sequence (166 amino acids, methionine at #1, cysteine at #17) as the natural fibroblast-derived IFNB from which it is physicochemically indistinguishable. The carbohydrate moiety within the protein confers high polarity, hydrophilicity and a highly negative potential, factors which may well be critical for receptor recognition and attachment and thus biological activity. In addition, rIFNB-1a has the same pharmacological profile as natural human interferon in healthy volunteers (Liberati *et al.*, 1992; 1994), and more than 10 times higher specific activity than IFNB-1b (i.e. > 300 Miu/mcg for IFNB-1a compared with 32 Miu/mcg for rIFNB-1b) (Chernajovsky *et al.*, 1984; IFNB Multiple Sclerosis Study Group, 1993; Table 4.1).

The actions of interferons are multiple and extraordinarily complex. They are known to induce or suppress about 20 gene products *in vitro* and clinical studies have demonstrated that IFNB can increase the production of many critical immunological mediators. As well as affecting auto-immunity, IFNB has antiviral and antiproliferative actions. The induction of the intracellular enzyme $2'$-$5'$-oligoadenylate (2-5A) synthetase may contribute to these actions by degrading viral RNA. Other relevant biological activity may be reflected by increased production of beta 2-microglobulin, a protein involved in the activation of cytotoxic lymphocytes, neopterin, which indexes monocyte activation and the human Mx protein (Liberati *et al.*, 1992). IFNB is induced by viruses or polynucleotides, by cytokines released from activated T-cells and macrophages, particularly interleukin-2 (IL-2), IL-1 and tumour necrosis factor (TNF). Although secreted locally, IFNB spreads throughout the lymphatic system (Bocci *et al.*, 1988) to produce systemic effects without the need for high concentrations in the blood

Table 4.1 Currently available interferon beta products

	Rebif®	Avonex™	Betaseron®
Type	IFNB-1a	IFNB-1a	IFNB-1b
Cell origin	CHO	CHO	E. coli
Amino acids	166	166	165*
Glycoprotein	Yes	Yes	No
Specific activity**	27×10^7	27×10^7	2×10^7
Formulation	Liquid PFS	FD	FD
Weekly dose (mcg)	66–132	30	875
Route of administration	Subcutaneous	Intramuscular	Subcutaneous

*Absent N-Methyl, position 17 Cys→Serine

**IU/mcg by bioassay

CHO, Chinese hamster ovary cells; PFS, pre-filled syringe; FD, freeze-dried.

(Revel et al., 1981; Schonfield et al., 1984). In experimental models of MS such as experimental allergic encephalomyelitis, IFNB upregulates MHC Class I immune expression to increase the effectiveness of T-cell antiviral action. It has numerous immune modulating functions, including the upregulation of IL-10 expression, the secretory functions of T-cells and monocytes, the inhibition of IL-12 and T-cell migration and the suppression of Class II proteins.

How IFNB favourably affects the clinical course of MS remains unclear (see reviews by Arnason and Reder, 1994; Arnason, 1996; Hartung and Kieseier, 1996; Hohlfeld, 1997). Various theories are supported by in vitro and/or in vivo observations. The original rationale for its use in MS trials came from the observation that INFB stimulates the production of several antiviral products. However, whereas exacerbations may be triggered by a number of different viruses (Sibley et al., 1985; Panitch, 1994; Edwards et al., 1998), there is little evidence to support antiviral actions per se as a major mechanism of action of IFNB in MS. It is generally considered that the main effects on disease activity may be brought about by a reduction of cellular proliferation and modulation of the immune response (Rudick et al., 1993). The antiproliferative effect could operate on either side of the blood–brain barrier (BBB), although it is not yet certain whether IFNB can enter the central nervous system in MS. In addition, IFNB upregulates depressed suppressor T-cell function (Weinstock-Guttman et al., 1995) and has a direct effect on matrix metallo-proteinases to inhibit trafficking of activated T-cells (Stuve et al., 1996). At the present time it is not known whether the striking suppression of disease activity by rIFNB-1a in MS is brought about mainly by reduced T-cell proliferation or trafficking, downregulation of the immune response within the CNS, a combination of multiple actions, or by some other unknown mechanism.

There are currently two commercial formulations of rIFNB-1a, Rebif® and Avonex® (Table 4.1). The two doses of Rebif® (22 mcg and 44 mcg) are available in either a lyophilized powder form, which includes mannitol, serum albumin and sodium acetate, or a liquid formulation in a syringe. Avonex™ is a 30 mcg single powder formulation, which contains serum albumin, sodium chloride and phosphate (Alam *et al.*, 1997). While manufacturing processes, formulations and methods of administration clearly differ, the molecular structure, pharmacokinetics and pharmacodynamics of these two products appear to be identical. Any apparent differences can be attributed to dose and dosing schedules.

After intravenous injection, the serum levels of rIFNB-1a increase over several minutes and then show a biphasic reduction over several hours, characteristic of a two-compartment distribution model (Salmon *et al.*, 1996; Alam *et al.*, 1997). By contrast, subcutaneous or intramuscular injections result in a monophasic decline in serum concentrations (Alam *et al.*, 1997). Intramuscular or subcutaneous injections of a single dose of rIFNB-1a in the range of 22–66 mcg result in the same maximum serum concentration and pharmacokinetic profile (Munafo *et al.*, 1998; Figure 4.1). Studies of biological markers, such as the production of neopterin and 2-5A synthetase activity, show no differences between subcutaneous and intramuscular administration. The peak biological action after a single injection occurs within 1–2 days (Alam *et al.*, 1997) but, unlike serum levels, can persist for up to 6 days (Alam *et al.*, 1997). However, the maintenance of maximal biological responses requires alternate day regimens (Witt *et al.*, 1993; Salmon *et al.*, 1996; Munafo *et al.*, 1997).

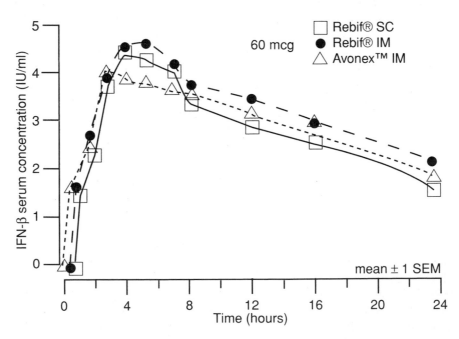

Figure 4.1 Comparison in 30 healthy subjects between pharmacokinetics of 60 mcg of Rebif® given either intramuscularly or by subcutaneous injection with the same dose of intramuscular Avonex™. The three curves are fully superimposable. (Reproduced with permission from Munafo *et al.*, 1998).

This review will concentrate on the clinical evidence for the use of recombinant interferon beta-1a (rIFNB-1a) in RRMS.

Pilot studies and phase II clinical trials

Natural human fibroblast-derived interferon beta (nIFNB) was first administered by intramuscular injection to three patients with chronic progressive MS, with no apparent benefit (Verveken *et al.*, 1979). The subsequent studies, which provided the first insights into the potential benefits of this treatment, used the intrathecal route. The first was an open pilot study of nIFNB (Jacobs *et al.*, 1981, 1982), in which 20 patients with either chronic progressive or relapsing–remitting MS (RRMS) were treated for 5 months (Table 4.2). Clinical improvements were confined to those with RRMS, the overall relapse rate falling from a mean pre-trial rate of 1.8 to 0.25 on trial ($P < 0.01$). A similar effect was observed in the control patients when they were switched to active treatment in the second phase of the study. The double-blind, placebo-controlled study of 69 RRMS patients that followed compared intrathecal nIFNB with monthly sham lumbar punctures over a 6-month period (Jacobs *et al.*, 1986, 1987). There was a 58 per cent lower annual relapse rate in those receiving nIFNB (1.79 relapses for placebo versus 0.76 for nIFNB; $P < 0.04$). The in-trial relapse rate was significantly lower than the pre-trial rate ($P < 0.001$) in the actively treated patients.

Another double-blind, placebo-controlled trial of intrathecally administered nIFNB reported an apparent increase in progression rate and frequency of exacerbations in 16 patients with MS (Milanese *et al.*, 1990; Table 4.2). Interpretation is complicated by the small mixed cohort of patients with either RRMS or chronic progressive MS and possibly by the slightly different nIFNB resulting from the use of the synthetic polymer (PICLC) to induce interferon in the manufacturing process. An apparent lack of effectiveness was also reported from another small un-blinded study of intravenous nIFNB in patients with RRMS (Huber *et al.*, 1988).

Positive benefits of treatment with nIFNB were demonstrated in a multicentre, randomized, placebo-controlled phase II study of RRMS (Fernandez *et al.*, 1995; Table 4.2). The 58 patients enrolled had higher than average levels of disease activity (two attacks in 2 years). Half the patients ($n = 29$) were treated with 9 Miu of nIFNB three times weekly by subcutaneous injection for 1 year and the other half with placebo for 6 months followed by 9 Miu of nIFNB for a further 6 months. The primary endpoints were changes in lesions on PD/T2 scans and gadolinium-enhanced lesions on monthly T1-weighted MRI scans (Gd-lesions). Treated patients showed a 67 per cent reduction in the median number of active lesions (i.e. the combined numbers of Gd-lesions and new PD/T2-lesions); 4 vs 12 ($P < 0.05$). The clinical assessments in this trial were not blinded, but comparisons of the pre-treatment and on-trial relapse rates showed a 52 per cent reduction with nIFNB. Active treatment conferred a 38 per cent reduction in the mean exacerbation rate compared with placebo (1.24 ± 1.7 for 9 Miu nIFNB vs 2.0 ± 1.7 for placebo; $P < 0.05$). The proportion of exacerbation-free patients was also

Table 4.2 Pilot studies and phase II treatment trials of nIFNB* and rIFNB-1a

Ref	Trial design	Dosage	Trial duration (months)	n	MS type	Results
Verveken et al., 1979	*Open	5×10^4 iu/kg IM	0.5	3	CP	No effect
Jacobs et al., 1982	*Open	1 Miu IT; 2/wk (4 wks), 1/mth (5 mths)	6	20	RR, CP	Reduced attacks in RR cases
Confavreux et al., 1986	*Open	0.1/0.64 Miu IT; 1/wk	2	11	CP	No effect
Jacobs et al., 1986	*DB, PC	1 Miu IT; 1/wk (4 wks), 1 mth (5 mths)	6	69	RR	Reduced attacks
Baumhefner et al., 1987	Open	3 Miu IV; 1/wk	3	6	CP	Four cases improved
Huber et al., 1988	*Open	3 Miu IV; 2/wk to 2/mth	5	9	RR	No effect
Milanese et al., 1990	DB, PC	1 Miu IT; 2/wk (1 wk), 1/wk (3 wks), 1/mth (4 mths)	5	16	RR, CP	Relapses increased, disability worse
Fernandez et al., 1995	*Open (MRI DB)	9 Miu SC 3/wk	12	60	RR	Reduced relapses
Pozzilli et al., 1996	Open (MRI DB)	3 or 9 Miu 3/wk	6	68	RR	Reduced relapses and MRI activity

RR, relapsing–remitting multiple sclerosis; CP, chronic progressive multiple sclerosis; DB, double-blind; PC, placebo-controlled; IM, intramuscular; IV, intravenous; IT, intrathecal; SC, subcutaneous; wk, week; mth, month.

in favour of active treatment, with 17 (59 per cent) patients on nIFNB free of attacks versus nine (31 per cent) on placebo ($P = 0.03$). In addition, there were 4/29 (14 per cent) cases with moderate or severe exacerbations in the nIFNB-treated group compared with 11/29 (38 per cent) in the placebo group ($P < 0.05$).

All subsequent studies have used recombinant interferon beta-1a (rIFNB-1a) preparations produced commercially from stimulated mammalian cells (Table 4.2). A small phase II/III trial of rIFNB-1a in 68 patients (four dropouts occurred after the enrolment of 72 patients) with RRMS (less than 10 years' duration, an EDSS of 1–5 inclusive and at least two attacks in the previous 2 years) used two dose levels for 6 months after a 6-month run-in period (Koudriatseva et al., 1996,

1998; Pozzilli *et al.*, 1996) (Table 4.2). Patients were randomized to either 11 mcg or 33 mcg of a glycosylated rIFNB-1a (Rebif®) three times weekly by subcutaneous injection. The primary endpoint was the mean number and volume of Gd-lesions on monthly T1-weighted MRI (Table 4.3). Compared with baseline, a weekly dose of 33 mg reduced the mean 6-monthly activity (number of Gd-lesions per patient per scan) by 49 per cent (3.5 vs 1.8) and; the reduction was 62 per cent (2.4 vs 0.9) for 99 mcg weekly (both $P < 0.001$). The Gd-lesion volumes were also significantly reduced (by 61 per cent and 74 per cent for the low and high doses, respectively). The comparable reductions for activity on T2-weighted MRI were 65 per cent and 69 per cent, respectively ($P < 0.05$). In addition, there were reductions of 65 per cent (33 mcg weekly) and 70 per cent (99 mcg weekly) in the mean number of new T2 lesions. Individual analysis of Gd-lesions during the treatment period of the trial showed that 78 per cent of the 68 patients had reduced numbers of lesions (including 18 per cent with complete disappearance of lesions) and 12 per cent an increased number of lesions. The remaining 10 per cent had no Gd-lesions throughout the study period.

Table 4.3 Mean (SD) 6-monthly MRI data in patients treated with IFNB-1a 33 mcg and 99 mcg weekly

	No. Gd-lesions	Volume enhancement (cm^3)	No. new T2 lesions
Baseline for 33 mcg group	3.5 (5.0)	0.56 (0.82)	5.7 (5.6)
33 mcg weekly	**1.8 (2.6)**	**0.22 (0.36)**	**2.0 (2.6)**
Baseline for 99 mcg group	2.4 (3.5)	0.38 (0.18)	3.9 (5.0)
99 mcg weekly	**0.9 (1.7)**	**0.1 (0.2)**	**1.2 (1.9)**

Values in bold differ significantly from respective baseline values ($P < 0.001$). (Adapted from Pozzilli *et al.*, 1996.)

The two treatment arms achieved 54 per cent (33 mcg weekly) and 70 per cent (99 mcg weekly) reductions in the rate of clinical relapses (i.e. pre-treatment rates per 6 months of 0.93 and 0.79 were reduced to 0.43 and 0.24 respectively, $P < 0.001$ for both doses). In addition, the percentage of patients who were exacerbation-free increased from 43 per cent to 66 per cent on the low dose and from 52 per cent to 79 per cent on the high dose ($P < 0.01$). In the 2-year extension phase of this study (Pozzilli *et al.*, 1997) the difference between the two doses of rIFNB-1a became more apparent, with significant effects emerging for the relapse rate, the proportions of patients free of attacks and those with no Gd-lesions. A comparison of the 2 years pre-study and the 2 years on trial in the 62 completers showed relapses falling from a mean of 3.46 to 1.56 (55 per cent reduction) for the low dose and from 3.14 to 0.84 (73 per cent reduction) for the high dose. After 24 months' follow-up, the burden of disease on T2-weighted images was reduced by 15 per cent and 14 per cent for 33 mcg and 99 mcg doses, respectively.

Treatment with rIFNB-1a may usefully prolong the beneficial effects of intravenous steroids on blood–brain barrier permeability (Gasperini *et al.*, 1998). In patients treated with rIFNB-1a, the low rate of new enhancement seen on MRI after intravenous steroids was more persistent than with steroids alone. There appear to be no disadvantages to combining rIFNB-1a treatment and intermittent steroids.

Phase III clinical trials

Multiple Sclerosis Collaborative Research Group Trial (MSCRG) (Avonex®, Biogen)

The MSCRG trial of rIFNB-1a involved 301 patients with relatively early RRMS who were mildly impaired (EDSS range 1.0–3.5). Although the terminology has been variously reported as 'exacerbating–remitting' (Jacobs *et al.*, 1995) or 'relapsing multiple sclerosis' (Jacobs *et al.*, 1996), the inclusion criteria specifically excluded patients with secondary progression. The patients were aged 18–55 years and had suffered at least two documented attacks (with or without complete remission) in the previous 3 years. The actual pre-treatment attack rate was approximately 0.7 per annum. Patients were required to be free of attacks for the 2 months prior to trial entry. The patients were randomized to receive either 30 mcg of rIFNB-1a or placebo by once-weekly intramuscular injection. There were initially 143 patients in the placebo group and 158 in the active treatment group. Enrolment was stopped at a stage that left the trial significantly underpowered, with 42 per cent of patients completing less than the originally planned 24 months.

The main findings were a significant ($P = 0.02$) delay in the progression of disability (the primary endpoint) as defined by a deterioration of at least one point on the EDSS, confirmed 6 months later. Of those completing 2 years in the study, 29/87 (33 per cent) on placebo and 18/85 (21 per cent) of those actively treated developed progression. Most treatment failures occurred in the first year, but there was no analysis as to how reliable this endpoint was (i.e. how many patients subsequently improved and became 'erroneous treatment failures'). Subsequently it has been reported that 7/15 patients who were progressors in the first year improved during follow-up and were therefore erroneous treatment failures (Rice and Ebers, 1998).

While clearly showing treatment effects, the clinical interpretation of such findings is not straightforward. The demonstration of benefits of active treatment on disease progression also depends on the behaviour of the placebo group. In the MSCRG trial, the placebo group deteriorated at an unexpectedly high rate (Noseworthy, 1997). Apparent efficacy may be largely if not entirely due to the behaviour of these placebo patients, whatever the stringency of the definitions of confirmed progression (Rudick *et al.*, 1997). Why the MSCRG placebo patients did so poorly compared with placebo patients in other similar trials and why deterioration occurred at more or less regular 6-monthly intervals on a survival-type analysis (Noseworthy, 1997) are questions that have yet to be satisfactorily explained.

Treatment effects of this relatively low dose rIFNB-1a on disease activity (i.e. relapse-related parameters and MRI) were less impressive than those seen in other trials. Active treatment with 30 mcg of rIFNB-1a weekly did not significantly reduce the relapse rate in the first year of the MSCRG trial (the reduction compared with placebo was only 9.6 per cent; FDA, 1996). By 2 years there was an overall 18 per cent reduction of relapses ($P < 0.05$), but neither the proportion of patients rendered free of relapses nor the time to the first in-trial exacerbation were significantly reduced. Nevertheless, the annual relapse rate fell from 0.90 per patient year in the placebo group to 0.61 per patient year in the active treatment group ($P = 0.002$) and high relapse rates (three or more exacerbations) occurred in 12/85 (14 per cent) treated patients compared with 28/87 (32 per cent) controls ($P = 0.03$). Unfortunately, no data were provided on exacerbation severity, steroid use or hospitalization rates.

The reduction of disease activity on Gd-enhanced MRI was modest. Neither the proportion of active scans at the end of year one (30 per cent on treatment compared with 42 per cent on placebo) nor year two attained significance. Similarly, the proportion of patients free of activity on their MRI scans at 2 years was not significantly increased. However, the number and volume of Gd-lesions was reduced for both year one and year two ($P < 0.05$). The percentage change in T2 lesion volume (BOD), while just significant in favour of treatment with rIFNB-1a in the first year (–13.1 per cent on active therapy versus –3.3 per cent on placebo, $P = 0.02$), was not significantly different by the end of year two. This was probably due to the paradoxical reduction of T2 lesion volume in the placebo group (–13.2 per cent for rIFNB-1a and –6.5 per cent for placebo, $P = 0.36$).

A *post hoc* analysis of the 2-year MRI data from this trial has shown significant reductions in the number of new ($P = 0.006$) and enlarging T2 lesions ($P = 0.024$) with treatment, with differences particularly for those patients whose scans showed Gd-lesions at baseline (Simon *et al.*, 1998).

The Once-Weekly Interferon for MS Trial (OWIMS) (Rebif®, Ares-Serono)

This trial investigated the effects of once-weekly subcutaneous injections of two relatively low doses of rIFNB-1a on monthly MRI (Freedman *et al.*, 1998). It involved 293 patients with RRMS from 11 centres in five countries, randomized to receive either 22 mcg or 44 mcg weekly for 1 year. Inclusion criteria were similar to the PRISMS study, except that patients with one relapse in the last 2 years were included, a pre-study MRI was required to show at least three lesions 'consistent with MS' and 'neurological stability' was required for 21–35 days prior to study entry.

The primary outcome measure was the number of combined active lesions (new/enlarging lesions on PD/T2 images and/or Gd-lesions on T1-weighted images) on monthly MRI during the first 24 weeks of treatment. The secondary measures included numbers of active PD/T2 lesions, percentage of scans with combined active lesions, change in the burden of disease (total area of lesions on PD/T2 scans), relapse count, time to first relapse, percentage of relapse-free patients and the need for steroids and hospitalization. The study was not powered to detect clinical endpoints.

Of the 293 patients enrolled, 287 (98 per cent) and 269 (92 per cent) completed 24 and 48 weeks of therapy, respectively. The 44 mcg/week (–53.5 per cent, $P < 0.01$) but not the 22 mcg/week dose (–29.6 per cent) resulted in a significant reduction of combined active MRI lesions. In addition, the median percentage of MRI scans showing combined active lesions was reduced, compared to placebo (50 per cent), to 33 per cent ($P < 0.05$) with 44 mcg and to 45 per cent with 22 mcg once weekly (NS). The median percentage change in the burden of disease was reduced, compared with placebo (5.9 per cent), to –2.0 ($P < 0.005$) and –1.4 ($P < 0.01$) by the 22 mcg and 44 mcg doses, respectively. The 22 mg dose had no effect on relapse rates when compared with placebo, whereas there was a mean reduction of 19 per cent for the 44 mcg dose (NS).

The results will be discussed in more detail in the section comparing dose-responsiveness below.

The Prevention of Relapses and Disability by Interferon Beta-1a (Rebif®, Ares-Serono) Subcutaneously in Multiple Sclerosis (PRISMS Trial)

The largest phase III trial of RRMS (PRISMS Study Group, 1998) involved 560 patients (389 females and 171 males) from 22 centres in nine countries across Europe, Canada and Australia. The PRISMS trial studied the safety and efficacy of rIFNB-1a given in two relatively high doses (22 mcg and 44 mcg, three times weekly by subcutaneous injection) to patients with higher than average disease activity (two attacks in the last 2 years). In addition, the inclusion criteria required an EDSS of 0–5.0 (effectively including disabled patients as well as the merely impaired), the ability to walk without assistance and 'neurological stability' at baseline (no attacks in the 2 months prior to study entry). The primary efficacy endpoint was the number of relapses per patient. Secondary endpoints included duration and severity of exacerbations, time to first exacerbation, progression of disability on the EDSS, need for hospitalization, intravenous steroids, disease activity and burden of disease on MRI.

Only 10 per cent of the patients (58/560) failed to complete the planned 2 years of treatment and follow-up data were available on 533/560 patients (95 per cent) at 2 years. There were 1094/1120 (98 per cent) patient–years of the theoretical total possible data available for the final analysis.

There were significant beneficial effects in all three major disease domains (relapses, disability and MRI) for all primary and secondary outcomes, almost invariably favouring the high dose (Tables 4.4, 4.5). There was a highly significant reduction of relapses after both 1 and 2 years and an increased proportion of patients were free of attacks (Table 4.4). At 2 years, the likelihood of freedom from attacks was increased by 69 per cent with the weekly dose of 66 mcg and by

119 per cent with 132 mcg (a significant difference in favour of the high dose). In addition, there was a highly significant increase in the time to the first exacerbation (prolonged by 69 per cent with 66 mcg and 113 per cent with 132 mcg) and to the second exacerbation (prolonged by 56 per cent with 66 mcg and not reached at 2 years with 132 mcg). The numbers of moderate and severe attacks were also significantly decreased by both doses. Accordingly, hospitalization (a significant 48 per cent lower than placebo with the high dose) and steroid use (30 per cent and 46 per cent lower than placebo for low and high doses, respectively) were reduced by rIFNB-1a (Table 4.4).

Table 4.4 Clinical outcomes (at 2 years) from the PRISMS study

Endpoints	Placebo (n = 187)	66 mcg weekly (n = 189)	132 mcg weekly (n = 184)
Primary			
Mean number of excerbations over 2 years	2.56	1.82 (P = 0.0002)	1.73 (P = <0.0001)
Secondary			
Percentage of patients free of exacerbations	14.6	26 (P = 0.0022)	32 (P < 0.0001)
Median time to first exacerbation (months)	4.5	7.6 (P = 0.0008)	9.6 (P < 0.0001)
Time to confirmed progression of disability (months)	11.8	18.2 (P – 0.0398)	21 (P = 0.0136)
Percentage of patients hospitalized one or more times	25	23	18 (P = 0.0382)
Percentage of patients receiving steroids one or more times	56	42 (P = 0.0129)	39 (P = 0.0002)

Disability worsening on the EDSS was assessed in two different ways. First, using the conventional outcome measure of an increase of one point on the EDSS confirmed at 3 months ('confirmed progression'), there was a significant delay induced by both doses (Table 4.4). The time to this endpoint (first quartile) was 11.9 months in the placebo group, 18.5 months in the group treated with 66 mcg weekly and 21 months in those treated with 132 mcg. Secondly, using the area under the EDSS/time plots (AUC), the median 'accumulated' total disability (both transient and permanent changes in EDSS) was significantly less in both actively treated groups than for the placebo group (a 77 per cent reduction for 66 mcg weekly, $P = 0.0157$ and 88 per cent reduction for 132 mcg weekly, $P = 0.0003$). In addition, the proportion of patients progressing by two points on the Ambulation Index was reduced compared with placebo by 46 per cent ($P < 0.05$) with 132 mcg weekly and by 7.7 per cent (NS) with 66 mcg weekly.

Table 4.5 MRI outcomes at 2 years from the PRISMS study

Endpoints	Placebo	66 mcg weekly		132 mcg weekly	
Median no. active lesions/patient/scan					
Total cohort (*n* = 560)	2.25	0.75	(*P*<0.0001)	0.5	(*P*<0.0001)
Monthly cohort for 9 months (*n* = 205)	0.88	0.17	(*P*<0.0001)	0.11	(*P*<0.0001)
Monthly cohort for 2 years (*n* = 39)	0.90	0.10	(*P*<0.0905)	0.02	(*P*<0.0105)
Burden of disease	10.9%	−1.2% (*P*<0.0001)		−3.8% (*P*<0.0002)	

The MRI results were more impressive than the clinical results (Table 4.5). 551/560 complete data sets were available for analysis. The analysis included a study of the burden of disease (BOD) on five proton density/T2 weighted (PD/T2) MRI scans carried out twice yearly (at baseline and at 6, 12, 18 and 24 months). In the first 6 months, a reduction of BOD associated with treatment persisted to trial end at 24 months. At 24 months, the median increase in BOD in the placebo group was 10.9 per cent compared with −1.2 per cent and −3.8 per cent for those actively treated with 66 mcg and 132 mcg weekly, respectively ($P < 0.0001$ for both arms versus placebo and $P = 0.0537$ for 66 mcg versus 132 mcg). In addition, the median number of T2 active lesions per patient per scan was reduced from 2.25 to 0.75 and 0.5 (both $P < 0.0001$ vs placebo, and $P = 0.0003$ in favour of 132 mcg versus 66 mcg). In addition, the number of active scans (T2 weighted scans with new or enlarging lesions) was reduced from 75 per cent to 50 per cent and 25 per cent by the low and high doses, respectively ($P < 0.0001$ and, for 66 mcg vs 132 mcg, $P = 0.0002$). The proportion of patients who had no T2 activity throughout the study was 8 per cent on placebo, 19 per cent on 66 mcg ($P < 0.0001$) and 31 per cent on 132 mcg ($P < 0.0001$; 66 mcg versus 132 mcg, $P < 0.009$).

The median number of new enhancing lesions was reduced from 8.0 in the placebo group to 1.4 and 1.3 for the 66 mcg and 132 mcg doses, respectively (both $P < 0.0001$ versus placebo). This treatment effect was seen within 2 months of treatment initiation and was persistent. A sub-cohort of 205 patients from seven centres had monthly PD/T2 and Gd-enhanced T1 MRI at baseline (1 month before and 1 day before treatment started) and then monthly for 9 months. Of these, 198/205 data sets were available for analysis. rIFNB-1a significantly reduced the combined unique activity (as reflected by both T2-active lesions and Gd-lesions), by 89 per cent and 98 per cent for 66 mcg and 132 mcg, respectively, compared with placebo. This treatment effect commenced early and persisted throughout the study period. In addition, the percentage of patients with no T2 or T1 Gd activity was increased from 11 per cent in the placebo group to 31 per cent and 41 per cent by the low and high doses respectively (thus representing an increase of 182 per cent and 272 per cent in those with no MRI activity).

In a cohort of patients scanned monthly throughout the trial, the proportion of active scans per patient was 2 per cent (132 mcg weekly) and 10 per cent (66 mcg weekly) in the treated groups and 52 per cent in the placebo group.

Safety

There is no evidence that treatment with rIFNB-1a causes a significant deterioration of MS by perhaps increasing disease activity or progression. One early study that reported possible worsening with an artificially produced nIFNB was, although well conducted, so small that the observations may have been no more than chance (Milanese et al., 1990). Although there was a concern that initiation of IFNB-1b treatment could be associated with a transient increase in relapse frequency (Rudge et al., 1995), this suggestion was also based on an insufficient sample size and has not been confirmed by larger studies specifically addressing this question (Khan and Hebel, 1998). rIFNB-1a has an almost immediate beneficial effect on MRI activity overall, although, on monthly imaging, a minority of patients with RRMS may show apparently increased activity on gadolinium-enhanced MRI during the early months of treatment (Pozzilli et al., 1996).

While flu-like symptoms, headaches, myalgia, lethargy, fever and inflammatory cerebrospinal fluid reactions were reported as common adverse events in early studies of intrathecally administered nIFNB (Jacobs et al., 1981, 1982), the treatment was nevertheless considered well tolerated in 95 per cent of the recipients (Jacobs et al., 1986, 1987). With subcutaneous administration of nIFNB, adverse events were noted mainly within the first few weeks of treatment initiation and reported to be mostly self-limiting or controlled by paracetamol, without the need for termination or dose alteration (Fernandez et al., 1995; Table 4.6). The most common adverse events were flu-like symptoms, fever, injection site reactions and myalgia. The most frequent laboratory abnormality was lymphopenia and, less commonly, mild leucopenia, neutropenia or slightly elevated hepatic transaminases (Fernandez et al., 1995). These observations are consistent with those reported for rIFNB-1a to date (Table 4.6), although mere counts of single occurrences do not take account of the transient nature of the symptoms.

In the phase II study by Pozzilli and colleagues (1996), adverse events (Table 4.6) were generally only mild and transient. No patient developed injection site necrosis.

rIFNB-1a has been well tolerated in all recent major phase III trials, with few serious adverse events. In the MSCRG trial, the relatively low-dose intramuscular rIFNB-1a was associated with a significant incidence of flu-like symptoms, muscle aches and chills (Table 4.6), but no significant laboratory abnormalities were reported. In the PRISMS study the most frequent adverse events were local injection site reactions, which were similar for the two doses (Table 4.6). The few patients who experienced skin reactions generally noted only mild skin redness or swelling, which lessened with time. Dose reduction or termination of treatment was not necessary.

Necrosis of the skin at injection sites did not occur with nIFNB (Fernandez et al., 1995), or with rIFNB-1a given either by the intramuscular route (Jacobs et al.,

Table 4.6 Percentage occurrence of common adverse events with nIFNB and rIFNB-1a

Adverse event	Fernandez (1995) (nIFNB) (n = 58)	Pozzilli (1996) (rIFNB-1a) 11 mcg, 33 mcg (n = 68)	MSCRG (1996) (rIFNB-1a) 30 mcg (n = 204)	PRISMS† (1998) (rIFNB-1a) 66 mcg, 132 mcg (n = 560)
Injection site reaction	53	40, 61	nil	61*, 62*
Flu-like syndrome	20	31, 42	61**	25, 27
Headache	20	26	67	47, 45
Fever	37	21	23	13
Chills	na	na	21**	12
Aesthenia	33	15	21	14, 19
Muscle aches	20	na	34*	13, 14
Lymphopenia:				
Grade II	50	na	nil	5, 13
Grade III	10	na	nil	na
Neutropenia	27	na	nil	4, 8
SGOT	43	na	nil	5, 7
SGPT	47	21	nil	2, 3

†(first 3 months' data); *$P<0.05$; **$P<0.01$ from placebo.

1996) or with low and/or infrequent doses (Pozzilli *et al.*, 1996; Freedman, 1998). In the PRISMS trial, only eight skin necroses occurred in more than 150 000 injections. Each was a single event and healed spontaneously, requiring no specific treatment or dose change and with no subsequent recurrences. Experience suggests that serious skin reactions can largely be avoided with a careful plan of rotating injection sites.

Laboratory abnormalities were more common on high doses and generally reduced in prevalence in the second year of treatment. There were no differences in the pattern of adverse events between high and low disability patients. Eleven patients (2 per cent) dropped out because of adverse events, one from the placebo arm, three from the low-dose arm and seven from the high-dose arm. Asymptomatic increases in hepatic enzymes caused dropout in two cases, injection site reactions in two, flu-like symptoms in two and lymphopenia in one case.

Despite the reduction of white cells by rIFNB-1a, there is no evidence of an increased risk of infection. Infections in the PRISMS trial, whether viral, fungal or bacterial, were invariably *less* frequent in the active treatment arms (with a consistent trend in favour of high dose).

There is no evidence that the incidence of depression is increased by rIFNB-1a treatment. There was an equal incidence of depression in the active and placebo treated arms of the MSCRG trial. Suicidal ideation or suicide attempts were evenly balanced across the three treatment arms of the PRISMS trial, the only successful suicide occurring in the placebo group.

Autoantibodies

Although interferons have been shown to enhance antibody production and exacerbate some autoimmune diseases (Arnason and Reder, 1994), an increased incidence of autoantibodies has not been reported in the major phase III trials of rIFNB-1a. Data from one small, short-duration trial provided no evidence that rIFNB-1a causes any significant increase in antinuclear, antithyroid or anticardiolipin antibodies compared with untreated patients (Colosimo et al., 1997).

Neutralizing antibodies (NABs)

Neutralizing antibodies to IFNs typically appear several months after starting treatment, and their prevalence generally increases with time (Antonelli et al., 1998), although their detection in different trials varies with the route of administration of the treatment, type of assay and definitions (Table 4.7). In 334 patients with RRMS or SPMS receiving rIFNB-1a subcutaneously in two different trials, 3 per cent became NAB-positive in 3 months, 14 per cent in 12 months and 16–18 per cent in 2 years (Abdul-Ahad et al., 1997). However, the majority of patients subsequently reverted to sero-negativity; although 48 (14 per cent) were positive at any time point, only 7 per cent had 'sustained' NAB activity on two or more consecutive tests 6 months apart.

In the study reported by Pozzilli and colleagues (1996), NABs (defined as serum titres of 1 : 20 or more) were detected in 3 per cent, 14 per cent and 16 per cent at 3, 6 and 24 months, respectively (Antonelli et al., 1998). In addition, there is no evidence of any clear relationship between NAB incidence and dose. Positive sera occurred in 5/30 (17 per cent) patients on the low dose (3 Miu) and 5/33 (15 per cent) patients on the high dose.

During the course of the PRISMS study, there was a reduction in the proportion of patients with NABs and a differential dose effect; after 2 years there were significantly less NAB-positive patients on the high dose (132 mcg weekly) than on the low dose (66 mcg weekly) ($P < 0.05$; Table 4.7). The phenomenon of high-zone tolerance is one possible explanation for this interesting observation. The incidence of NABs in both the PRISMS and MSCRG trials was much lower than

Table 4.7 Proportion (%) of patients with neutralizing antibodies in trials of nIFNB and rIFNB-1a

	Fernandez (1995) (nIFNB)	OWIMS (1998) (rIFNB-1a) 22 mcg, 44 mcg	MSCRG (1996) (rIFNB-1a) 30 mcg	PRISMS (1998) (rIFNB-1a) 66 mcg, 132 mcg
1 year	5.3	14	16.3	15.8, 13.6
2 years	12	na	22	23.8, 12.5

that reported for the rIFNB-1b trial of RRMS (27 per cent, 33 per cent and 38 per cent, confirmed on two samples several months apart, for 1, 2 and 3 years, respectively and 45 per cent if detected on one occasion only) (IFNB Multiple Sclerosis Study Group, 1993, 1995), suggesting that the rIFNB-1a molecule is less immunogenic. Furthermore, unlike the controversial conclusions arising from the report of NABs in the IFNB-1b RRMS trial, there is no evidence that NABs to nIFNB or rIFNB-1a are clinically relevant. Thus in one study, although 12 per cent of patients had neutralizing serum activity to nIFNB by the end of the second year, no association with either clinical or MRI activity could be demonstrated (Fernandez et al., 1995). Similarly, in the MRI study of rIFNB-1a (Pozzilli et al., 1996) there was no relationship between NAB formation and the loss of either clinical or MRI response (Antonelli et al., 1998). The PRISMS investigators found no relationship between NABs and relapse frequency (PRISMS Study Group, 1998).

Clinical issues on the use of IFNb-1a for RRMS

The currently available evidence from phase III trials leaves no doubt of the efficacy of rIFNB-1a for reducing disease activity in patients with RRMS. Major areas of interest that require further clarification include the identification of responders and non-responders, dose–response effects and long-term efficacy in preventing or reducing permanent disability.

Heterogeneity

There is a challenge in maximizing treatment efficacy. It is apparent from the IFNB trials to date that not all patients appear to benefit, or to benefit to the same degree, although studies of prognostic and predictive factors are still lacking. RRMS includes an extraordinary heterogeneity of outcomes, ranging from benign MS, in which there is little functional impairment after 10, 15 or more years, to malignant MS, with death or severe disability arising from relapses within a matter of several months or years. Trial investigators have understandably selected patients with above average disease activity as reflected by relapse rates. Nevertheless, apart perhaps from the MSCRG study with its narrower inclusion criteria, cases covering a wide range of disability outcomes will have been included in the PRISMS and OWIMS trials. Apart from the *post hoc* analysis of the IFNB-1b trial of RRMS, in which no significant effects on 'disability progression' could be demonstrated for subgroups above and below an EDSS of 4, the possibility of response heterogeneity has been given scant attention in the trial analyses to date.

Several reports suggest that patients with high levels of disease activity and an EDSS of 3.5 or above are at high risk of rapid and permanent progression to serious levels of disability (Weinshenker et al., 1989, 1995; Weinstock-Guttman et al., 1997). Such patients were excluded from earlier trials of rIFNB-1a, but the PRISMS cohort contained a significant sample above EDSS 3.5. As the ITT analysis of the overall PRISMS cohort demonstrated significance for all primary and secondary endpoints, and as the high risk subgroup is clinically relevant and important, an analysis of this subgroup can be considered both appropriate and statistically inferential (Koch, 1997).

Comparison of the 'low' and 'high' EDSS subgroups at baseline showed that patients with an EDSS > 3.5 had longer disease durations, worse mean scores on the Ambulation Index and SNRS and significantly higher mean BOD on PD/T2 MRI (Blumhardt et al., 1998). The high EDSS subgroup was well balanced and matched across treatment arms, with no evidence that randomization balances had been compromised. For the placebo patients in the high EDSS subgroup, the worst on-trial course for all clinical endpoints confirmed the natural history studies. In this subgroup, the high mean number of relapses was reduced by 40 per cent with 66 mcg weekly and by 60 per cent for those on 132 mcg weekly (Table 4.8). Only the higher dose significantly increased the number of patients free of exacerbations, prolonged the time to the first relapse and reduced the number of moderate or severe attacks to the same degree as did active treatment (with either dose) in the low EDSS cohort. Furthermore, the high dose (27 per cent vs 56 per cent, $P = 0.027$) but not the low dose (41 per cent vs 56 per cent, NS) significantly reduced the percentage of patients with 'confirmed progression' and prolonged the time to either a one-point ($P = 0.0481$) or two-point increase

Table 4.8 PRISMS trial: major clinical endpoints for sub-cohort with baseline EDSS > 3.5

Clinical endpoint	Placebo ($n = 28$)	66 mcg weekly ($n = 35$)	132 mcg weekly ($n = 31$)
Mean number of relapses/patient in 2 year study (% reduction)	3.07	1.83** (40%)	**1.22* (60%)**
Mean number of moderate and severe relapses (% reduction)	1.8	1.0 (44%)	**0.9** (50%)**
Mean number of steroid courses	2.5	1.2	**0.9****
Mean number of hospitalizations (MS-related only)	0.86	0.54	0.48
Median time to first relapse (months)	2.8	7.5	**10.8***
Patients relapse-free at 2 years (%)	7	18	**32****
Time to confirmed disability progression (Q1 – month) (% increase)	7.3	7.5 (3%)	**21.3** (192%)**
Median % change in MRI BOD	5.4	−2.3	**−6.9****
Median number active lesions/patient/scan (PD/T2; 6-monthly)	1.9	0.9	**0.5***

Significant values in bold; *$P<0.05$; **$P<0.005$.
BOD, burden of disease (T2 lesion load).

($P = 0.042$) in the EDSS. The low dose had no significant effect on either end-point.

For MRI in the high EDSS cohort, the median lesion area on PD/T2 images increased by 5.4 per cent in placebo-treated patients and decreased by 2.3 per cent and 6.9 per cent in those on 66 mcg (NS) and 132 mcg ($P = 0.0207$) respectively. Although both doses significantly reduced MRI disease activity on PD/T2 scans, the higher dose (132 mcg weekly) was significantly more effective (a 74 per cent vs 55 per cent reduction, $P < 0.0001$) than the lower dose (66 mcg weekly).

These findings are not an artefact of selecting a 'cutpoint' of EDSS 3.5; a sensitivity analysis (effects of different doses at different levels of disability) showed dose–response effects across the whole range of disabilities in the trial, with even greater differences present when subgroups were defined by an EDSS of 4.0. However, natural history studies suggest that an EDSS > 3.5 is of greater clinical relevance.

This study of a high-risk cohort with RRMS confirms the concept that patients with active RRMS and an EDSS > 3.5 have a more aggressive disease course than those with similar clinical evidence of disease activity but lower EDSS scores. The data strongly suggest that higher doses of rIFNB-1a are required to produce similar levels of benefit in more disabled patients with RRMS (Table 4.8).

Dose–response effects of rIFNB-1a

There appears to be a widespread notion that there is little to choose in terms of efficacy between currently available interferons. This is surprising, given the accumulating evidence of dose-responsive effects of interferons and the practicalities of administering increasing doses.

Many pharmacodynamic effects and immunomodulatory actions of IFNB that may be clinically relevant have been shown to be dose-dependent *in vitro*. The effects on interferon gamma release (Panitch, 1987a, 1987b), proliferation of T-cells (Noronha, 1993), MHC Class II expression (Miller *et al.*, 1996), production of matrix metalloproteinase and T-cell migration (Leppert *et al.*, 1996; Stuve *et al.*, 1998), production of NO (Hua *et al.*, 1998), astrocyte secretion of NGF (Boutros *et al.*, 1997) and IL-10 production (Rudick *et al.*, 1996) have been demonstrated to show dose responsiveness. In addition, EAE lesions and the severity of the inflammatory response in rats (Abreu *et al.*, 1983), and the T-cell response, relapse rate, clinical scores, delay in disease progression and mortality in mice with EAE, are all dose-dependent (Yu *et al.*, 1996).

Early dose-ranging studies of IFNB demonstrated greater efficacy of 8 Miu and 16 Miu of IFNB-1b on annualized relapse rates compared with 0.8 Miu and 4 Miu (Knobler *et al.*, 1993). Although the best results were obtained with 16 Miu, the maximum dose used in the phase III trial that followed was 8 Miu due to the adverse events associated with the higher dose. This trial showed dose–response effects on all clinical and MRI outcome measures (IFNB Multiple Sclerosis Study Group, 1993; Paty *et al.*, 1993). Similarly, differences in the effects of rIFNB-1a on biological markers have been reported across doses ranging from 0.09–45 Miu (Witt *et al.*, 1993). MRI-related dose–response effects of rIFNB-1a have also been shown in phase II studies (Pozzilli, 1996; Koudretseva *et al.*, 1998). In addition to the effect of an absolute weekly dose, more sustained pharmacological effects have been demonstrated in a number of studies using a three times a week regimen, compared with once-weekly, for both rIFNB-1b and rIFNB-1a preparations (Witt *et al*, 1993; Khan and Dhib-Jalbut, 1998; Munafo *et al.*, 1998; Williams and Witt, 1998).

Comparisons between the results of phase III trials of rIFNB-1a might appear to show a similar degree of partial effectiveness, in that clinical evidence of disease activity is reduced by about a third, with less certain effects on 'disease progression' outcomes. However, such superficial comparisons ignore the dose–response effects that are clearly present. The results of treatment with low once-weekly doses of rIFNB-1a (22 mcg in OWIMS and 30 mcg in MSCRG) show less consistent, delayed and smaller effects across multiple endpoints than the higher doses used in PRISMS, despite between-trial differences in disability, which may well be working in the opposite direction. On the other hand, in the PRISMS study, despite more disabled patients, the primary endpoint and most secondary endpoints were significant for both the higher doses (66 mcg and 132 mcg weekly).

Within the PRISMS trial there were dose–response effects, which favoured the highest dose, on steroid courses, hospitalization rates, the time to reach the sustained progression endpoint (1.0 EDSS sustained for 3 months) and the proportion of patients who reached this endpoint (despite the greater disability levels). Furthermore, outcomes in all three major disease domains favoured the higher dose (132 mcg weekly). In the PRISMS trial, 132 mcg weekly but not 66 mcg had a significant effect on mobility as reflected by the Ambulation Index. The reduction in progression (defined as a two-point change on this scale) was 7.7 per cent (NS) for the lower dose and 46 per cent ($P < 0.05$) for the higher dose. As previously mentioned above, the highest available dose of rIFNB-1a (132 mcg) appears to be essential for comparable efficacy in patients with higher disability.

For clinical trials with many endpoints, O'Brien (1984) proposed a global assessment of efficacy using a rank sum test on multiple outcome measures. This method was applied to the PRISMS data using five endpoints covering the major disease domains (exacerbation count, time to first progression on the EDSS, the percentage change in BOD, mean number of PD/T2 active lesions and the integrated area under the EDSS time plots). For a theta of 3.77 (the number of endpoints for which a patient will respond better), the 132 mcg weekly dose was significantly better than the 66 mcg dose ($P = 0.0248$).

The methodological similarities between the OWIMS and PRISMS trials, the similarities of the patient cohorts (Table 4.9) despite slight differences in recruitment criteria and the identical molecular nature and activity of the two currently available rIFNB-1a products have allowed studies of dose–response effects to be made across trials for both clinical and MRI endpoints (Freedman, 1998; Blumhardt, 1999; O'Connor, 1999). For relapse counts in the first year of the three trials, there are graded effects of increasing weekly doses in the range 22–132 mcg, with reductions varying between 0 per cent and 37 per cent and significant results occurring only at 66 mcg and above (Figure 4.2). At the end of 2

Table 4.9 Demographic characteristics of patients in phase III treatment trials of rIFNB-1a

| | MSCRG (Avonex™) | | PRISMS (Rebif®) | | | OWIMS (Rebif®) | | |
	Placebo	30	Placebo	66	132	Placebo	22	44
n	143	158	187	189	184	100	95	98
Females (%)	72	75	75	67	66	74	73	71
Age (years)	36.9	36.7	34.7	34.8	35.2	34.9	35.4	35.5
Symptom duration (years)	6.4	6.6	6.1	7.7	7.8	6.3	6.9	6.7
Pre-study relapse rate	1.2	1.2	1.5	1.5	1.5	1.2	1.2	1.3
Baseline EDSS	2.3	2.4	2.4	2.5	2.5	2.6	2.7	2.4

EDSS, Expanded Disability Status Scale.

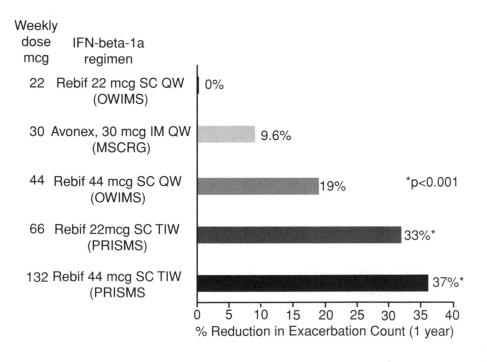

Figure 4.2 Effects of different weekly dose regimes on the percentage reduction of exacerbation rates at 1 year compared with placebo (from OWIMS and PRISMS trials and Summary Basis of Approval for Avonex™).

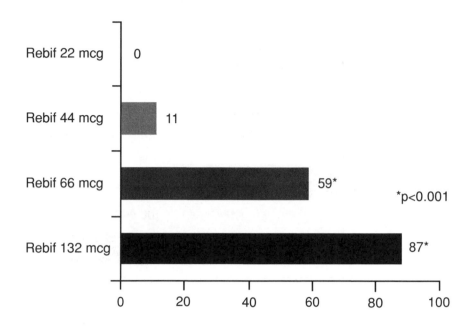

Figure 4.3 Effects of different weekly dose regimens on the percentage increase in patients free of exacerbations at 1 year (from the OWIMS and PRISMS trials).

years, the size of the treatment effect over placebo with 30 mcg weekly was nearly doubled by the 132 mcg weekly dose. The proportion of patients rendered attack-free at the end of the first year was improved by more than five-fold over placebo by 66 mcg weekly, and by more than eight-fold by 132 mcg weekly (Figure 4.3). By 2 years, there was a more than 2.5-fold advantage to 132 mcg weekly compared with 30 mcg weekly (Figure 4.4). Compared with 30 mcg rIFNB-1a weekly, the higher Rebif® dose of 66 mcg weekly delayed the next attack by more than 2.5 times, and 132 mcg weekly delayed it by nearly four times (Figure 4.5). In terms of preventing moderate to severe attacks, the 66 mcg dose was 3.85 times more effective than 44 mcg weekly, whereas 132 mcg was more than 4.5 times more effective than 44 mcg weekly, and more than 10 times more effective than 22 mcg weekly (Figure 4.6). For MRI endpoints, disease activity in the first year of therapy (albeit assessed by different but highly correlated parameters) showed a more than two-fold advantage in favour of 66 mcg weekly over 44 mcg, and a more than three-fold advantage with 132 mcg (Figure 4.7). By contrast, the effects of 22 mcg weekly were insignificant. Once-weekly 30 mcg of rIFNB-1a did not increase the proportion of patients free of MRI activity at 2 years, whereas 66 mcg and 132 mcg weekly achieved highly significant effects on this outcome (Figure 4.8). Similarly, the modest effects of 22 mcg or 44 mcg weekly on achieving a reduction in the mean percentage of T2 active scans in the first year of the trials were improved by nearly four-fold (over 22 mcg) by 66 mcg, and nearly

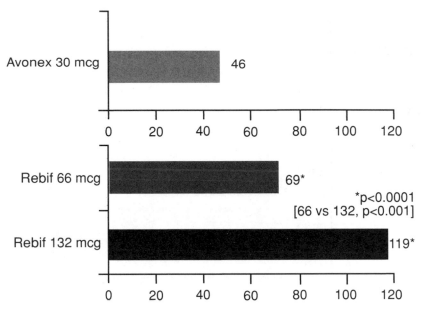

Figure 4.4 Comparison between the effects of 30 mcg weekly (MSCRG trial) (NS), and 66 mcg and 132 mcg weekly dose regimes (PRISMS trial) on the percentage increase in patients free of exacerbations at 2 years compared with placebo.

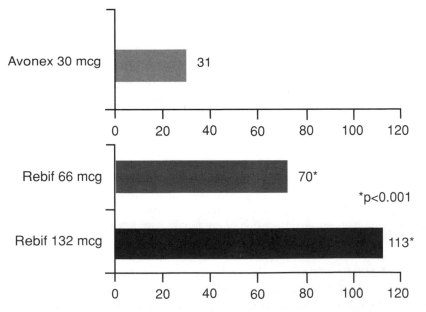

Figure 4.5 Comparison between 30 mcg weekly of rIFNB-1a (Avonex™) in the MSCRG trial (NS) and 66 mcg and 132 mcg in the PRISMS trial, for percentage delay to the first in-trial attack.

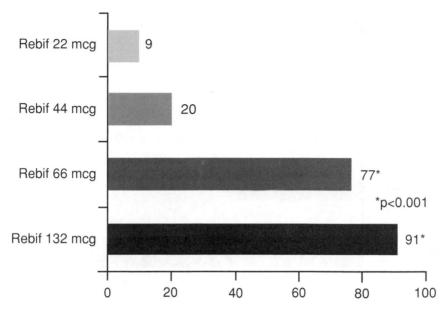

Figure 4.6 Comparison between weekly dose regimes in OWIMS and PRISMS trials for percentage increase in time to the first 'moderate or severe' exacerbation. Only the PRISMS doses were significant compared with placebo (N.B. to first quartile for OWIMS and median for PRISMS).

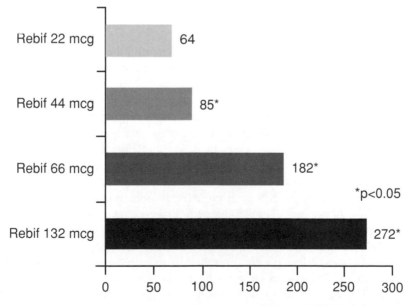

Figure 4.7 Comparison between weekly dose regimes in OWIMS and PRISMS trials for percentage increase in proportion of patients free of MRI activity in the first year of the trials (note that the outcome measures are T2 activity for OWIMS and T2 activity plus T1-Gd lesions for PRISMS).

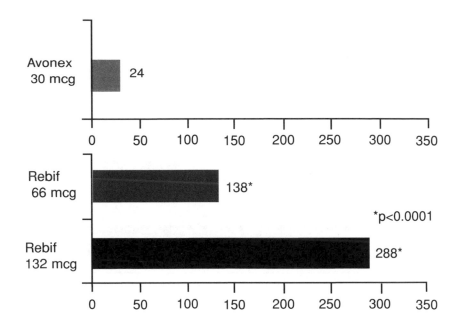

Figure 4.8 Comparison between MSCRG and PRISMS results for the percentage of patients with no active lesions on MRI at 2 years (N.B. T1-Gd for MSCRG/Avonex and T2 activity for PRISMS/Rebif).

five-fold by 132 mcg. By 2 years, the improvement in the median number of T2 active lesions obtained with 30 mcg was doubled by 66 mcg weekly and significantly improved even further with 132 mcg (Figure 4.9).

Within PRISMS, there were significant advantages of the highest dose (132 mcg weekly) over 66 mcg weekly for new and enlarging T2 lesions, an MRI outcome that best indexes all activity in the preceding month. The end result of all the inflammatory activity was seen in the accumulating BOD. This was not significantly affected by 30 mcg, but was reduced by 12.1 per cent by 66 mcg weekly and 14.7 per cent by 132 mcg weekly, compared with placebo.

The percentage of patients with no active lesions on their MRI at 2 years increased by 24 per cent over placebo with 30 mcg weekly, and by 138 per cent and 288 per cent with 66 mcg and 132 mcg, respectively (66 mcg versus 132 mcg, $P < 0.0001$). For a similar endpoint (the reduction in the median number of active lesions at 2 years), 30 mcg weekly resulted in an increase of 33 per cent, versus 67 per cent and 78 per cent increases for 66 mcg and 132 mcg, respectively (66 mcg vs 132 mcg, $P < 0.001$). BOD was not significantly affected by 30 mcg, but was reduced by 12.1 per cent and 14.7 per cent ($P = 0.054$) by 66 mcg and 132 mcg weekly, respectively. There was a significant difference in favour of the highest dose (132 mcg weekly) for new T2 lesions (median number of new lesions/year was 1.3 on 66 mcg and 0 on 132 mcg, $P < 0.001$).

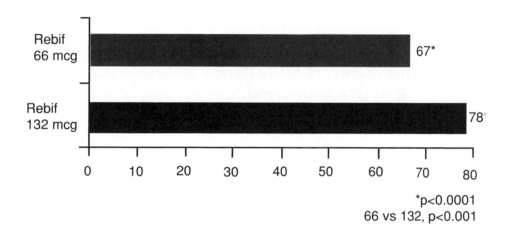

Figure 4.9 Comparison between effects of different weekly doses (MSCRG and PRISMS trials) on reduction of median number of T2 active lesions at 2 years.

It is clear from the OWIMS study that once-weekly rIFNB-1a in doses up to 44 mcg are insufficient to significantly reduce the relapse rate in the first year of treatment. The dose–response effects were particularly clear for the time to the first moderate or severe attack and the percentage increase in relapse-free patients in the first year, endpoints not affected by doses of 44 mcg weekly or less in the OWIMS trial, but significantly reduced by 66 mcg and 132 mcg weekly in the PRISMS trial. The percentage increase in relapse-free patients at 2 years was not affected by 30 mcg weekly in the MRCG trial, but was significant for both doses in the PRISMS trial ($P < 0.0001$). Again, there was a significant advantage of 132 mcg weekly over 66 mcg weekly in the PRISMS trial (119 per cent vs 69 per cent, $P < 0.001$).

Hospitalization rates in the PRISMS trial were significantly reduced only by the 132 mcg dose, an indication of the effectiveness of the high dose in preventing or reducing the severity of the more disabling attacks. Again, although both doses significantly increased the time to 'progression of disability' on the EDSS, the significant reduction in progression on the Ambulation Index was only achieved with 132 mcg weekly.

A meta-analysis of the individual data from the OWIMS and PRISMS trials suggests that the dose–response relationship for rIFNB-1a approximates reasonably to a linear model, predicting that for each additional 22 mcg increment of rIFNB-1a there is an approximately 10 per cent improvement for clinical outcome measures and 20 per cent for MRI measures (Blumhardt, 1999). Overall, there are clear and significant treatment advantages in favour of the higher weekly dose regimen (132 mcg) for many endpoints and, as yet, no significant downside in terms of increased adverse events. The risk–benefit ratio therefore clearly favours the maximum dose for all RRMS patients, and particularly for the high risk, high EDSS cohort, where it is essential to obtain equivalent benefits to those achieved in patients with less marked disability or mainly impairment (Blumhardt et al., 1998).

Clinical relevance of rIFNB-1a therapy for long-term disability

Despite clear short-term benefits of IFNB, there is a continuing debate about its value for the prevention of long-term disability (Rice and Ebers, 1998). This stems partly from the limitations of the outcome measures for so-called 'disease progression' in the clinical trials, and partly from the unrealistic expectations of investigators (and their critics) that significant effects of treatment on *irreversible* worsening of disability can be detected in 2-year trials of RRMS. Natural history studies show that it takes some 15 years or more on average for 50 per cent of such cohorts to reach firm endpoints such as an EDSS of 6.0 (Runmarker and Andersen, 1993). Over shorter periods the disease course is highly variable, and endpoints for 'progression' are either insensitive due to their low incidence, or have a high false-positive rate (Liu and Blumhardt, 1999). The appropriate use of such endpoints requires much larger and/or longer trials than those performed to date. In the meantime, an appropriate assessment of the value of rIFNB-1a therapy needs to take into account the main aim of rIFNB-1a therapy, which should be axonal protection.

Short-term benefits that arise from immediate reductions in disease activity are the easiest to quantify. The reduction in the number and severity of relapses alone justifies early treatment, not only because relapses are unpredictable and unpleasant in their own right (with important social and employment impact), but also because the sequelae of many relapses that fail to fully resolve contribute to accumulating, irreversible disability. In addition, recurrent episodes of inflammation are more likely to be followed by permanent disability as damage accumulates and repair mechanisms become increasingly compromised. As clinical relapses represent only one-tenth to one-thirtieth (Thompson et al., 1991) of the underlying, ongoing, acute disease activity on MRI, the major anti-inflammatory effects of the higher doses of rIFNB-1a can be expected to be relevant for long-term disability well beyond the durations of recent trials. Clinical observations (Muller, 1949; Alexander, 1958), epidemiological (Weinshenker et al., 1989) and MRI (Morrissey et al., 1993; Filippi et al., 1994; O'Riordan et al., 1998) studies all testify to the relationship between the levels of disease activity at or near disease onset and the disability reached 5–10 years later.

There are direct and highly significant correlations between acute inflamma-tory lesions and irreversible axonal transection (Ferguson *et al.*, 1997; Trapp *et al.*, 1998). The evidence from several pathological studies suggests that much axonal damage and loss occurs as an episodic, relapse-related phenomenon. Pathological studies have clearly demonstrated that axonal damage is a feature of early acute inflammatory lesions (Ferguson *et al.*, 1997; Mews *et al.*, 1998; Trapp *et al.*, 1998). In studies of RRMS, reduced N-acetylaspartate (NAA) levels on MRI spectroscopy have been found both in acute lesions and normal-appearing white matter (Matthews *et al.*, 1996; Fu *et al.*, 1998; de Stefano *et al.*, 1999). Changes in NAA in the normal-appearing white matter over periods of months, which correlate with increasing disability (Fu *et al.*, 1998), imply that a more or less continuous process of axonal damage and loss is occurring in RRMS. In addition, quantitative MRI studies suggest that high rates of irreversible tissue atrophy are occurring early in the disease, probably from the onset of the inflam-matory lesions that result in RRMS (Liu *et al.*, 1999).

The evidence from several different sources linking acute inflammatory axonal damage to disability provides a clear rationale for initiating early treatment. A significant reduction of clinical and MRI disease activity in the early stages may well slow the accumulating axonal and oligodendrocyte burden and delay the clinical threshold for secondary progression, the main stage of permanent dis-ability worsening in MS (Runmarker and Andersen, 1993; Andersen, 1999). As disabled RRMS patients require higher doses of rIFNB-1a to achieve significant effects (Blumhardt *et al.*, 1998), and as SPMS patients continue to progress despite treatment (IFNB Multiple Sclerosis Study Group, 1993, 1995), a more aggressive 'prophylactic' treatment strategy using treatments with proven anti-inflammatory (and thus axon-protective) effects should be urgently considered.

The PRISMS trial shows that the total disability experienced by patients rela-tively early in the disease course can now be reduced by a median 88 per cent (AUC analysis), and new inflammatory (Gd-enhancing) lesions by 84 per cent, by using the highest available dose of rIFNB-1a (132 mcg weekly). On current evi-dence this must be the most sensible treatment option, with the best risk–benefit ratio for the patient with active RRMS, at least until further data (or better treat-ments) are available.

New clinical trials

At the time of writing, the results of a major multicentre Phase III trial of rIFNB-1a (Rebif®, Ares-Serono) 66 mcg and 132 mcg weekly in secondary progressive MS have been reported at the European Neurological Society meeting in Milan, Italy, but have not yet been published. This 3-year trial of 618 patients with clin-ically definite SPMS is particularly pertinent, given the criticisms of the prema-ture termination (at 2 years) of the European rIFNB-1b treatment trial of SPMS (Betaseron, Schering). Importantly, the trial showed that rIFNB-1a is safe and well tolerated in the most advanced and disabled cohort of SPMS patients yet studied with IFNB. The overall results were positive for major endpoints. Both doses (66 mcg and 132 mcg weekly) resulted in a significant reduction in relapse rate, use of steroids and disease activity, and a change in the burden of disease on MRI. The high dose also had significant beneficial effects on all other relapse-related outcomes, including hospitalization. Effects on disability progression appear less than for the PRISMS study, with significant effects resulting only when multiple covariants were taken into account ($P < 0.046$). An unexpected finding was the effect of gender, with significant beneficial effects on disability progression for females at both doses, but no significant effects for males. The results overall are consistent with the hypothesis that early treatment is likely to be more effective in preventing permanent disability in MS.

Further dose-ranging studies of rIFNB-1a (Avonex™, Biogen) are currently comparing the effects of weekly intramuscular doses of 6 Miu and 12 Miu in RRMS and SPMS cohorts.

At the other end of the disease spectrum, two trials are investigating the effects of treatment with rIFNB-1a in patients with single clinical attacks and abnormal MRI. The Early Treatment of MS (ETOMS, Rebif®, Ares-Serono) trial has enrolled 308 patients with a single attack and is following patients to the primary endpoint of 'conversion to clinical MS' (Comi *et al.*, 1998). The North American study (CHAMPS Trial), which has randomized 383 patients to date (Jacobs *et al.*, 1999), is also investigating the role of rIFNB-1a in preventing or delaying clinical conversion from an isolated clinical syndrome to CDMS.

The results of these current trials are eagerly awaited, as they are likely not only to extend the spectrum of patients for whom rIFNB-1a is a valuable therapy but also to re-define our strategies for targeting patients for maximal benefits. While it seems counterintuitive at the present time not to expect at least some benefit for most patients who receive IFNB, it also seems likely that new long-term follow-up data will eventually support the concept that the really worthwhile benefits will arise in cohorts where the most effective (high-dose) treatment regimens have been initiated as soon as possible after the onset of the disease.

References

Abdul-Ahad, A. K., Galazaka, A. R., Revel, M. *et al.* (1997). Incidence of antibodies to interferon-B in patients treated with recombinant human interferon-B1a from mammalian cells. *Cyto. Cell. Mol. Ther.*, **3**, 27–32.

Abreu, S. L., Tondreau, J., Levine, S. *et al.* (1983). Inhibition of passive localized experimental allergic encephalomyelitis by interferon. *Int. Arch. Appl. Immunol.*, **72**, 30–33.

Alam, J., McAllister, A., Scaramucci, J. *et al.* (1997). Pharamacokinetics and pharmacodynamics of interferon beta-1a (IFNB-1a) in healthy volunteers after intravenous, subcutaneous or intramuscular administration. *Clin. Drug Invest.*, **14**, 35–43.

Alexander, L., Berkeley, A. W. and Alexander, A. M. (1958). Prognosis and treatment of multiple sclerosis; quantitative nosimetric study. *J. Am. Med. Assoc.*, **166**, 1943.

Andersen, O. (1999). Treatment alternatives in relapsing–remitting multiple sclerosis. In: *Frontiers in Multiple Sclerosis* (A. Siva, J. Kesselring and A. J. Thompson, eds), pp. 173–94. Martin Dunitz.

Antonelli, G., Bagnato, F., Pozzilli, C. *et al.* (1998). Development of neutralizing antibodies in patients with relapsing-remitting multiple sclerosis treated with IFNB-1a. *J. Int. Cyt. Res.*, **18**, 345–50.

Arnason, B. G. W. and Reder, A. T. (1994). Interferons and multiple sclerosis. *Clin. Neuropharm.*, **17**, 495–547.

Arnason, B. G. W., Dayal, A., Xiang, Z. *et al.* (1996). Mechanism of action of interferon beta in multiple sclerosis. *Springer Sem. Immunopathol.*, **18**, 125–48.

Baumhefner, R. W., Tourtellotte, W. W., Syndulkok, P. *et al.* (1987). Effect of intravenous natural interferon beta on clinical neurofunction, magnetic resonance imaging plaque burden, intrablood brain barrier IgG synthesis, blood and cerebrospinal fluid cellular immunology, and visual evoked responses. *Ann. Neurol.*, **22**, 171.

Blumhardt, L. D. (1999). Interferon beta-1a in relapsing-remitting multiple sclerosis: a meta-analysis. *Neurology*, **52A**, 498.

Blumhardt, L. D., Paty, D. W., Hughes, R. A. C. *et al.* (1998). Dosage effect of interferon B-1a (Rebif®) in preventing relapses and progression of disability in relapsing–remitting multiple sclerosis with baseline EDSS > 3.5. *J. Neurol.*, **245**, 371.

Bocci, V., Pessina, G. P., Paulescu, L. *et al.* (1988). The lymphatic route. V. Distribution of natural interferon-beta in rabbit plasma and lymph. *J. Interferon Res.*, **8**, 633–40.

Boutros, T., Croze, E. and Yong, V. W. (1997). Interferon beta is a potent promoter of nerve growth factor production by astrocytes. *J. Neurochem.*, **69**, 939–46.

Chernajovsky, Y., Mory, Y., Chen, L. *et al.* (1984). Efficient constitutive production of human fibroblast interferon by hamster cells transformed with the IFN-B1 gene fused to an SV40 promoter. *DNA*, **3**, 297–308.

Colosimo, C., Pozzilli, C., Frontoni, M. *et al.* (1997). No increase of serum antibodies during therapy with recombinant human interferon beta-1a in relapsing-remitting multiple sclerosis. *Acta Neurol. Scand.*, **96**, 372–4.

Comi, G. and ETOMS Study Group (1998). ETOMS study: baseline characteristics of the included population. *J. Neurol.*, **245**, 443.

Confavreux, C., Chapuis-Cellier C., Arnaud, P. *et al.* (1986). Oligoclonal 'fingerprint' of CSF IgG in multiple sclerosis patients is not modified following intrathecal administration of natural beta-interferon. *J. Neurol. Neurosurg. Psychiatr.*, **49**, 1308–12.

De Stefano, N., Narayanan, S., Pelletier, D. *et.al.* (1999). Evidence of early axonal damage in patients with multiple sclerosis. *Neurology*, **52** (suppl. 2), A 378.

Edwards, S. G. M., Zvartau, M., Clark, H. *et al.* (1998). Clinical relapses and disease activity on magnetic resonance imaging (MRI) associated with viral upper respiratory tract infection (URTI) in multiple sclerosis (MS). *J. Neurol. Neurosurg. Psychiatr.*, **64**, 736–41.

Ferguson, B., Matyszak, M. K., Esiri, M. M. *et al.* (1997). Axonal damage in acute multiple sclerosis. *Brain*, **120**, 393–9.

Fernandez, O., Antiquedad, A., Arbizu T. *et al.* (1995). Treatment of relapsing-remitting multiple sclerosis with natural interferon beta: a multicentre, randomized clinical trial. *Multiple Sclerosis*, **1**, S67–S69.

Filippi, M., Horsfield, M. A., Morrissey, S. P. *et al.* (1994). Quantitative brain MRI lesion load predicts the course of clinically isolated syndromes suggestive of multiple sclerosis. *Neurology*, **44**, 635–41.

Freedman, M. S. and Once-Weekly Interferon for MS (OWIMS) Study Group (1998). Dose-dependent clinical and magnetic resonance imaging efficacy of interferon beta-1a (Rebif®) in multiple sclerosis. *Ann. Neurol.*, **44**, 992.

Fu, L., Matthews, P. M., de Stefano, N. *et al.* (1998). Imaging axonal damage of normal-appearing white matter in multiple sclerosis. *Brain*, **121**, 103–13.

Gasperini, C., Pozilli, C., Bastianello, S. *et al.* (1998). Effect of steroids on Gd-enhancing lesions before and during recombinant beta interferon-1a treatment in relapsing–remitting multiple sclerosis. *Neurology*, **50**, 403–6.

Hartung, H. P. and Kieseier, B. C. (1996). Targets for the therapeutic action of interferon-beta in multiple sclerosis. *Ann. Neurol.*, **40**, 825–6.

Hohlfeld, R. (1997). Biotechnical agents for the immunotherapy of multiple sclerosis. Principles, problems and perspectives. *Brain*, **120**, 865–916.

Hua, L. L., Liu, J. S., Brosnan, C. F. *et al.* (1998) Selective inhibition of human glial inducible nitric oxide synthase by interferon-b: implications for MS. *Ann. Neurol.*, **43**, 384–7.

Huber, M., Bamborschke, S., Assheur, J. *et al.* (1988). Intravenous natural beta interferon treatment of chronic exacerbating-remitting multiple sclerosis: clinical response and MRI/CSF findings. *J. Neurol.*, **235**, 171–3.

IFNB Multiple Sclerosis Study Group (1993). Interferon beta-1b is effective in relapsing-remitting multiple sclerosis. I. Clinical results of a multicentre, randomized, double-blind, placebo-controlled trial. *Neurology*, **43**, 655–61.

IFNB Multiple Sclerosis Study Group and the University of British Columbia MS/MRI Analysis Group (1995). Interferon beta-1b in the treatment of multiple sclerosis: final outcome of the randomized controlled trial. *Neurology*, **45**, 1277–85.

Jacobs, L., O'Malley, J., Freeman A. *et al.* (1981). Intrathecal interferon reduces exacerbations of multiple sclerosis. *Science*, **214**, 1026–8.

Jacobs, L. D., O'Malley, J., Freeman, A. and Ekes, R. (1982). Intrathecal interferon in multiple sclerosis. *Arch. Neurol.*, **39**, 609–15.

Jacobs, L., Herndon, R., Freeman, A. *et al.* (1986). Multicentre double-blind study of effect of intrathecally administered natural human fibroblast interferon on exacerbations of multiple sclerosis. *Lancet*, **2**, 1411–13.

Jacobs, L. D., Salazar, A. M., Herndon, R. *et al.* (1987). Intrathecally administered natural human fibroblast interferon reduces exacerbations of multiple sclerosis: results of a multicentre double-blind study. *Arch. Neurol.*, **44**, 589–95.

Jacobs, L. D., Cookfair, D. L., Rudick, R. A. *et al.* (1995). A phase III trial of intramuscular recombinant interferon beta as treatment for exacerbating-remitting multiple sclerosis: design and conduct of study and baseline characteristics of patients. *Multiple Sclerosis*, **1**, 118–35.

Jacobs, L. D., Cookfair, D. L., Rudick, R. A. *et al.* (1996). Intramuscular interferon beta-1 for disease progression in relapsing multiple sclerosis. *Ann. Neurol.*, **39**, 285–94.

Jacobs, L. D., Beck, R. W., Brownscheidle, C. M. *et al.* (1999). A profile of patients at high risk for the development of clinically definite MS (CDMS): the first report of the CHAMPS study. *Neurology*, **52A**, 495.

Khan, O. A. and Dhib-Jalbut, S. S. (1998). Serum interferon-beta-1a (Avonex) levels following intramuscular injection in relapsing–remitting MS patients. *Neurology*, **51**, 738–42.

Khan, O. A. and Hebel, J. R. (1998). Incidence of exacerbations in the first 90 days of treatment with recombinant human interferon beta-1b in patients with relapsing–remitting multiple sclerosis. *Ann. Neurol.*, **44**, 138–9.

Knobler, R. L., Greenstein, J. L., Johnstone, K. P. *et al.* (1993). Systemic recombinant human interferon beta treatment of relapsing–remitting multiple sclerosis: pilot study and 6-year follow-up. *J. Interferon Res.*, **13**, 333–40.

Koch, G. (1997). Discussion of '*P* value adjustments for subgroup analyses'. *J. Biopharm. Stat.*, **7**, 323–31.

Koudriavtseva, T., Fiorelli, M., Bastianello, S. *et al.* (1996). Profile of clinical responders to interferon beta-1a treatment in relapsing–remitting multiple sclerosis. *Eur. J. Neurol.*, **3**, 90–91.

Koudriavtseva, T., Pozzilli, C., Fiorelli, M. *et al.* (1998). Determinants of Gd-enhanced MRI response to IFNB-1a treatment in relapsing-remitting multiple sclerosis. *Multiple Sclerosis*, **98**, 403–7.

Leppert, D., Waubant, E., Burk, M. R. *et al.* (1996). Interferon beta-1b inhibits gelatinase secretion and *in vitro* migration of human T cells: a possible mechanism for treatment efficacy in multiple sclerosis. *Ann. Neurol.*, **40**, 846–52.

Liberati, A. M., Horisberger, M. A., Palmisano, L. *et al.* (1992). Double-blind randomized phase I study on the clinical tolerance and biological effects of natural and recombinant interferon-beta. *J. Interferon Res.*, **12**, 329–36.

Liberati, A. M., Garofani, P., De Angelis, V. *et al.* (1994). Double-blind, randomized phase I study on the clinical tolerance and pharmacodynamics of natural and recombinant interferon-beta given intravenously. *J. Interferon Res.*, **14**, 61–9.

Liu, C. and Blumhardt, L. D. (1999). Analysis of disability endpoints in placebo cohorts from relapsing–remitting multiple sclerosis treatment trials. *J. Neurol.* **246** (suppl. 1); 35.

Liu, C., Li Wan Po, A., Blumhardt, L. D. (1998). 'Summary measure' statistic for assessing the outcome of treatment trials in relapsing-remitting multiple sclerosis. *J. Neurol. Neurosurg. Psychiatr.*, **64**, 726–9.

Liu, C., Edwards, S., Gong, C. *et al.* (1999). Three-dimensional MRI estimates of brain and spinal cord atrophy in multiple sclerosis. *J. Neurol. Neurosurg. Psychiatr.*, **66**, 323–30.

Matthews, P. M., Pioro, E., Narayanan, S. *et al.* (1996). Assessment of lesion pathology in multiple sclerosis using quantitative MRI morphometry and magnetic resonance spectroscopy. *Brain*, **119**, 715–22.

Mews, I., Bergmann, M., Bunkowski, S. *et al.* (1998). Oligodendrocyte and axon pathology in clinically silent multiple sclerosis lesions. *Multiple Sclerosis*, **4**, 55–62.

Milanese, C., Salmaggi, A., La Mantia, L. *et al.* (1990). Double-blind study of intrathecal beta-interferon in multiple sclerosis: clinical and laboratory results. *J. Neurol. Neurosurg. Psychiatr.*, **53**, 554–7.

Miller, A., Lanir, N., Shapiro, S. *et al.* (1996). Immunoregulatory effects of interferon-beta and interacting cytokines on human vascular endothelial cells. Implications for multiple sclerosis and other autoimmune diseases. *J. Neuroimmunol.*, **64**, 151–61.

Morrissey, S. P., Miller, D. H., Kendall, B. E. *et al.* (1993). The significance of brain magnetic resonance imaging abnormalities at presentation with clinically isolated syndromes suggestive of multiple sclerosis. *Brain*, **116**, 135–46.

Muller, R. (1949). Studies on disseminated sclerosis, with special reference to symptomatology, course and prognosis. *Acta Med. Scand.*, **133**, 1–214.

Munafo, A., Spertini, F., Rothuisen, L. *et al.* (1997). Phamacodynamic response to r-IFN beta administered subcutaneously once a week (QW) or three times a week (TIW), over one month. *Multiple Sclerosis*, **3**, 343.

Munafo, A., Trinchard-Lugan, I., Nguyen, T. X. Q. *et al.* (1998). Bioavailability of recombinant human interferon beta-1a after intramuscular and subcutaneous administration. *Eur. J. Neurol.*, **5**, 187–93.

Noronha, M. J., Toscas, A. and Jensen, M. A. (1993). Interferon beta decreases T-cell activation and interferon gamma production in multiple sclerosis. *J. Neuroimmunol.*, **46**, 145–54.

Noseworthy, J. (1997). Are placebo-controlled trials still ethical in multiple sclerosis? In: *Multiple Sclerosis: Clinical Challenges and Controversies* (A. J. Thompson, C. Polman and R. Hohfield, eds), pp. 177–94. Martin Dunitz.

O'Brien, P. C. (1984). Procedures for comparing samples with multiple endpoints. *Biometrics*, **40**, 1079–87.

O'Connor, P. (1999). Comparison of outcome measures in interferon beta studies in relapsing multiple sclerosis. *Neurology*, **52A**, 498.

O'Riordan, J. I., Thompson, A. J., Kingsley, D. P. E. *et al.* (1998). The prognostic value of brain MRI in clinically isolated syndromes of the CNS. A 10-year follow-up. *Brain*, **121**, 495–503.

Panitch, H. S. (1994). Influence of infection on exacerbations of multiple sclerosis. *Ann. Neurol.*, **36**, S25–S28.

Panitch, H. S., Folus, J. S. and Johnson, K. P. (1987a). Recombinant beta interferon inhibits gamma interferon production in multiple sclerosis. *Ann. Neurol.*, **22**, 139.

Panitch, H. S., Hirsch, R. L., Haley, A. S. *et al.* (1987b). Exacerbations of multiple sclerosis with gamma interferon. *Lancet*, **i**, 893–5.

Paty, D. W., Li, D. K. B., UCB MS/MRI Study Group *et al.* (1993). Interferon beta-1b is effective in relapsing–remitting multiple sclerosis. II . MRI analysis results of a multicenter, randomized, double-blind, placebo-controlled trial. *Neurology*, **43**, 662–7.

Pozzilli, C., Bastianello, S., Koudriatseva, T. *et al*. (1996). Magnetic resonance imaging changes with recombinant human interferon beta-1a: a short-term study in relapsing–remitting multiple sclerosis. *J. Neurol. Neurosurg. Psychiatr.*, **61**, 251–8.

Pozzilli, C., Bastianello, S., Koudriatseva, T. *et al*. (1997). An open randomised trial with two different doses of recombinant interferon beta 1a in relapsing–remitting multiple sclerosis: clinical and MRI results at 24 months. *J. Neurol.*, **244**, S25.

PRISMS Study Group (1998). Randomized, double-blind, placebo-controlled study of interferon beta-1a in relapsing–remitting multiple sclerosis: clinical results. *Lancet*, **352**, 1498–1504.

Revel, M., Schattner, A. and Wallach, D. (1981). Monitoring of interferon therapy, diagnosis of viral diseases and detection of interferon deficiencies by assay of an interferon-indiced enzyme in human peripheral white blood cells. In: *The Clinical Potential of Interferons* (R. Kono and J. Vilcek, eds), pp. 353–67. University of Tokyo Press.

Rice, G. and Ebers, G. (1998). Interferons in the treatment of multiple sclerosis. Do they prevent the progression of the disease? *Arch. Neurol.*, **55**, 1578–80.

Rudge, P. R., Miller, D. H., Crimlisk, H. *et al*. (1995). Does interferon beta cause initial exacerbations of multiple sclerosis? *Lancet*, **345**, 580.

Rudick, R. A., Carpenter, C. S., Cookfair, D. L. *et al*. (1993). *In vitro* and *in vivo* inhibition of nitrogen-driven T-cell activation by recombinant interferon beta. *Neurology*, **43**, 2080–87.

Rudick, R. A., Ransohoff, R. M., Peppler, R. *et al*. (1996). Interferon beta induces interleukin-10 expression: relevance to multiple sclerosis. *Ann. Neurol.*, **40**, 618–27.

Rudick, R. A., Goodkin, D. E., Jacobs, L. D. *et al*. (1997). Impact of interferon beta-1a on neurologic disability in relapsing multiple sclerosis. *Neurology*, **49**, 358–63.

Runmarker, B. and Andersen, O. (1993). Prognostic factors in a multiple sclerosis incidence cohort with twenty-five years of follow-up. *Brain*, **116**, 117–34.

Salmon, P., Le Cotonnec, J.-Y., Galazaka, A. *et al*. (1996). Pharmacokinetics and pharmacodynamics of recombinant human interferon-beta in healthy male volunteers. *J. Interferon Res.*, **16**, 759–64.

Schonfeld, A., Nitke, S., Schatter, A. *et al*. (1984). Intramuscular human interferon beta injections in treatment of condylomata acuminata. *Lancet*, **i**, 1038–42.

Sibley, W. A., Bamford, C. R. and Clark, K. (1985). Clinical viral infections and multiple sclerosis. *Lancet*, **i**, 1313–15.

Simon, J. H., Jacobs, L. D., Campion, M. *et al*. (1998). Magnetic resonance studies of intramuscular interferon β-1a for relapsing multiple sclerosis. *Ann. Neurol.*, **43**, 79–87.

Stuve, O., Dooley, N. P., Uhm, J. H. *et al.* (1996). Interferon beta-1b decreases the migration of T-lymphocytes *in vitro*: effects on matrix metalloproteinase-9. *Ann. Neurol.*, **40**, 853–63.

FDA (1996). *Summary Evidence for FDA Approval: Interferon Beta-1a, Avonex®, Biogen, Inc.* PLA 95-0979; ELA 95-0975.

Thompson, A. J., Kermode, A. G. and Wicks, D. (1991). Major differences in the dynamics of primary and secondary progressive multiple sclerosis. *Ann. Neurol.*, **29**, 53–62.

Trapp, B. D., Peterson, J., Ransohoff, R. M. *et al.* (1998). Axonal transection in the lesions of multiple sclerosis. *N. Engl. J. Med.*, **338**, 278–85.

Verveken, D., Carton, H. and Billiau, A. (1979). Intrathecal administration of interferon in MS patients. In: *Humoral Immunity in Neurological Disease* (D. Karcher, A. Lowenthal and A. D. Strosberg, eds), pp. 625–7. Plenum Press.

Weinshenker, B. G. (1995). The natural history of multiple sclerosis. *Neurol Clin.*, **1**, 119–46.

Weinshenker, B. G., Bass, B., Rice, G. P. A. *et al.* (1989). The natural history of multiple sclerosis: a geographically based study. 1. Clinical course and disability. *Brain*, **112**, 133–46.

Weinstock-Guttman, B., Kinkel, R. P., Cohen, J. A. *et al.* (1997). Treatment of 'transitional MS' with cyclophosphamide and methylprednisolone (CTX/MP) followed by interferon beta. *Neurology*, **48A**, 341.

Williams, G. J. and Witt, P. L. (1998). Comparative study of the pharmacodynamic and pharmacologic effects of Betaseron and Avonex. *Interferon Cyt. Res.*, **18**, 967–75.

Witt, P. L., Storer, B. E., Bryan, G. *et al.* (1993). Pharmacodynamics of biological response *in vivo* after single and multiple doses of interferon-beta. *J Immunother.*, **13**, 191–200.

Yu, M., Nishuyawa, A., Trapp, B. D. *et al.* (1996). Interferon-b inhibits progression of relapsing–remitting experimental autoimmune encephalomyelitis. *J. Neuroimmunol.*, **64**, 91–100.

5

Glatiramer acetate

Introduction

The rationale for the use of glatiramer acetate (formerly copolymer 1; trade name Copaxone®) in multiple sclerosis (MS) derives directly from studies of experimental allergic encephalomyelitis (EAE). Investigators at the Weizmann Institute initially speculated that the interaction of the highly positively charged myelin basic protein (MBP) with myelin lipids might render the lipids immunogenic (Arnon, 1996). To test the hypothesis, several copolymers of amino acids whose composition was based on the crude amino acid composition of MBP were fabricated. One of these, recently designated as glatiramer, was composed of glutamic acid, lysine, alanine and tyrosine. While not encephalitogenic as anticipated, this copolymer suppressed acute EAE in guinea pigs (Teitelbaum *et al.*, 1971, 1973). Subsequent studies showed that glatiramer could block both acute and chronic EAE in a number of species, and also effectively suppressed EAE when treatment was begun after initial clinical signs were evident (Teitelbaum *et al.*, 1997). Details of the molecular and immunological mechanisms that form the bases for these effects are only now beginning to crystallize. However, the consistent findings in the EAE model led to the preliminary and definitive trials of glatiramer that support its beneficial modification of the course of relapsing MS. Studies are now underway to determine if glatiramer will also benefit patients with the primary progressive form of the disease.

This chapter will review the current understanding of the mechanisms of action of the drug, its basis for current use in relapsing MS in the clinic, and the rationale for new studies that may extend its use to the most recalcitrant form of the disease.

Biochemistry

Glatiramer acetate consists of the acetate salts of polypeptides formed from the controlled synthesis of four naturally occurring amino acids, glutamic acid, alanine, tyrosine and lysine, in their levorotatory forms:

$$\text{Poly}\{\text{L-Glu}^{13-15}, \text{L-Lys}^{30-37}, \text{L-Ala}^{39-46}, \text{L-Tyr}^{8.6-10}\}, n\text{CH}_3\text{COOH}$$

The average molar fraction of the four amino acids is 0.14, 0.34, 0.43 and 0.1, respectively. The molecular weight of the average resultant copolymer is within the range of 4700–13 000 daltons (Lobel *et al.*, 1996). Attempts to define digestion fragments of glatiramer acetate with biological activity have been unsuccessful. Further, monoclonal antibodies reactive with intact glatiramer do not bind to these controlled proteolytic digests. Copaxone® is currently formulated only for subcutaneous injection as a lyophilized powder in single-use vials that contain 22 mg glatiramer and 40 mg mannitol, to be reconstituted with 1 ml sterile water. The reconstituted drug is given at 20 mg single doses at a calculated overfill of 10 per cent. The lyophilized material is stable at room temperature, but it is currently licensed for storage under refrigerated conditions. Following subcutaneous injection into animals, radio-iodinated glatiramer acetate is rapidly degraded into smaller molecular-weight fragments. After a very high-dose subcutaneous injection glatiramer can be transiently detected in the blood, but intact glatiramer acetate cannot be detected systemically when administered at clinically effective doses in humans (Lea and Goa, 1996).

Mechanisms of action

Fundamental to the development of an antigen-specific T-cell dependent immune response is the processing and presentation of a fragment of the antigen by an antigen-presenting cell to a T-cell precursor. This occurs when an appropriately processed antigen is bound by physicochemical interactions within the antigen-binding cleft of the major histocompatibility antigen of an antigen-presenting cell. The resulting unique structure is presented on the cell surface of the antigen-presenting cell, where it can interact with the complementary hypervariable portions of the T-cell receptors of appropriate T-cells. Formation of this trimolecular complex is a critical, though by itself not necessarily a sufficient prerequisite to provide required stimulating signals that activate and condition the behaviour of the T-cell (for details see the comprehensive review of Hohlfeld, 1997).

Intact glatiramer binds directly to major histocompatibility class II antigens (MHC) displayed on intact or fixed antigen-presenting cells (Fridkis-Kareli *et al.*, 1994). This binding can be blocked with anti-DR, but not anti-DQ or anti-class I, antibodies. The binding of glatiramer to class II must occur at (or very near to) the peptide-binding cleft. When isolated DR molecules are exposed to glatiramer, covalently linked complexes are formed (Fridkis-Hareli and Stromoinger, 1998), and this molecular interaction is not easily blocked by Staphylococcal B antigen. Staphylococcal B antigen has a known binding site to the class II antigen, which resides outside the antigen-binding cleft. The binding of glatiramer to class II antigen is of high avidity, and has been demonstrated for all common MS-associated DR haplotypes. Based on the recently resolved crystallographic structure of the immunodominant peptide of MBP and DR2 (Gauthier *et al.*, 1998), theoretical arguments suggest that repeated alanines and tyrosines in glatiramer may facilitate anchoring of the copolymer within binding pockets of the class II binding cleft. Furthermore, the variation in amino acid sequence inherent to glatiramer could account for its ability to bind efficiently to a wide array of different class II haplotypes. However, the high affinity interaction of glatiramer with class II is in itself insufficient to explain the mechanism of action of the drug, as the immunobiologically inert dextrorotatory form of copolymer-1 binds with similar avidity to DR.

In contrast to most T-cell dependent antigens, neither glatiramer nor intact MBP require intracellular processing for their binding to class II antigens and subsequent presentation to T-cells. Earlier *in vitro* studies demonstrated that T-cell lines and clones generated to either glatiramer or MBP were frequently inhibited when cross-stimulated by either antigen (Teitelbaum *et al.*, 1988, 1992). More recent studies have shown that glatiramer competitively inhibits and displaces MBP and MBP peptides from antigen-presenting cells (Fridkis-Hareli *et al.*, 1995). This is because the glatiramer-MHC class II binding constant is substantially higher than that of MBP and the putative immunodominant peptides of MBP. In the same tissue culture systems, glatiramer appears to displace other nominal antigens from the antigen-binding cleft of antigen-presenting cells, to competitively inhibit the expected proliferative responses of T-cell lines and clones reactive with the antigens in question. These include a number of putative autoantigens of potential relevance to MS, including proteolipid protein (PLP) (Teitelbaum *et al.*, 1996), myelin oligodendrocyte glycoprotein (MOG) (Ben-Nun *et* al., 1996) and alpha-B-crystallin (van Sechel and van Noort, 1996). However, this blocking activity extends to a number of cognate antigen systems that involve antigens with no restriction of expression to either oligodendroglial cells or other tissues of the central nervous system (Racke *et al.*, 1992). It is therefore uncertain whether the high avidity binding of glatiramer to class II antigen is central to its mechanism of action *in vivo*, but this seems unlikely. Nonetheless, this property assures concentration of glatiramer on class II molecules of antigen-presenting cell surfaces for presentation to T-cells at the site of subcutaneous injection of the drug in humans.

Glatiramer can prevent EAE induction, not only with spinal cord homogenates or MBP but also with PLP (Teitelbaum *et al.*, 1996) and MOG (Ben-Num *et al.*, 1996). Other as yet unpublished data suggest that glatiramer has little effect on model systems of autoimmunity that do not target the central nervous system (Arnon *et al.*, 1996). Superficially, these data imply that glatiramer could exert its effects through the induction of organ-specific immunoregulatory T-cells. However, studies done thus far have usually mixed glatiramer with the inciting antigen and injected both at the same site in the test animals. Therefore, it is quite possible that the displacement by glatiramer of most antigens from class II molecules of antigen-presenting cells demonstrated *in vitro* occurs in these models *in vivo*. If so, the animals in these experiments may never have been adequately challenged by the inciting autoantigen. Until these studies are repeated with injection of glatiramer and the inciting autoantigens at different sites or at different times, the importance of these observations in describing a potential mechanism of action of the drug remains uncertain.

There are some data available that suggest a shared similarity of molecular shape between glatiramer and MBP, which is recognized by the immune system at both the humoral and cellular level. This is primarily based upon limited monoclonal antibody-defined cross-reactivity (Teitelbaum *et al.*, 1991). However, while selected monoclonal antibodies developed against either MBP or glatiramer can bind to either, polyclonal antibodies do not share this cross-reactivity. This distinction is probably important. When either animals or humans are repetitively injected with glatiramer, they develop polyclonal antibodies that bind to glatiramer in solid-phase, enzyme-linked binding assays. These antibodies do not cross-react in the assays when MBP is substituted as the target antigen. This suggests that the anti-glatiramer antibody response, which is a marker for T-cell induction, is unlikely to bind to native or degraded myelin in the treated animal. The data at the cellular level are more difficult. Most evidence for cross-recognition between glatiramer and MBP derives from competitive inhibition of T-cell clones and lines studied *in vitro*. As discussed above, the high affinity of glatiramer for the MHC class II binding cleft makes it likely that these earlier studies reflected nominal antigen displacement, rather than definite cross-reactive immune recognition. Recent studies have suggested that there may be partial complementarity of recognition between T-cell receptors used by both glatiramer-specific T-cell lines and certain MBP-specific T-cell lines in a manner that implies that TCR antagonism may occur (Aharoni *et al.*, 1999). This important observation requires independent confirmation.

Notwithstanding the above concerns, there are compelling data to suggest that the mechanism of action of glatiramer in modifying the course of EAE and MS may depend upon the induction of antigen-specific regulatory T-cells and the current tenets of organ-specific autoimmunity. Conceptually, organ-specific autoimmunity requires that the putative target autoantigen is a molecule expressed only in a single organ or organ system (Romagnani *et al.*, 1992). Central to the destructive immunopathology of organ-specific autoimmune diseases are autoantigen-specific CD4$^+$ T-cells of the Th1 type. When stimulated by their cognate antigen, Th1 cells secrete a variety of cytokines, including interleukin-2 (IL-2), interferon gamma (IFN-γ) and tumour necrosis factor alpha (TNF-α). To regulate this response, a target organ antigen-specific subset of T-cells of the CD4$^+$ Th2 type must be induced or expanded. On activation, CD4$^+$ Th2 type T-cells have cytokine secretory profiles that are generally inhibitory, including IL-4, IL-6, IL-10 and transforming growth factor beta (TGFβ), among others (Morel and Oriss, 1998). When present in adequate number, these regulatory T-cell subsets can be rapidly recruited to the organ in question, attracted by chemokines (the products of activated organ-specific CD4$^+$ Th1 T-cells) and the consequences of early immune-mediated damage. On contact with their specific antigen, newly released at the site of immune-mediated damage, the modulating T-cells then release regulatory cytokines that act to end organ-specific immune damage. This concept was suggested by early workers to explain an observed apparent paradoxical dissociation between the clinical and histopathologic outcomes in glatiramer-treated EAE models (Lisak *et al.*, 1993). This type of regulatory, glatiramer-specific Th2 cell has been identified in both animals and humans, and these cells may in large part be responsible for the protective effects of the drug (Aharoni *et al.*, 1997, 1998; Miller *et al.*, 1998). The data supporting this proposed mechanism of action of glatiramer are briefly reviewed below.

Perhaps the most clinically relevant experiments in understanding the potential mechanisms of glatiramer's action are those demonstrating that cells harvested from glatiramer-treated donor animals adoptively transfer protection from active EAE challenge to naive recipients. Early experiments harvested rather crude spleen cell preparations from glatiramer-treated animals, and showed that this cell population could adoptively transfer protection from acute challenge with highly encephalitogenic spinal cord homogenates (Lando *et al.*, 1979). Protection could be abrogated by pre-treatment with low dose cyclophosphamide, an immunological manipulation recognized to selectively deplete suppressor cell populations. Subsequent refinements of this experiment confined the effect of adoptive transfer to glatiramer-specific T-cell lines and hybridomas, and provided *in vitro* evidence that the effect might in part be related to soluble factors secreted by the protective cells (Aharoni *et al.*, 1993). More recent experiments have isolated the protective effect to glatiramer-specific T-cell lines and clones with secretory properties that define them as of the $CD4^+$ Th2 type (Aharoni *et al.*, 1998).

In summary it appears that, following injection, glatiramer is rapidly bound to class II molecules present on the antigen-presenting cells that are found in subcutaneous tissues. These cells, either locally or following circulation to draining lymph nodes or spleen, present unprocessed glatiramer to $CD4^+$ T-cells. This results in the induction of a population of glatiramer-specific and MBP cross-reactive $CD4^+$ T-cells, which rapidly develop secretory profiles that identify them as being of the Th2 or regulatory type. Once expanded to adequate numbers, these cells can then be rapidly and efficiently recruited to sites of MBP and other myelin-associated antigen-specific $CD4^+$ Th1 type T-cell mediated damage. In the presence of MBP and MBP breakdown products, these cross-reactive regulatory T-cells limit immune-mediated damage through local downregulation of the immune response. Whether glatiramer has any direct or indirect effect in rendering MBP-specific T-cells anergic remains speculative, and this is an issue that requires further study. However, it is quite possible that the putative autoreactive T-cells that orchestrate the damage seen in MS may be regulated systemically, as well as within developing and evolving central nervous system lesions.

Relapsing multiple sclerosis

Based on the effectiveness of glatiramer in suppressing EAE and the similarities between EAE and MS, several preliminary and major clinical trials of glatiramer were initiated in humans. Initial studies involved small doses of glatiramer given to three patients with acute disseminated encephalomyelitis (the direct equivalent of acute monophasic EAE in animals) and four patients in the terminal stages of MS (Abramsky *et al.*, 1977). In another early open trial, Bornstein and co-workers found that 20 mg of glatiramer given as daily subcutaneous injections was well tolerated by 16 chronic progressive and relapsing–remitting MS patients (Bornstein *et al.*, 1982). While efficacy could not be evaluated in these early trials, treatment was well tolerated, with no drug toxicity noted and no adverse effects on the clinical disease recognized.

The first double-blind, placebo-controlled trial

The first double-blind, placebo-controlled trial of glatiramer involved 50 well defined relapsing–remitting MS patients treated for 24 months with daily subcutaneous injections of 20 mg of glatiramer or placebo (Bornstein et al., 1987). The outcomes evaluated included the absence of new relapses, the number of relapses during treatment, and progression of neurological disability – evaluated as a change in disability status scale (DSS) from baseline, and the time to progression by 1 point on the DSS (Kurtzke, 1989). The patients entered into this trial were similar in baseline characteristics to those entered into more recent studies of relapsing disease, with a mean disability score of ~3.0, average disease duration ~5 years and prior 2-year exacerbation rate of ~4. The pre-planned primary outcome analysis, the proportion of exacerbation free subjects, was based on a matched pairs trial design. Two of the entered patients remained unmatched. Of the 24 matched pairs, only 22 were available for inclusion in the primary outcome analysis; this was because two patients randomized to placebo were removed early from the study for psychological reasons. When their data were dropped from the analysis, their active treatment-matched subjects were no longer matched. Two patients in the placebo group had no exacerbations when their matched treatment-paired partners did, and 10 patients in the active treated group had no exacerbations when their placebo-matched pairs did. The remaining pairs had concordant results. Based on the pre-planned data analysis, the results were significant ($P = 0.039$). An unmatched analysis of all exacerbation-free patients retained in the trial was also significant, favouring glatiramer (56 per cent glatiramer vs 26 per cent placebo, $P = 0.045$) (Bornstein et al., 1987).

The analyses of all other planned secondary endpoints in this trial were significant, in favour of treatment with glatiramer. Specifically, the average number of clinical relapses over 2 years was reduced in the glatiramer treated group (0.6) compared to those treated with a placebo (2.7). The proportion of patients who worsened on the DSS was of borderline significance, favouring treatment (20 per cent glatiramer vs 48 per cent placebo, $P = 0.064$), but Kaplan–Meier analysis of time to progression of 1 point on the DSS sustained for 90 days favoured glatiramer ($P = 0.05$). Although there were limited subjects available for any of the planned subgroup analyses, it appeared that all differences observed were more pronounced for those with the least disability as measured on the DSS at entry into the study. The side effects that were observed were mild, consisting of local reactions at the injection site and occasional curious transient reactions (flushing, sweating, palpitations, a feeling of chest tightness, a perception of difficulty in breathing and associated anxiety) that appeared during or shortly after administering the drug.

While the rationale for the exclusion of two of the placebo-randomized patients from the planned statistical evaluation was reasonable, the analysis presented in the paper by Bornstein was of an evaluable rather than a more rigorous intention to treat (ITT) cohort. The data were subsequently re-analysed using a strict ITT analysis that included both placebo-randomized subjects dropped from the original evaluation. This re-analysis of the data was adjusted for the baseline covariates originally used to match pairs, based on the expectation that these demo-graphic factors influence disease outcome (gender, prior 2-year relapse rate, base-line DSS score). The ITT analysis did not change the overall study impression that active treatment was favoured over placebo and most, but not all, analyses remained statistically significant. The addition of two rejected subjects to this analysis increased the number of patients in the placebo-randomized group with no relapses on study. As a result, the proportion of patients without relapse on trial shifted (56 per cent glatiramer vs 32 per cent placebo, $P = 0.131$), and signifi-cance was lost for the primary outcome measure. The 2-year relapse rates changed slightly (0.64 ± 1.54 glatiramer vs 2.36 ± 2.41 placebo), as did the distri-bution of the frequency of exacerbations between groups, with only one glati-ramer-treated patient experiencing three or more exacerbations compared to 11 of the placebo-randomized subjects (both $P = 0.01$). Active treatment significantly delayed the median time to first exacerbation (glatiramer could not be calculated, 156 days for placebo, $P = 0.01$). In the ITT analysis, secondary endpoints related to progression remained strong. The mean change in DSS from baseline favoured active treatment (–0.08 glatiramer, 0.80 placebo, $P < 0.03$), as did the proportion of patients who were progression-free (80 per cent glatiramer, 52 per cent placebo, $P = 0.03$), and the time to confirmed progression of 1 point on the DSS sustained for at least 90 days (glatiramer could not be calculated, 656 days for placebo, $P = 0.03$).

Thus, the original controlled study by Bornstein and his colleagues strongly suggested that glatiramer could reduce the frequency of relapses in relapsing MS and this, at least in the short term, could be translated into reduced accumulated disability. The data also suggested that patients treated with glatiramer were more likely to show measurable improvement on the drug (32 per cent glatiramer, 13 per cent placebo). As such, this was the first study to show that continuous self-administered treatment with any drug could beneficially alter the behaviour of patients with relapsing MS. However, the relatively small numbers of patients studied rendered the robustness of the results sensitive to the type of analysis per-formed.

The American multicentre study

The need to confirm or reject the results of the preliminary data, that glatiramer was both safe and effective when used early in MS, led to the American multicentre study. Before this study could be initiated, a problem that had complicated clinical studies of glatiramer required solving. Material used in the early clinical trials was initially produced by investigators at the Weizmann Institute of Science and later by the Bio-Yeda Company, both located in Rehovot, Israel. Some variability in the performance of drug batches produced for the clinical trials in their ability to suppress EAE occurred (Bornstein *et al.*, 1987). Teva Pharmaceutical Industries, Ltd licensed glatiramer in 1985, and con-siderable effort was then made to produce the copolymer in a rigorously bio-chemically defined manner and with consistent performance in bioassays, including limited variation in the drug's ability to block clinical disease in the acute EAE model. All clinical trials conducted since 1991 have used glatiramer produced under these conditions.

In the pivotal American trial involving 11 centres, 251 subjects with clinically definite relapsing–remitting MS and mild to moderately severe disability (extended DSS (EDSS) ≤ 5.0) were randomized to receive either 20 mg glatiramer by daily subcutaneous injection or placebo (Johnson *et al.*, 1995a). The exacerbation rate in the 2 years before entry into the study was 1.45 per year, and the mean duration of disease was ~7 years in both arms of the study (Table 5.1). As a group, the patients selected for the study were slightly older, had been diagnosed somewhat longer, and had similar entry disability levels to those studied by Bornstein and his colleagues. The patients in the two studies primarily differed in the frequency of reported relapses in the 2 years prior to entry, with prior relapses being about 30 per cent more frequent in the Bornstein cohort of relapsing patients. In the American pivotal study, disability (as judged by entry EDSS score) favoured the placebo-randomized subjects (2.8 ± 1.2 glatiramer vs 2.4 ± 1.3 placebo, $P = 0.01$). However, this singular difference in demographic characteristics was accounted for by the type of analysis planned for the study.

Table 5.1 Entry characteristics of the major trials in relapsing multiple sclerosis

	American pivotal		European–Canadian MRI	
	Glatiramer	Placebo	Glatiramer	Placebo
n	125	126	119	120
Mean age (years)	34.6 ± 6.0	34.3 ± 6.5	34.1 ± 7.4	34.0 ± 7.5
Disease duration (years)	7.3 ± 4.9	6.6 ± 5.1	7.9 ± 5.5	8.3 ± 5.5
Prior 2-year relapse rate	2.9 ± 1.3	2.9 ± 1.1	2.8 ± 1.8	2.5 ± 1.4
EDSS	2.8 ± 1.2	2.4 ± 1.3	2.3 ± 1.1	2.4 ± 1.2
Ambulation Index	1.2 ± 1.0	1.1 ± 0.9	1.1 ± 0.9	1.2 ± 1.1

The primary study outcome in this trial was the mean number of confirmed relapses that occurred during the 2 years of therapy, using a strict ITT cohort analysis of covariance (ANCOVA) that included predefined covariates of sex, duration of disease, prior 2-year relapse rate and entry EDSS. Relapses were rigidly defined and required examination for confirmation. Withdrawal rates were comparable in the two arms of the study (15.2 per cent glatiramer vs 13.5 per cent placebo), as were the times to individual patient withdrawals. The mean number of relapses was reduced 29 per cent by glatiramer (1.19 ± 0.13 glatiramer vs 1.68 ± 0.13 placebo, $P = 0.007$). When stratified by entry EDSS, the number of relapses was reduced in the glatiramer-treated cohort by 33 per cent among those least affected (EDSS 0–2), and by 22 per cent in those more disabled at entry. The median time to first exacerbation was extended by 31 per cent by active treatment (287 days on glatiramer vs 198 days on placebo). A trend for a greater reduction in the number of relapses over time on treatment was also seen, with 30 per cent fewer attacks over the last 6 months of the 2-year study, and fewer patients on active treatment experiencing three or more relapses ($P = 0.023$). As anticipated for the subjects recruited for this trial, few patients in either arm of the study showed progression sustained for at least 90 days of ≥ 1 point on the EDSS (21.6 per cent glatiramer vs 24.6 per cent placebo). While small, the mean change in EDSS seen from entry over the trial was significantly reduced by active treatment (−0.09 units glatiramer vs +0.22 units placebo, $P = 0.023$). Additionally, the percentage of patients who improved by ≥ 1 point on the EDSS was increased by glatiramer (24.8 per cent glatiramer vs 15.2 per cent placebo, $P = 0.037$).

The trial was extended for a total blinded and placebo-controlled observation period of 35 months (Johnson *et al.*, 1998). This planned extension allowed the last patient enrolled to complete 2 years of active treatment, and the entire database to be locked prior to the analysis of the trial results and before the loss of the placebo-treated arm of the study. Most (94 per cent) of the patients who completed the 24-month study consented to continued treatment with study medication under the double-blind trial. There was no difference between the baseline characteristics of those patients who entered the extension phase and those who did not. Overall, patients remained on assigned treatment for an additional 1–11 months (mean of 5.2 additional months for those on glatiramer and 5.9 additional months for those on placebo). Only nine patients failed to complete the extension study; seven of those randomized to placebo and two randomized to glatiramer.

During the extension, no further relapses occurred in those glatiramer-treated patients who had been relapse free over the first 2 years of the trial. The final relapse rate over the entire study was 1.34 ± 0.15 for the glatiramer and 1.98 ± 0.14 for the placebo groups ($P = 0.002$); a 32 per cent reduction in favour of the active treatment. More patients on glatiramer were relapse free over the entire study than were those on placebo (33.6 per cent vs 24.6 per cent, $P = 0.035$), and multiple relapses were more frequent among the placebo-treated group ($P = 0.008$). In comparison to the earlier Bornstein study, there was a trend for those patients with the highest relapse rates in the 2 years before entry to have a better reduction of attacks while on glatiramer. However, this may simply reflect the improved sensitivity to any drug effect when the events measured occur more frequently. The accumulated mean number of relapses on study is shown in Figure 5.1. There was little change in the apparent trajectory or slope of the curve for the patients randomized to placebo; in contrast, the trajectory of the curve for the glatiramer-treated patients appeared to progressively flatten with time. The two curves first diverged at about 3 months, and they continued to diverge over time.

The difference in the percentage of patients who improved by ≥ 1 point on the EDSS from baseline to the end of the extension study between glatiramer and placebo widened (27.2 per cent glatiramer vs 12.0 per cent placebo, $P = 0.001$). Similarly, the difference in the mean change in EDSS seen from entry to the trial's end also increased during the extension (−0.11 points glatiramer vs +0.34 points placebo, $P = 0.006$). A Kaplan–Meier analysis of time to progression of either ≥ 1.0 or a more stringent ≥ 1.5 units on the EDSS in the absence of a recent exacerbation-associated deterioration favoured glatiramer ($P = 0.008$ and $P = 0.004$,

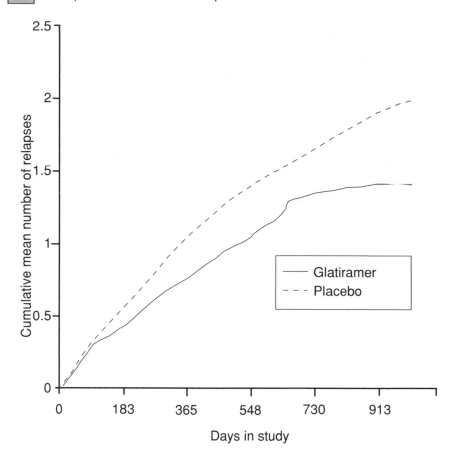

Figure 5.1 The cumulative mean number of relapses observed for patients entered and continuing in the multicentre, randomized, placebo-controlled trial of glatiramer in the pivotal American trial of relapsing MS is shown for the 2 years and the preplanned extension. The curves for the glatiramer (solid line) and placebo (dashed line) began to separate at about 90 days following randomization. The slope of the curve for the placebo arm of this study shows little change in its slope after the first year of the trial, while the slope of the curve for the glatiramer arm becomes less steep with time.

respectively). The proportion of patients who reached the ≥ 1.5 unit milestone by the end of the trial was reduced by nearly 50 per cent for the glatiramer-treated group. The effect of glatiramer on disability was also supported by an analysis of the area under the EDSS disability curve (IDSS), which measures both transient disability during relapses and accumulated disability over time (Liu *et al.*, 1998). The IDSS scores were calculated as the change in the EDSS score from baseline multiplied by the duration of the change in months. The mean IDSS scores differed significantly (0.42 ± 24.8 glatiramer, 6.4 ± 21.3 placebo, $P < 0.05$). These data from the extension phase are consistent with persistence, if not improvement, of the treatment effect over time.

At the conclusion of the placebo-controlled extension study all patients were offered open-label drug therapy, and 190 accepted treatment with continued close monitoring (Ford *et al.*, 1998). The overwhelming majority remain on the drug under close follow-up, and there are plans to follow this critical cohort of patients for a full 10 years on therapy. The absence of a concomitant control group and the potential bias of patient dropout during follow-up complicate interpretation of the findings on this vanguard cohort of patients (Goodkin *et al.*, 1999). Nevertheless, they represent the best opportunity to understand the potential long-term safety and benefit profile of glatiramer. Clinical data are now available on 76 of the 125 patients originally randomized to glatiramer, and these 76 patients have a mean continuous treatment exposure to glatiramer of 5.93 ± 0.20 years. Their behaviour can be considered either as an evaluable cohort of 76 patients, or by ITT analysis based on the original 125 patient cohort. Their annualized relapse rate is significantly reduced from baseline using either type of analysis (annualized relapse rate 0.37 ± 0.41 evaluable, 0.54 ± 0.62 ITT; reduction from baseline 1.14 ± 0.75 evaluable, 0.91 ± 0.82 ITT; Figure 5.2). Remarkably, 27.6 per cent of the evaluable cohort remain free of relapses since originally randomized. The mean change from entry EDSS for the evaluable cohort after 6 years of treatment is 0.14 ± 1.43, and 75 per cent of these patients remain stable or have improved from their original trial baseline EDSS. Just under 70 per cent of the patients in the evaluable long-term treated cohort remain unchanged or improved despite their experiencing at least one relapse on study; slightly over 90 per cent of those patients who have remained relapse free since randomization are either stable or have improved from their entry condition. Those subjects who entered the long-term open-label follow-up from the placebo group have shown a similar stabilization of disease to that in the evaluable long-term treated cohort.

All patients in this vanguard cohort were recently evaluated by quantitative magnetic resonance imaging (MRI). These data are still under analysis and require correlation with the clinical status of the patients, and no baseline MRI data exist for any patients except those studied at the University of Pennsylvania. However, the volume of enhanced tissues found appears to be remarkably low in this cohort of subjects compared to other untreated relapsing MS cohorts (unpublished observations).

Since publication of the original Bornstein study there has been a keen and growing interest in understanding the effect of glatiramer on MRI-measured disease parameters (Weiner, 1987), but until recently little was known of the effect of glatiramer on MRI-monitored disease parameters. A subset of patients studied at the University of Pennsylvania as part of the American trial underwent gadolinium-enhanced MRI at variable intervals. Trends were seen that favoured active treatment, but the results were far from conclusive in this small cohort (Cohen *et al.*, 1995). Ten relapsing MS patients were followed with monthly gadolinium-enhanced MRI at the University of Genoa for a year or more as part of a natural history study. They were then given glatiramer in open-label fashion for another year with monthly imaging (Mancardi *et al.*, 1998). Significant reduc-

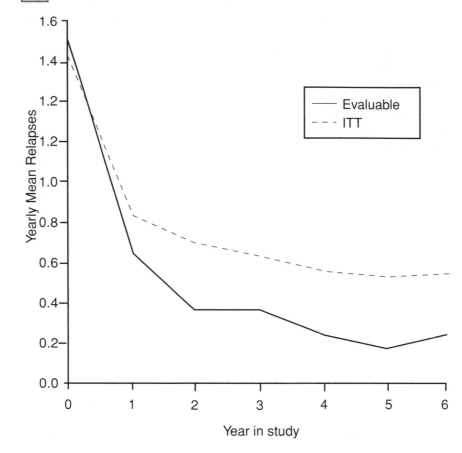

Figure 5.2 The yearly mean relapse rate for patients originally randomized to glatiramer in the multicentre, randomized, placebo-controlled trial of glatiramer in the pivotal American trial of relapsing MS and continued on close follow-up into the open label phase of the trial. Of the original 125 patients in the active treatment arm, 76 have remained on continuous treatment for 6 years. The annualized or yearly relapse rate is shown calculated either as an evaluable cohort of patients still on treatment in the sixth year of follow-up (solid line), or analysed as an intention to treat cohort (ITT, dashed line).

tions were seen in the proportion, number and volume of new enhancing lesions following the initiation of therapy. The mean number of new enhanced lesions in the pre-treatment period was reduced by 57 per cent during the treatment period (2.20 vs 0.92). However, some form of regression to the mean could account for a proportion of this difference.

European–Canadian Study

In order to address conclusively whether glatiramer has any measurable effect on

MRI-monitored activity, a randomized, placebo-controlled and blinded, multicentred European and Canadian study was initiated in early 1997. This study was specifically designed to determine if, in a patient population with similar clinical characteristics to that enrolled in the American pivotal trial, glatiramer could be shown to have any effect on the inflammatory component of the disease as measured by gadolinium (Gd)-enhanced activity on monthly MRI. If such an effect could be found, the second question to be considered was what was the time course of its appearance. These two issues were addressed in a patient population with one or more Gd-enhanced lesions at the time that they were formally pre-screened for entry into the trial using combined clinical and MRI activity measures. Given the known clinical benefits of the drug in relapsing MS, long-term exposure of the placebo group could not be justified. Therefore, the controlled phase of the study was limited to 9 months (36 weeks), after which all patients received glatiramer under open-label conditions with continued MRI monitoring at 3-monthly intervals for an additional 9 months to determine the persistence of any effects observed during the placebo-controlled phase of the trial. Enrolment into this study was concluded in November 1997, and all patients entered the open-label phase of the trial by September 1998. Trial results from the placebo-controlled phase were recently presented (Comi *et al.*, 1999).

Altogether, 485 subjects were pre-screened for entry into the trial. Of these, 239 had one or more Gd-enhanced lesions and met all clinical entrance criteria. Patients entered into the trial, as anticipated by the pre-planned entry criteria, were very similar in their baseline characteristics to those enrolled in the American pivotal trial (Table 5.1). At the time the study was planned, sample size projections were based upon an early understanding of the behaviour of patients followed with monthly MRI monitoring for Gd-enhanced lesion activity (Nauta *et al.*, 1994; Andersen *et al.*, 1996). However, the extent to which the presence or absence of Gd-enhanced activity on MRI might influence differences in the behaviour of clinical activity in otherwise similar patient populations was less well understood (Stone *et al.*, 1995; Simon *et al.*, 1998). Also, it was not clear to what extent selecting patients for Gd-activity at a particular point in time would assure continued activity over the course of a two-phased 18-month trial. In retrospect, the selection criteria used culled out an otherwise clinically indistinguishable subset of patients destined to have substantial clinical and MRI measurable events over a relatively short period of time, with little evidence of regression to the mean.

The primary endpoint, the total number of Gd-enhancing lesions, was analysed as the sum of these lesions counted in all nine serial scans performed during the 36 weeks of the double-blind treatment period for each patient. A baseline-adjusted ANCOVA, incorporating terms for treatment and centre as main effects, and pre-randomization Gd-enhancing lesions, baseline EDSS score, number of relapses in the 2 years prior to trial entry, disease duration, age and gender as additional covariates was used to compare the two groups. For other predetermined quantitative MRI secondary outcome measures, the particular measure at baseline was used as a covariate. Based on projections from the North American study, clinical measures of efficacy were not expected to be informative; these were therefore relegated exploratory endpoint status. Nevertheless, collection of data on all clinical measures was prospectively held to a rigorous standard.

The baseline clinical (Table 5.1) and MRI-defined (Table 5.2) characteristics at baseline were similar in patients randomized to initial therapy with glatiramer or placebo. The quantitative MRI characteristics were similar to relapsing MS patient cohorts entered into other trials, with the exception of Gd-based measures, which as expected were enriched in this study population (Simon *et al.*, 1998; Wolinsky *et al.*, 1998). Over 95 per cent of all planned MRI data in the controlled phase of the trial were collected and available for analysis.

Table 5.2 Entry MRI characteristics of European–Canadian trial

		Glatiramer			Placebo	
	n	Mean	Median	*n*	Mean	Median
Total Gd-enhanced lesions	119	4.2 ± 4.8	3.0	120	4.4 ± 7.1	2.0
New Gd-enhanced lesions	115	2.5 ± 3.5	1.0	118	2.6 ± 4.1	1.0
Volume Gd-enhanced tissue (ml)	119	0.57 ± 0.71	0.33	120	0.73 ± 2.20	0.23
New T2 lesions	115	1.0 ± 1.0	1.0	118	1.2 ± 1.7	1.0
T2 disease burden (ml)	119	20.0 ± 17.2	14.1	120	20.5 ± 18.8	16.3
T1 hypodense disease burden (ml)	119	3.4 ± 3.9	1.8	120	4.0 ± 4.9	2.9

The mean number of accumulated lesions per patient was substantially reduced by 32 per cent for those patients treated with glatiramer (25.96 glatiramer, 36.8 placebo; a reduction of 10.84 enhanced lesions over 9 months; 95 per cent confidence interval (CI) –17.97, –3.71; $P = 0.003$). The median number of accumulated lesions per patient was reduced by 35 per cent (11 glatiramer, 17 placebo). When evaluated over time, there was little change in the behaviour of any Gd-defined parameter for the placebo group over the course of the 9-month study. In contrast, an effect on the rate of accumulation of Gd-enhanced lesions could be discerned as early as 2 months following initiation of treatment, and this became statistically significant by 6 months of therapy. The percentage reduction in the mean number of Gd-enhanced lesions per subject fell progressively over each trimester of the trial for the group on glatiramer, from a 17 per cent reduction in the first trimester to a 26 per cent reduction in the second trimester and a 45 per cent reduction in the third trimester. The accumulated effect of treatment over time is illustrated in Figure 5.3, which shows the median change in Gd-enhanced tissue volume from baseline for the two treatment groups.

All other pre-planned secondary outcome measures favoured treatment with glatiramer, were of similar magnitude of treatment effect to that observed for Gd-enhanced MRI parameters, and followed a similar time course of development. Of these, only the change from baseline T1-measured hypointense lesion volume

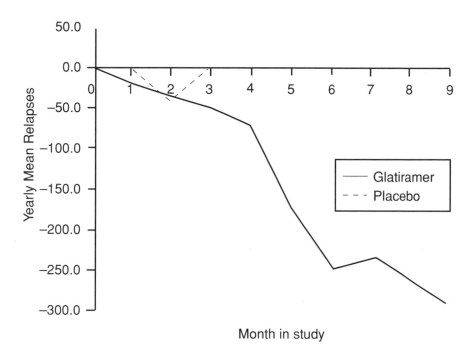

Figure 5.3 The change in the median Gd-enhanced tissue volume in cubic mm from baseline in the European–Canadian MRI-monitored trial by month in study. The median values for the placebo randomized arm of the study (dashed line) changed very little over the entire trial with all of the 2-month on-study values superimposed on the X-axis. In contrast, the median amount of Gd-enhanced tissue found in the glatiramer treated arm of the study (solid line) fell progressively from baseline and achieved statistically significant differences from month 7 and beyond ($P < 0.05$ months 7 and 8, $P < 0.01$ month 9).

failed to reach statistical significance (mean change 0.86 ml glatiramer, 1.33 ml placebo, $P = 0.095$). The change in T2-measured disease burden increased in both groups from baseline to the month nine MRI, but the change was substantially contained by active therapy (mean change 16.5 per cent glatiramer, 31.7 per cent placebo, $P = 0.001$; median change 12.3 per cent glatiramer, 20.6 per cent placebo). The magnitude of the change seen over this relatively short interval in the placebo group is substantial when compared to most recently reported MRI-monitored trials in relapsing MS (Paty *et al.*, 1993; Ebers *et al.*, 1998; Simon *et al.*, 1998). This presumably reflects the enrichment for patients with very MRI active disease in the European–Canadian trial. Nevertheless, the magnitude of the effective treatment in reducing the burden of disease is at least comparable to the beta interferon trials.

Remarkably, the relapse rate was reduced by 33 per cent in treated patients over the course of this short 9-month trial (mean relapse rate 0.51 glatiramer, 0.76 placebo, $P = 0.012$). The curves for the cumulative number of relapses were surprisingly similar to those for the MRI-measured parameters, with a slowing of the trajectory of the curve for glatiramer-treated patients with time that was most prominent in the third trimester. There were only five relapses in the glatiramer-treated group during the last trimester, compared to 26 for those randomized to placebo. The apparent magnitude of the effect of treatment in this cohort of patients appeared to be greater than that found over the same time interval for the cohort followed in the American pivotal study. Despite the clinical similarity of these two study cohorts at baseline, it is possible that the addition of the MRI selection criteria in the European–Canadian cohort isolated a sub-population of patients likely to show the greatest benefit from treatment with glatiramer over a short interval.

Summary

Taken together, the data from the major controlled trials of glatiramer in MS patients with relapsing disease suggest that treatment can be expected to reduce the relapse rate by at least one-third over the first 2 years of treatment, and that protection from relapses may steadily increase with time thereafter. Approximately 70–75 per cent of treated patients can expect stabilized disease disability for at least 2 years, and probably for at least 7 years. It appears unlikely that there is a clinically or MRI-defined identifiable subgroup of relapsing patients who will not derive benefit from treatment. Finally, the early MRI signature of glatiramer's effect on the disease process differs substantially from that reported for the beta interferons, possibly reflecting differences in the probable mechanisms of action of these two different classes of immunomodulatory drugs.

Progressive multiple sclerosis

A single trial of glatiramer in chronic progressive MS patients with moderately severe disability was conducted at two centres (Bornstein *et al.*, 1991). Patients were selected for the study based on evidence of a chronic progressive course over at least 18 months, no more than two exacerbations in the previous 2 years, and entry disability between 2.0 and 6.5 points inclusive on the EDSS. The study was unique in that 169 eligible patients were entered into a pre-trial observation period during which they were formally evaluated for evidence of neurological progression every 3 months for a minimum of 6 and a maximum of 15 months. In order to be randomized to treatment, otherwise eligible patients were required to demonstrate worsening during the pre-trial observation as defined by either a two-grade deterioration in one of the functional systems, a one-grade worsening in two unrelated functional systems of the EDSS, a full-grade change in the EDSS, or a two-unit change in the Ambulation Index sustained for 3 months. Patients were also allowed only a single exacerbation during the pre-trial observation. Ultimately, 106 patients were randomized either to treatment with 15 mg glatiramer administered subcutaneously twice daily, or to placebo injections. Randomization was stratified according to EDSS at the time of randomization. The primary outcome measure of this study was the time to confirmed progression of disability, where progression was defined as a worsening of one full unit from baseline EDSS for those patients with an entry EDSS ≥ 5.0, or 1.5 units for those with an entry EDSS < 5.0. Patients were continued in trial until they demonstrated confirmed progression or had completed 24 months of treatment. While some attempt was made to examine all trial patients 24 months after entry, only the primary outcome measure could be viewed as fulfilling ITT analysis criteria.

There were 23 confirmed progressions on study, nine in the glatiramer-treated group and 14 in the placebo group. Analysis of the Kaplan–Meier progression survival curves showed that they began to diverge after month nine. Fewer patients progressed in the glatiramer-treated arm, with a 24-month probability of progression of 20.4 per cent for glatiramer and 29.5 per cent for the control group $(P = 0.09)$. When a proportional hazards model was applied to correct for baseline characteristics of the subjects, no statistically significant differences were found. Using less stringent criteria of confirmed progression, the survival curves of the two study arms began to diverge after 6 months, with a 24-month probability of progression of 15.4 per cent for glatiramer and 27.8 per cent for the control group $(P = 0.026)$. Interestingly, the proportion of placebo patients showing confirmed progression was more than twice as high at one of the two centres that contributed to the study. This and a number of other subgroup analyses suggested that the promising, but statistically negative results might reflect intercentre differences in patient behaviour and the rather small sample of patients studied.

The former categorization of patients into a chronic progressive type of disease could be expected to include patients that now would be considered to have both secondary progressive as well as primary progressive disease types (Lublin et al., 1996). Therefore, the original data from this study were revisited for the purpose of planning a trial of glatiramer in primary progressive MS. A subgroup of patients was defined based on no previous record of relapses, or a single relapse that occurred at least 10 years prior to the onset of progressive disability (Table 5.3). Fortunately, the quality of the data from this secondary progressive trial was exceptionally high, with detailed clinical histories that allowed these distinctions to be made. The data were reanalysed based on criteria proposed for the planned primary progressive trial. The subcohort randomized to glatiramer showed an apparent prolongation of the time to progression (twenty-fifth percentile: 328 days glatiramer, 204 days placebo; fiftieth percentile: never reached glatiramer, 556 days placebo; odds ratio 1.69, CI 0.59–4.89), and an increased number of progression-free subjects (62.5 per cent glatiramer, 42.9 per cent placebo; odds ratio 2.22, CI 0.51–9.61). These results provide some assurance that the sample size projection for the planned primary progressive trial is appropriate, and that there is reasonable hope for a positive trial outcome.

Table 5.3 Chronic progressive trial subgroup

	All	Subgroup	
		Glatiramer	Placebo
n	106	16	14
No prior relapse (%)	21.7	75.0	78.6
Single remote relapse (%)	6.6	25.0	21.4
Age (years)	42.0	41.3	43.4
Males (%)	45.3	25.0	50.0
EDSS	5.6	5.9	5.6
EDSS $\leq$ 5.0 (%)	30.2	12.5	21.4
EDSS $\geq$ 5.5 (%)	69.8	87.5	78.6

Side effect profile

The largest and longest placebo-controlled database on side effects comes from the American multicentre trial. Few side effects were encountered. Most glatiramer recipients (90 per cent overall, with 2 per cent consequently stopping treatment), and 59 per cent of placebo patients reported local injection site reactions. Pain at the injection site was nearly twice as common among those on glatiramer (66 per cent vs 37 per cent). However, all local injection site reactions diminished markedly with time, and no skin necrosis was encountered. As in earlier and all subsequent studies of glatiramer, the systemic post-injection reaction was seen. This was reported from one to five times in 15.2 per cent of the glatiramer-treated patients, and from one to four times in 3.2 per cent of the placebo-treated subjects. The symptoms usually resolved in a few minutes, and rarely lasted several hours. They were temporally associated with injection of the drug, were not seen with the first injection, and did not occur on successive injections. These unusual reactions appeared to be benign. The mechanism of induction of the systemic post-injection reaction remains uncertain. Other side effects were evenly distributed between the study groups.

All patients who received glatiramer developed binding antibodies to the copolymer. These levels peaked between months three and six of treatment, and then persisted at lower levels (Johnson *et al.*, 1995b). The presence of these antibodies did not appear to compromise the drug's clinical effect or its activity as measured *in vitro* or in the EAE model.

Importantly, pre-clinical studies in animals have suggested that glatiramer is neither toxic nor teratogenic when administered parenterally. Data from open-labelled studies conducted in Israel, Italy and Germany, and a treatment investigational new drug (IND) programme in the United States, further support the safety of glatiramer. More than 900 patients have been exposed to glatiramer in pre-marketing studies, with nearly 1200 patient years and > 500 000 doses of the polymer given.

Prospects for the future

Much has already been learned about glatiramer acetate and its role in the treatment of relapsing MS, the likely mechanisms that underlie its mode of action, and the signature of its effect on MRI-monitored pathology. Further refinement in these three areas is expected to be forthcoming in the near future from the open-label phase of the European–Canadian MRI trial, the extended open-label phase of the American pivotal trial, and further basic and clinical investigations of the immunobiological effects of glatiramer. Two recently initiated trials and another planned new avenue of investigation should provide important additional information over the next 2–5 years.

In March 1999, recruitment and entry of patients into a multicentre, double-blind, placebo-controlled trial of glatiramer in primary progressive multiple sclerosis was initiated in North America, France and the United Kingdom. More than 50 centres are participating in this study, which is designed to randomize 900 patients with relentlessly progressive disease in the absence of prior or ongoing relapses and an entry EDSS of 3.0–6.5 inclusive. Subjects will be randomized at a two to one ratio to receive either glatiramer or placebo at 20 mg daily by subcutaneous injection. They will be stratified according to EDSS for purposes of randomization and primary outcome analysis. The study is designed to determine whether glatiramer slows the confirmed progression of disease. For the purposes of this study, progression is defined as the time to confirmed disease progression demonstrated by an increase of > 1 point in EDSS sustained for at least 3 months for patients with a baseline EDSS < 5.5, or a sustained increase of > 0.5 point in EDSS patients with an entry EDSS ≥ 5.5. Secondary endpoints will explore if treatment with glatiramer acetate is associated with beneficial outcomes in cerebral MRI, quality of life, and overall neurological course. More details of this study and its progress can be found at a web site developed for this purpose (www.promisetrial.com).

Limited *in vitro* data suggest that the combination of an interferon beta and glatiramer may have additive effects (Milo and Panitch, 1995). Given differences in the presumed mechanisms of action of these two classes of drugs, it is attractive to anticipate that a similar combination might improve the outcome for MS patients treated with both drugs. However, data developed in mice have suggested that combinations of an interferon alpha and glatiramer at doses where either one is individually effective in blocking the induction of EAE are ineffective when combined (Brod *et al.*, 2000). To what extent these laboratory observations have relevance to humans is uncertain; however, they do suggest caution in evaluating combined therapy in MS (Lublin and Reingold, 1998). A trial has recently been initiated in which relapsing MS patients who have been taking interferon beta-1a for at least 6 months will be followed on continued interferon for an additional 3 months of monitoring by monthly Gd-enhanced MRI, and then have glatiramer added for another 6 months of MRI monitoring. The goal of this multicentre trial is to determine if the combination is safe, before more complex and larger studies are initiated to determine if the combination is additive or synergistic in benefits.

Finally, recent studies suggest that feeding glatiramer orally to rats by gavage beginning 10 days before the active induction of EAE protects animals from disease, and that this protection may be better than when rats are fed MBP (Teitelbaum *et al.*, 1999). These results and extensive studies performed in both rodents and subhuman primate species by Dr Riven-Kreitman and her colleagues at Teva Pharmaceuticals have suggested that oral administration of glatiramer might be beneficial. Definitive dose-finding studies in patients with relapsing forms of MS are underway.

References

Abramsky, O., Teitelbaum, D. and Arnon, R. (1977). Effect of a synthetic polypeptide (Cop I) on patients with multiple sclerosis and with acute disseminated encephalomyelitis. *J. Neurol. Sci.*, **31**, 433–8.

Aharoni, R., Teitelbaum, D. and Arnon, R. (1993). T-suppressor hybridomas and interleukin-2-dependent lines induced by copolymer 1 or by spinal cord homogenate down-regulate experimental allergic encephalomyelitis. *Eur. J. Immunol.*, **23**, 17–25.

Aharoni, R., Teitelbaum, D., Sela, M. and Arnon, R. (1997). Copolymer 1 induces T-cells of the T-helper type 2 that crossreact with myelin basic protein and suppress experimental autoimmune encephalomyelitis. *Proc. Natl. Acad. Sci. USA*, **94**, 10821–6.

Aharoni, R., Teitelbaum, D., Sela, M. and Arnon, R. (1998). Bystander suppression of experimental autoimmune encephalomyelitis by T-cell lines and clones of the Th2 type induced by copolymer 1. *J. Neuroimmunol*, **91**, 135–46.

Aharoni, R., Teitelbaum, D., Arnon, R. and Sela, M. (1999). Copolymer-1 acts against the immunodominant epitope 82-100 of myelin basic protein by T-cell receptor antagonism in addition to major histocompatibility complex blocking. *Proc. Natl. Acad. Sci. USA*, **96(2.2)**, 634–9.

Andersen, O., Lycke, J., Tollesson, P. O. *et al.* (1996). Linomide reduces the rate of active lesions in relapsing–remitting multiple sclerosis. *Neurology*, **47**, 895–900.

Arnon, R. (1996). The development of Cop 1 (Copaxone®), an innovative drug for the treatment of multiple sclerosis: Personal reflections. *Immunol. Lett.*, **50**, 1–15.

Arnon, R., Sela, M. and Teitelbaum, D. (1996). New insights into the mechanism of action of copolymer-1 in experimental allergic encephalomyelitis and multiple sclerosis. *J. Neurol.*, **243(4 Suppl. 1)**, S8–13.

Ben-Nun, A., Mendel, I., Bakimer, R. *et al.* (1996). The autoimmune reactivity to myelin oligodendrocyte glycoprotein (MOG) in multiple sclerosis is potentially pathogenic: effect of copolymer 1 on MOG-induced disease. *J. Neurol.*, **243(Suppl. 1),** S14–22.

Bornstein, M. B., Miller, A. I., Teitelbaum, D. *et al.* (1982). Multiple sclerosis: trial of a synthetic polypeptide. *Ann. Neurol.*, **11,** 317–19.

Bornstein, M. B., Miller, A., Slagle, S. *et al.* (1987). A pilot trial of Cop 1 in exacerbating–remitting multiple sclerosis. *N. Engl. J. Med.*, **317,** 408–14.

Bornstein, M. B., Miller, A., Slagle, S. *et al.* (1991). A placebo-controlled, double-blind, randomized, two-centre, pilot trial of Cop 1 in chronic progressive multiple sclerosis. *Neurology*, **41,** 533–9.

Brod, S. A., Lindsey, J. W. and Wolinsky, J. S. (2000). Combined therapy with glatiramer acetate (copolymer –1) and a type I interferon (IFNα) does not improve experimental allergic encephalomyelitis. *Ann Neurol*, **47,** 127–31.

Cohen, J. A., Grossman, R. I., Udupa, J. K. *et al.* (1995). Assessment of the efficacy of copolymer-1 in the treatment of multiple sclerosis by quantitative MRI. *Neurology*, **45(Supppl. 4),** A418.

Comi, G., Filippi, M., for the Copaxone MRI Study Group (1999). The effect of glatiramer acetate (Copaxone®) on disease activity as measured by cerebral MRI in patients with relapsing–remitting multiple sclerosis (RRMS): a multicentre, randomized, double-blind, placebo-controlled study extended by open-label treatment. *Neurology*, **52, (suppl. 2), A 289**.

Ebers, G. C., Rice, G., Lesaux, J. *et al.* (1998). Randomised double-blind placebo-controlled study of interferon beta-1a in relapsing/remitting multiple sclerosis. *Lancet*, **352,** 1498–504.

Ford, C. C., Brooks, B. R., Cohen, J. A. *et al.* (1998). Sustained efficacy of glatiramer acetate for injection in a 5+ year trial of relapsing–remitting MS. *MS J. Clin. Lab. Res.*, **4,** 521.

Fridkis-Hareli, M. and Strominger, J. L. (1998). Promiscuous binding of synthetic copolymer 1 to purified HLA-DR molecules. *J. Immunol.*, **160,** 4386–97.

Fridkis-Hareli, M., Teitelbaum, D., Gurevich, E. *et al.* (1994). Direct binding of myelin basic protein and synthetic copolymer 1 to class II major histocompatibility complex molecules on living antigen-presenting cells: Specificity and promiscuity. *Proc. Natl. Acad. Sci.*, **91,** 4872–6.

Fridkis-Hareli, M., Teitelbaum, D., Arnon, R. and Sela, M. (1995). Synthetic copolymer 1 and myelin basic protein do not require processing prior to binding to class II major histocompatibility complex molecules on living antigen-presenting cells. *Cell Immunol.*, **163,** 229–36.

Gauthier, L., Smith, K. J., Pyrdol, J. *et al.* (1998). Expression and crystallization of the complex of HLA-DR2 (DRA, DRB1*1501) and an immunodominant peptide of human myelin basic protein. *Proc. Natl. Acad. Sci. USA*, **95,** 11828–33.

Goodkin, D. E., Reingold, S., Sibley, W. *et al.* (1999). Guidelines for clinical trials of new therapeutic agents in multiple sclerosis: reporting extended results from phase III clinical trials. *Neurology*, **46,** 132–4.

Hohlfeld, R. (1997). Biotechnological agents for the immunotherapy of multiple sclerosis – principles, problems and perspectives. *Brain*, **120(5),** 865–916.

Johnson, K. P., Brooks, B. R., Cohen, J. A. *et al.* (1995a). Copolymer 1 reduces relapse rate and improves disability in relapsing–remitting multiple sclerosis: Results of a phase III multicentre, double-blind, placebo-controlled trial. *Neurology*, **45**, 1268–76.

Johnson, K. P., The Phase III Copolymer 1 Study Group *et al.* (1995b). Antibodies to copolymer 1 do not interfere with its clinical effect. *Ann. Neurol*, **38**, 973.

Johnson, K. P., Brooks, B. R., Cohen, J. A. *et al.* (1998). Extended use of glatiramer acetate (Copaxone) is well tolerated and maintains its clinical effect on multiple sclerosis relapse rate and degree of disability. *Neurology*, **50**, 701–8.

Kurtzke, J. F. (1989). The Disability Status Scale for multiple sclerosis – Apologia Pro DSS Sua. *Neurology*, **39**, 291–302.

Lando, Z., Teitelbaum, D. and Arnon, R. (1979). Effect of cyclophosphamide on suppressor cell activity in mice unresponsive to EAE. *J. Immunol*, **123**, 2156–60.

Lea, A. P. and Goa, K. L. (1996). Copolymer: a review of its pharmacological properties and therapeutic potential in multiple sclerosis. *Clin. Immunother.*, **6**, 319–31.

Lisak, R. P., Zweiman, B., Blanchard, N. and Rorke, L. B. (1983). Effect of treatment with copolymer 1 (Cop-1) on the *in vivo* and *in vitro* manifestations of experimental allergic encephalomyelitis (EAE). *J. Neurol. Sci.*, **62**, 281–93.

Liu, C., Po, A. L. W. and Blumhardt, L. D. (1998). 'Summary measure' statistic for assessing the outcome of treatment trials in relapsing–remitting multiple sclerosis. *J. Neurol. Neurosurg. Psychiatr.*, **64**, 726–9.

Lobel, E., Riven-Kreitman, R., Amselem, A. and Pinchasi, I. (1996) Copolymer-1: agent for multiple sclerosis. *Drugs Fut.*, **21**, 131–4.

Lublin, F. D. and Reingold, S. C. (1996). Defining the clinical course of multiple sclerosis: results of an international survey. *Neurology*, **46**, 907–11.

Lublin, F. D. and Reingold, S. C. (1998). Combination therapy for treatment of multiple sclerosis. *Ann. Neurol.*, **44**, 7–9.

Mancardi, G. L., Sardanelli, F., Parodi, R. C. *et al.* (1998). Effect of copolymer-1 on serial gadolinium-enhanced MRI in relapsing remitting multiple sclerosis. *Neurology*, **50**, 1127–33.

Miller, A., Shapiro, S., Gershtein, R. *et al.* (1998). Treatment of multiple sclerosis with Copolymer-1 (Copaxone®): Implicating mechanisms of Th1 to Th2/Th3 immune-deviation. *J. Neuroimmunol.*, **92**, 113–21.

Milo, R. and Panitch, H. (1995). Additive effects of copolymer-1 and interferon beta-1b on the immune response to myelin basic protein. *J. Neuroimmunol.*, **61(2)**, 185–93.

Morel, P. A. and Oriss, T. B. (1998). Crossregulation between Th1 and Th2 cells. *Crit. Rev. Immunol.*, **18**, 275–303.

Nauta, J. J. P., Thompson, A. J., Barkhof, F. and Miller, D. H. (1994). Magnetic resonance imaging in monitoring the treatment of multiple sclerosis patients: Statistical power of parallel groups and crossover designs. *J. Neurol. Sci.*, **122**, 6–14.

Paty, D. W., Li, D. K. B., UBC MS-MRI Study Group and IFNB Multiple Sclerosis Study Group (1993). Interferon beta-1b is effective in relapsing–remitting multiple sclerosis. II. MRI analysis results of a multi-centre, randomized, double-blind, placebo-controlled trial. *Neurology*, **43**, 662–7.

Racke, M. K., Martin, R., McFarland, H. and Fritz, R. B. (1992). Copolymer-1-induced inhibition of antigen-specific T-cell activation: Interference with antigen presentation. *J. Neuroimmunol.*, **37**, 75–84.

Romagnani, S., Parronchi, P., D'Elios, M. M. *et al.* (1997). An update on human Th1 and Th2 cells. *Int. Arch. Allergy Immunol.*, **113**, 153–6.

Simon, J. H., Jacobs, L. D., Campion, M. *et al.* (1998). Magnetic resonance studies of intramuscular interferon beta-1a for relapsing multiple sclerosis. *Ann. Neurol.*, **43**, 79–87.

Stone, L. A., Smith, L. A., Albert, P. S. *et al.* (1995). Blood–brain barrier disruption on contrast-enhanced MRI in patients with mild relapsing–remitting multiple sclerosis: relationship to course, gender and age. *Neurology*, **45**, 1122–6.

Teitelbaum, D., Meshorer, A., Hirshfield, T. *et al.* (1971). Suppression of experimental allergic encephalomyelitis by a synthetic polypeptide. *Eur. J. Immunol.*, **1**, 242–8.

Teitelbaum, D., Webb, C., Meshorer, A. *et al.* (1973). Suppression by several synthetic polypeptides of experimental allergic encephalomyelitis induced in guinea pigs and rabbits with bovine and human encephalitogen. *Eur. J. Immunol.*, **3**, 379–86.

Teitelbaum, D., Aharoni, R., Arnon, R. and Sela, M. (1988). Specific inhibition of the T-cell response to myelin basic protein by the synthetic copolymer Cop 1. *Proc. Natl. Acad. Sci.*, **85**, 9724–8.

Teitelbaum, D., Aharoni, R., Sela, M. and Arnon, R. (1991). Cross-reactions and specificities of monoclonal antibodies against myelin basic protein and against the synthetic copolymer-1. *Proc. Natl. Acad. Sci.*, **88**, 9528–32.

Teitelbaum, D., Milo, R., Arnon, R. and Sela, M. (1992). Synthetic copolymer-1 inhibits human T-cell lines specific for myelin basic protein. *Proc. Natl. Acad. Sci.*, **89**, 137–41.

Teitelbaum, D., Fridkis-Hareli, M., Arnon, R. and Sela, M. (1996). Copolymer 1 inhibits chronic relapsing experimental allergic encephalomyelitis induced by proteolipid protein (PLP) peptides in mice and interferes with PLP-specific T cell responses. *J. Neuroimmunol.*, **64**, 209–17.

Teitelbaum, D., Sela, M. and Arnon, R. (1997). Copolymer 1 from the laboratory to FDA. *Isr. J. Med. Sci.*, **33**, 280–4.

Teitelbaum, D., Arnon, R. and Sela, M. (1999). Immunomodulation of experimental autoimmune encephalomyelitis by oral administration of copolymer-1. *Proc. Natl. Acad. Sci.*, **96**, 3842–7.

van Sechel, A. C. and van Noort, J. M. (1996). Copolymer-1 inhibits human T-cell responses to the major myelin antigen alpha B-crystallin. *J. Neurol.*, **243(Suppl. 2)**, S240.

Weiner, H. (1987). Cop 1 therapy for multiple sclerosis. *N. Engl. J. Med.*, **317**, 442–4.

Wolinsky, J. S., Narayana, P. A., the MRI-AC (Houston, TX) and the North American Linomide Trialists (1998). Phase III North American Linomide trial of roquinimex (Linomide) in relapsing–remitting (RR) and secondary progressive (SP) multiple sclerosis (MS): MRI findings. *Neurology*, **50,** 62.

6

Immunoglobulins

Introduction

The history of the therapeutic use of intravenous immunoglobulins (IVIg) is a telling example of how much empirical knowledge can contribute to medical progress, even in the realm of molecular medicine. When the advancement of protein purification technologies allowed the removal of aggregates and made immunoglobulins available for intravenous application (Drews, 1986; Schwartz, 1987), IVIg was first administered as replacement therapy in patients with primary immunodeficiency. In the early 1980s Imbach and colleagues observed by serendipity the recovery from severe thrombocytopenia in idiopathic thrombocytopenic purpura (ITP) after treatment with IVIg (Imbach *et al.*, 1981). This led to the discovery of the immunomodulatory potential of IVIg, and ever since the number of diseases with presumed autoimmune pathology treated with IVIg has steadily grown (Dwyer, 1992). This includes a variety of neurological disorders for which IVIg treatment has become increasingly recognized as an effective or promising therapeutic alternative (Voltz and Hohlfeld, 1996; Dalakas, 1997; Stangel *et al.*, 1998).

Immunological properties

Immunoglobulins are the mainstay of humoral immunity, and are capable of recognizing a broad spectrum of immunogenic structures (antigens). The immense variation in the spectrum of antibody-binding specificities is possible because of the contribution of germline diversity and somatic mutation (Klein and Horejsi, 1997). A prototypic immunoglobulin molecule is composed of four polypeptide chains, two identical heavy and two identical light chains, which are joined into a macromolecular complex by disulphide bonds (Figure 6.1). The exclusive use of one heavy chain and one light chain is the consequence of allelic exclusion. Based on experiments with proteolytic enzymes such as papain or trypsin, which cleave the immunoglobulin molecule at specific points, the molecule can be divided into two functional domains. The Fab fragment contains the antigen-binding capacity of the molecule and bears the 'recognition' function, and the remaining Fc portion (so named because it is easily crystallized) accomplishes the 'effector' functions. These biological effector functions include complement fixation or binding to

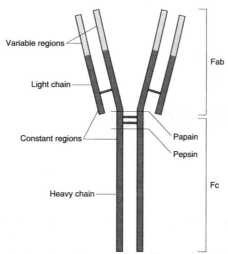

Figure 6.1 Schematic drawing of a prototypic immunoglobulin molecule.

respective Fc receptors (Deo *et al.*, 1997). Finally, immunoglobulins are glyco-proteins, and glycosylation is normally restricted to the constant region of the heavy chain.

The genetic events that generate and regulate the immunoglobulin gene rearrangement and the regulation of gene expression are complex. Human immunoglobulins are divided into five classes; IgA, IgD, IgE, IgG and IgM. IgM has a central function in a primary immune response. IgG, which makes up about 75 per cent of serum immunoglobulin, is the predominant antibody in a second-ary immune response. It has a molecular weight of 150 000 daltons, and is divided into four different subclasses that can activate the classical complement cascade, albeit with different efficiencies. By the interaction with specific subsets of T-cells and/or factors secreted by these cells, a class switch is mediated. Immunoglobulins can by themselves act as antigens that are recognized and neu-tralized by the immune system. Accordingly, antigenic markers found in only an individual member of a species, so called idiotypes, can be regulated by the anti-idiotypic network of the immune system (see below) (Abdou *et al.*, 1981).

Mechanisms of action

Therapeutic IVIg preparations are obtained from large plasma pools of several thousand donors. Despite some degree of variation between different manufac-turers, all IVIg preparations contain mainly IgG, with very small amounts of other immunoglobulins and fragments and also various other immunoactive pro-teins (Grosse–Wilde *et al.*, 1992; Blasczyk *et al.*, 1993; Kekow *et al.*, 1998). Many experimental studies, both *in vivo* and *in vitro*, have shown that IVIg can interfere with the immune system at several levels. In addition, IVIg may promote remyelination in demyelinating disease associated with viral infections

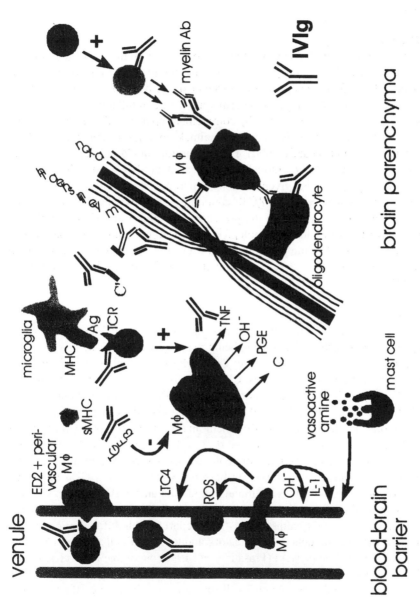

Figure 6.2 Possible mechanisms of action of immunoglobulins.

(Rodriguez and Lennon, 1990). At present, no single mode of action has been identified as being the crucial mechanism, which leads to the suggestion that at least some of the following effects of IVIg may act in concert.

Effects of immunoglobulins on components of the immune system

Complement

Immunoglobulins can bind complement components with their constant domain, and thus prevent tissue damage caused by the complement activation cascade. Evidence of the functionality of this mechanism in humans was demonstrated directly by serial muscle biopsies in dermatomyositis, an inflammatory disease of muscle (Dalakas *et al.*, 1993), and by complement uptake studies *in vitro*, where deposition of C3b and of the membrane attack complex disappeared on IVIg treatment (Basta and Dalakas, 1994). These inhibitory *in vitro* effects of sera from patients treated with IVIg gradually disappeared until day 30, when another course of IVIg had to be given. Recent experimental data also speak for an enhanced physiologic cleavage of C3b-containing complexes by IgG (Lutz *et al.*, 1996), which was dependent on the presence of factors I and H. The ability of high doses of IgG to stimulate complement inactivation is a novel regulatory role. This could also be of prime pathogenic importance in inflammatory demyelinating disorders, e.g. GBS, where complement deposition *in situ* has been demonstrated (Hartung *et al.*, 1998).

T-cells

The T-cell population can be divided into several subsets depending on the surface receptors expressed, the main division being made by the membrane glycoproteins CD4 and CD8. At present, most of our knowledge on the influence of IVIg on T-cells is derived from *in vitro* studies. Changes in both CD8$^+$ suppressor/cytotoxic and CD4$^+$ helper T-cells were demonstrated after IVIg treatment (Leung *et al.*, 1987; Macey and Newland, 1990). Antibodies directed against several T cell surface molecules are present in IVIg, including the T cell receptor (Marchalonis *et al.*, 1992), CD4, and MHC (Kaveri *et al.*, 1996). Neutralizing antibodies against bacterial/viral superantigens that stimulate T-cells nonspecifically are also contained in IVIg (Takei *et al.*, 1993). Furthermore, soluble CD4 or CD4-like activity and soluble HLA molecules are found in trace amounts in IVIg (Blasczyk *et al.*, 1993). The significance of these contaminations comigrating with IVIg is uncertain, because successful treatment trials were reported with different preparations containing variable amounts of these factors. Induction of T-cell apoptosis by components of the Fas/FasL system (Prasad *et al.*, 1998) or soluble HLA class I molecule (Zavazava and Krönke, 1996) included in therapeutic preparations of IVIg may also exert a regulatory role on T cell functions by eliminating effector cells.

B-cells

Many *in vitro* studies have shown the potential of IVIg to inhibit B-cell differentiation and antibody production (Kondo *et al.*, 1991, 1994). In some studies the effect was attributed to the Fc portion of the immunoglobulins (Kondo et al., 1994), whereas others showed it to be Fab dependent (Klaesson et al., 1996). This could be mediated by anti-idiotypic antibodies directed against the surface-bound idiotypes on B-cells producing pathogenic antibodies (see below), or by antibodies directed against the CD5 antigen (Vassilev et al., 1993) that is expressed on a sub-population of B-cells. These CD5-positive B-cells are thought to produce low affinity natural autoantibodies, which are detected in serum of healthy individuals (Lacroix-Desmazes et al., 1998). Anti-idiotypes have indeed been shown to be present in IVIg preparations. Finally, IVIg can inhibit the production of IL-6, a cytokine needed for the secretion of IgG by plasma cells (Andersson and Andersson, 1990).

Anti-idiotypes

Immunoglobulins that recognize and attach to the antigen-binding region of the F(ab) part of another immunoglobulin are called anti-idiotypic antibodies. The idiotypic diversity is greatly increased when IgG is pooled from a number of individuals (Rous and Jenkersly, 1990). These antibodies may occur naturally or may be driven by antigenic challenge with subsequent formation of autoantibodies. It is thought that a network of these various antibodies may play a role in the regulation of autoimmunity (Dietrich et al., 1992). The therapeutic relevance of this mechanism in human disease was demonstrated by the successful treatment of patients with autoantibodies to factor VIII (Sultan et al., 1984), or with systemic lupus erythematosus (Silvestris et al., 1996), using purified anti-idiotypic antibodies. Also, graft survival was prolonged by anti-idiotypic antibodies (Schussler et al., 1998). These effects are pertinent to autoimmune diseases of the nervous system as well, since anti-idiotypic mechanisms have been suggested to play a role in GBS and CIDP (van Doorn et al., 1988).

Fc receptor

The Fc portion of immunoglobulins interacts with many phagocytic cells of the reticuloendothelial system expressing appropriate Fc receptors on their cell surface. These Fc receptors link cellular and humoral immunity by serving as a bridge between antibody specificity and effector cell function (Deo et al., 1997). Pathogenic antibodies can bind to the Fc receptor and thereby target macrophages. Excessive amounts of immunoglobulins may compete with this binding, thus blocking the damaging effects of inflammatory effector cells. Modulation of Fc receptor-mediated functions has been shown in vitro (Kimberly et al., 1984; Kurlander and Hall, 1986) and administration of purified Fc fragments was indeed effective in children with idiopathic thrombocytopenic purpura (Clarkson et al., 1986; Debre et al., 1993). For neurological disorders, there is evidence from an experimentally induced inflammatory neuropathy in rats (EAN) that intact human IVIg, but not F(ab')$_2$ fragments can clearly reduce disease severity, suggesting that its effect is mediated via the Fc portion (Miyagi et al., 1997). In addition to the mere blockade of Fc receptors, immunoglobulins and complexes derived thereof can cross-link Fc receptors mediating apoptosis of B cells (Ashman et al., 1996).

Cytokines

Clinical studies have demonstrated that the cytokine profile of patients is altered by the administration of IVIg, and this is supported by studies showing that cytokine production can be modulated by IVIg in cultured mononuclear cells (Andersson *et al.*, 1996). However, so far it has not been proven that this mechanism plays a major role under pathologic conditions. Complementary to these *in vivo* studies are many *in vitro* studies suggesting that IVIg may influence the cytokine network by trace amounts of IFNγ (Lam *et al.*, 1993) and TGFβ (Kekow *et al.*, 1998) or by neutralizing antibodies directed against IL-1a, IL-6, and the class I interferons (IFNα, β) (Svenson *et al.*, 1993; Ross *et al.*, 1995). Immunoglobulins may also modulate the production and secretion of cytokines by lymphocytes or monocytes. Upregulation of IL-1 receptor antagonist (Aukrust *et al.*, 1997b; Ruiz de Souza *et al.*, 1995) and IL-8 secretion (Andersson *et al.*, 1996) has been induced by IVIg. In experimental autoimmune encephalomyelitis (EAE), human IVIg is thought to act via downregulation of TNFα secretion (Achiron *et al.*, 1994), whereas in HIV infection, IVIg therapy increased expression of the membrane-bound p75-TNF receptor (Aukrust *et al.*, 1997b). While all these observations attest to some modulation of the cytokine profile by IVIg, they do not yet lend themselves to formulating a unifying hypothesis regarding their pathophysiological consequences.

Effects of immunoglobulins on remyelination

The concept that IVIg may have the potential to remyelinate axons originated from the observation that polyclonal immunoglobulins against spinal cord homogenate were able to increase remyelination in the inflammatory model of Theiler's virus encephalitis (Rodriguez and Lennon, 1990). Further studies showed that more specific antibodies reactive with myelin basic protein also have the capacity to promote remyelination in this model (Rodriguez *et al.*, 1996). A monoclonal IgMk antibody was identified that could promote remyelination (Miller *et al.*, 1994), suppress inflammation, and also had some effect in a toxic model of demyelination (Miller *et al.*, 1997; Pavelko *et al.*, 1998). This monoclonal antibody was shown to be polyreactive, recognizing antigens present on the surface (Asakura *et al.*, 1996) and in the cytoplasm of oligodendrocytes and other glial cells. It is easiest to assume that the remyelination-promoting properties of these antibodies relate to the oligodendrocyte surface activity. Extrapolating from these experimental observations, IVIg may have a beneficial effect if containing such autoantibodies. This intriguing concept challenges the traditional view of classifying anti-myelin antibodies as being essentially detrimental. Thus IVIg may exert a protective or regenerative function independent from its other possible actions.

Immunoglobulin in MS

Following the first evidence of its immunomodulatory potential, IVIg was soon tested and proven effective in a variety of peripheral autoimmune neurological disorders including the Guillain-Barré syndrome, chronic inflammatory demyelinating polyneuropathy and multifocal motor neuropathy (Dalakas, 1997; PSGBS Trial Group, 1997; van der Meché and van Doorn, 1997; Stangel *et al.*, 1998). Early on, IVIg was also considered for the interval treatment of MS. Studies conducted by Rothfelder *et al.* (1982), Schuller and Govaerts (1983) and Soukop and Tschabitscher (1986) all reported some improvement in disability or a reduction in relapses of MS patients. However, these studies were carried out without randomization, lacked placebo controls, included patients with various patterns of MS, or were performed in combination with other therapies (Sørensen, 1994; Lisak, 1998). Further observations in small samples of patients with relapsing–remitting MS (Achiron *et al.*, 1992) or with progressive MS (Cook *et al.*, 1992) also did not meet the current requirements of conclusive drug trials. In the meantime, however, various prospective, randomized, double-blind, placebo-controlled studies have been completed that addressed the potential of IVIg both to reduce disease activity and accumulation of deficits in relapsing–remitting MS (Table 6.1), and to ameliorate fixed neurological deficits from MS.

Table 6.1 Published randomized, double-blind, placebo-controlled trials on IVIg in MS

	Fazekas *et al.* 1997a, 1997b (AIMS)	Achiron *et al.*, 1998	Sørensen *et al.*, 1998
Patient number	148	40	21
Study design	Parallel	Parallel	Crossover
Study duration	2 years	2 years	2×6 months
Primary endpoint	Disability	Relapses	MRI activity
IVIg dosage	0.15–0.2 g/kg per month	0.4 g/kg daily for 5 days 0.4 g/kg every 2 months	2g/kg per month

Interval treatment of relapsing–remitting MS

The Austrian Immunoglobulin in MS (AIMS) study compared a monthly dosage of 0.15–0.2 g/kg body weight of IVIg to physiological saline over a period of 2 years in 148 patients (Fazekas *et al.*, 1997a,b). Patients had to have a history of at least two clearly identified and documented relapses during the previous 2 years, and a baseline Kurtzke's Expanded Disability Status Scale (EDSS) score of between 1.0 (minor neurological signs without disability) and 6.0 (ambulatory with assistance). Patients were stratified with regard to centre, age, gender and deterioration rate by a centralized computer-generated randomization schedule. Primary outcome measures were the between-group differences in the absolute change of the EDSS score, and in the proportion of patients who improved, remained stable or worsened in disability, as defined by an increase or decrease of at least 1 point on the EDSS score by the end of the study. Secondary outcome measures were the number of relapses, the annual relapse rate, the proportion of relapse-free patients, and the time until first relapse during the study period. Sixty-four patients in the IVIg group and 56 in the placebo group completed 2 years of treatment, and demographic variables and disease characteristics were well balanced between both treatment groups.

Intention to treat analysis showed mild improvement of IVIg-treated patients over the study period from a baseline EDSS of 3.33 (95 per cent CI 3.01–3.65) to a final mean EDSS of 3.09 (CI 2.72–3.46). In contrast, the placebo group deteriorated slightly from a baseline EDSS of 3.37 (CI 2.96–3.76) to 3.49 (CI 3.06–3.92). This change in EDSS scores (IVIg –0.23, placebo 0.12) was significantly different ($P = 0.008$). A similar and significant difference was maintained when analysing only those patients who completed the study. There was an improvement of 1 point or more on the EDSS score in 23 (31 per cent) of the IVIg-treated patients compared with 10 (14 per cent) of the placebo-group patients. By contrast, deterioration of disability occurred in 12 (16 per cent) IVIg-treated patients and 17 (23 per cent) patients of the placebo group ($P = 0.041$). Overall, 24 per cent of patients did better on IVIg than on placebo when adding the differences in rate of improvement (17 per cent) and prevention of deterioration (7 per cent) between IVIg- and placebo-treated groups. Figure 6.3 shows the time course of the EDSS score in both patient groups.

The number of relapses in IVIg-treated patients was about half of that in the placebo group (62 vs 116). This resulted in a significantly higher proportion of relapse-free patients when receiving IVIg (53 per cent vs 26 per cent, $P = 0.03$). IVIg treatment reduced the annual relapse rate from a pre-study rate of 1.3 (95 per cent CI 1.09–1.51) to a mean of 0.52 (CI 0.32–0.72) during the study period. In placebo-treated patients, the annual relapse rate was 1.41 (CI

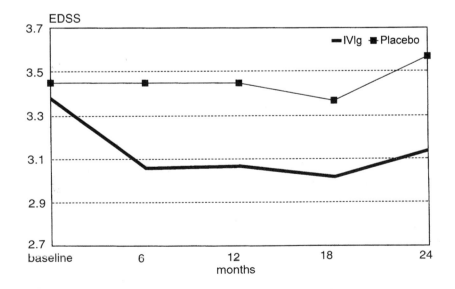

Figure 6.3 Time course of clinical disability (mean EDSS scores) in IVIg- and placebo-treated patients of the AIMS trial (from Fazekas *et al.*, 1997b).

1.21–1.61) before participating in the study and 1.26 (0.75–1.77) during the study. Hence, IVIg treatment was associated with a 59 per cent reduction of the annual relapse rate compared to placebo ($P = 0.0037$). Figure 6.4 shows the time course of the monthly relapse rates within 6-month intervals during the trial.

Similar clinical endpoints were tested in another study of 40 patients with clinically definite and MRI-confirmed relapsing–remitting MS over 2 years by Achiron *et al.* (1998). Their patients received IVIg at a loading dose of 0.4 g/kg body weight per day for five consecutive days. Subsequent booster doses of IVIg in a single dosage of 0.4 g/kg body weight were administered every 2 months. Again, physiological saline served as placebo. In IVIg-treated patients the annual exacerbation rate dropped from 1.85 ± 0.26 in the pre-study period to 0.75 ± 0.16 in the first year and 0.42 ± 0.14 in the second year ($P < 0.05$ compared with baseline). This compared with an annual exacerbation rate in the placebo group before the study of 1.55 ± 0.17, and rates of 1.8 ± 0.2 in the first year and 1.42 ± 0.23 in the second year of the trial, respectively. Overall, this corresponded to a 38.6 per cent reduction of the annualized exacerbation rate following IVIg treatment against a 4.2 per cent drop in the placebo group ($P = 0.0006$). The number of exacerbation-free patients and the probability of remaining exacerbation-free during the 2-year study period according to Kaplan–Meier analysis were significantly in favour of IVIg. Beneficial effects of IVIg were also noted concerning disability. The proportion of patients who improved by at least 1 point in the EDSS score was 23.5 per cent following IVIg, compared to 10.8 per cent in the placebo group. The proportions of patients worsening by at least 1 point were 13.7 per cent and 17.1 per cent, respectively ($P = 0.03$). Annually performed MRI examinations did not reveal significant differences in the change of lesion burden between both

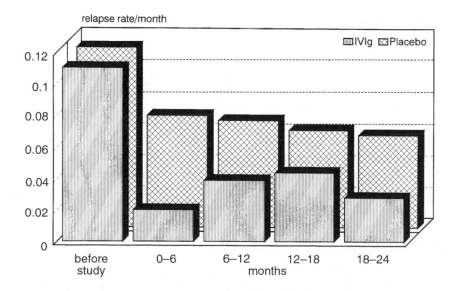

Figure 6.4 Monthly relapse rates of IVIg- and placebo-treated patients within 6-month intervals during the AIMS trial (from Fazekas *et al.*, 1997b).

groups. However, these data are weakened by the small number of patients who underwent the final MRI examination and a presumably low sensitivity of the MRI score used in the analysis (Achiron and Barak, 1999; Francis, 1999).

Apart from these clinical results, suppression of MS activity by repeated administration of IVIg has also been documented by using frequent gadolinium-enhanced magnetic resonance imaging in a cross-over study of 26 patients with relapsing–remitting or secondary progressive MS with relapses (Sørensen et al., 1998). IVIg treatment consisted of infusions of 1 g/kg body weight per day for two consecutive days at monthly intervals (total dose/month 2 g/kg). Human albumin (2 per cent concentration) served as placebo, and was administered with an identical regimen.

Overall, IVIg treatment reduced the mean number of new and total gadolinium-enhanced lesions significantly by approximately 60 per cent compared with placebo, both in the per-protocol population (baseline 3.8 ± 8.3; IVIg 1.2 ± 2.2; placebo 3.2 ± 5.9; $2P = 0.03$) and according to intention to treat analysis (baseline 3.6 ± 7.7; IVIg 1.3 ± 2.3; placebo 2.9 ± 5.4; $2P = 0.003$). Disease activity on MRI decreased after 1 month of treatment with IVIg and then remained stable, whereas no changes in activity were observed during treatment with placebo. The average percentage of per-protocol patients with active scans on 6-monthly serial MRIs was 37 per cent during IVIg treatment compared to 68 per cent when receiving placebo ($P < 0.01$). Four of 18 patients did not have any gadolinium-enhanced lesions during the whole IVIg treatment period, but none were free of new gadolinium-enhanced lesions while on placebo. In parallel, 15 patients remained free of exacerbations during IVIg treatment, compared to only seven receiving placebo ($P = 0.02$).

Reduction of fixed deficit

Based on the concept of remyelination, van Engelen et al. (1992) studied five MS patients with optic neuritis after a period of stable visual impairment and noted improvement in visual acuity and colour vision following 1–2 months of IVIg treatment. This improvement persisted over a follow-up period of 1.2–1.7 years. Noseworthy et al. (1997; 1998) attempted to confirm this observation of a reduction of fixed deficits by IVIg in two randomized, double-blind, placebo-controlled trials. IVIg was given in a dosage of 0.4 g/kg for 5 days and thereafter every 4 weeks, to a total of eight infusions, to patients with longstanding optic neuritis, and at a somewhat higher frequency to MS patients with recently acquired but stable muscle weakness. Neither of the trials, which have so far been reported only in abstract form, indicated a beneficial effect of IVIg.

Side effects

The reported side effects of IVIg are generally minor, and occur at a frequency of less than 5 per cent (see review in Stangel et al., 1997). Accordingly, side effects were rarely observed in both the AIMS trial (Fazekas et al., 1997) and the study by Achiron et al. (1998). They consisted of a transient rash or of fatigue, headaches and low-grade fever, which spontaneously resolved within a few hours. An unexpectedly high number of acute and chronic adverse events in association with IVIg treatment were seen by Sørensen et al. (1998). While the acute events (such as headaches, nausea and urticarial rashes) could be diminished by either reducing the infusion rate or administering antihistaminic drugs before the infusion, severe eczema was another major and long-lasting side effect, and this occurred in 11 of 23 patients during treatment with IVIg. In all patients the eczema eventually resolved after discontinuation of IVIg therapy, but in some patients it persisted for several weeks after the last infusion. According to the investigators, IVIg given rapidly in very high concentrations may have contained substances that were toxic to the skin (Sørensen et al., 1998). It should be noted, however, that these side effects have not previously been reported at such a frequency in other diseases, even with high doses of IVIg (Whitham et al., 1997). It may be that this unusual adverse effect profile can also in part be accounted for by differences in the concentration of cytokines between various commercially available IVIg preparations.

From general experience, it is known that the only strict contraindications for IVIg are selective IgA deficiency or an anaphylactic episode following previous infusions (Ratko et al., 1995). Further limitations include congestive heart failure and renal insufficiency, because administration of IVIg expands the plasma volume and increases blood viscosity (Dalakas, 1994; Tan et al., 1993), which may lead to decompensation in patients with compromised cardiac or renal function. The same mechanisms are considered responsible for the development of cerebral infarction and thrombembolic events, which are rather rare but severe neurological sequelae (Dalakas, 1994). Alternatively, encephalopathy could also be caused by arterial vasospasm (Voltz et al., 1996). To avoid these complications it is generally preferable to start the infusion at a slow rate of 30 ml/h for the first 15 minutes, and to slowly increase the flow to 120 ml/h, as recommended by the manufacturers.

In the past, intensive efforts have been made to increase the safety of blood products, including IVIg preparations. To minimize the transmission of infectious diseases, only selected donors are accepted; these are routinely screened for antibodies to HVC, HIV, syphilis and hepatitis B antigen. Furthermore, the specific purification processes eliminate high titres of infectious agents (Hamamoto et al., 1987; Uemura et al., 1989; Imbach et al., 1991; Kempf et al., 1991). With regard to HIV infection there is no well documented case of transmission by IVIg (Thornton, Ballow, 1993; Ratko et al, 1995). Only hepatitis C transmission by a single IVIg preparation had been reported (Healey et al., 1996; Barton, 1996) until the manufacturing process was improved (Schiff, 1994). Therefore high quality IVIg preparations appear to be safe, although the minimal residual risk inherent in every biological product can never be entirely excluded.

Current role of immunoglobulin in the treatment of MS

To date, three prospective, randomized, double-blind, placebo-controlled studies have indicated a beneficial effect of IVIg on disease activity and accumulation of deficits in patients with relapsing–remitting MS (Fazekas *et al.*, 1997a, b; Achiron *et al.,* 1998; Sørensen *et al.,* 1998). These effects are modest, but appear comparable to those reported for other accepted treatments for this indication, such as interferon-beta (IFNB MS Study Group, 1993, 1995; Paty *et al.*, 1993; Jacobs *et al.*, 1996; Pozzilli *et al.*, 1996; PRISMS Study Group, 1998) and glatiramer acetate (Johnson *et al.*, 1995, 1998). Clearly, the amount of supportive evidence for IVIg still lags far behind that for interferon beta. As in most other autoimmune disorders that are successfully treated with IVIg, it is not clear by which mechanism(s) IVIg preparations exert their therapeutic efficacy in MS (Lisak, 1998). Current evidence argues for a combination of immunomodulatory actions, but some contribution by enhancing remyelination is still under debate. Finally, the optimal dosage for IVIg in MS has not yet been determined. In view of the overall shortage of blood products and cost containment this issue will be of great relevance to further considerations on the use of IVIg in MS, and must be resolved by ongoing studies.

Despite these uncertainties, available scientific evidence for IVIg's action in relapsing–remitting MS appears to be consistent enough to allow consideration of its use in a number of settings even now. The frequency and routes of administration of interferon beta and glatiramer acetate are not acceptable to some patients, and local reactions at the injection site can become a problem. Moreover, concerns about antibody production following long-term interferon beta treatment have not yet been fully resolved (Cross and Antel, 1998). In these instances, IVIg could be considered as a further treatment option (Lisak, 1998; Fazekas *et al.*, 1999). The use of IVIg to prevent childbirth-associated relapses may also warrant consideration (Achiron *et al.*, 1996).

With many questions still unresolved, it is not yet possible to appreciate the final role of IVIg in the treatment of MS. Arguments for and against the use of IVIg are summarized in Table 6.2. Clearly there is not yet any scientific evidence for considering IVIg in other than a relapsing–remitting course of MS. In this respect, the results of a large European study with Canadian participation in more than 300 patients with secondary progressive MS are eagerly awaited.

Table 6.2 Current considerations on the use of IVIg for treating patients with relapsing–remitting MS

Possible concerns	Favourable aspects
• Efficacy proven in relatively small patient populations compared to IFNβ	• Well tolerated (at least at low dosages)
• No MRI data parallel to larger clinical trials available	• Application only once a month
• Dose–response relation not established	• Few contraindications
• Mechanisms of action unclear	• May act via mechanisms not activated by other drugs
• Limited availability and significant costs at high dosage	

References

Abdou, M. I., Wall, H., Lindsley, H. B. *et al.* (1981). Network theory in autoimmunity: *in vitro* suppression of serum anti-DNA antibody binding to DNA by anti-idiotypic antibody in systemic lupus erythematosus. *J. Clin. Invest.*, **67**, 1297–1304.

Achiron, A., Pras, E., Gilad, R. *et al.* (1992). Open controlled therapeutic trial of high-dose intravenous immunoglobulins in relapsing–remitting multiple sclerosis. *Arch. Neurol.*, **49**, 1233–6.

Achiron, A., Margalit, R., Hershkoviz, R. *et al.* (1994). Intravenous immunoglobulin treatment of experimental T-cell mediated autoimmune disease. Upregulation of T-cell proliferation and downregulation of tumor necrosis factor a secretion. *J. Clin. Invest.*, **93**, 600–605.

Achiron, A., Rotstein, Z., Noy, S. *et al.* (1996). Intravenous immunoglobulin treatment in the prevention of childbirth-associated acute exacerbations in multiple sclerosis: a pilot study. *J. Neurol.*, **243**, 25–8.

Achiron, A., Gabbay, U., Gilad, R. *et al.* (1998). Intravenous immunoglobulin treatment in multiple sclerosis. Effect on relapses. *Neurology*, **50**, 398–402.

Achiron, A. and Barak, Y. (1999). Intravenous immunoglobulin treatment in multiple sclerosis. *Neurology*, **52**, 214.

Andersson, J. P. and Andersson, U. G. (1990). Human intravenous immunoglobulin modulates monokine production in vitro. *Immunology*, **71**, 372–6.

Andersson, J., Skansén-Saphir, U., Sparrelid, E. *et al.* (1996). Intravenous immune globulin affects cytokine production in T-lymphocytes and monocytes macrophages. *Clin. Exp. Immunol.*, **104**, 10–20.

Asakura, K., Miller, D. J., Murray, K. *et al.* (1996). Monoclonal autoantibody SCH94.03, which promotes central nervous system remyelination, recognizes an antigen on the surface of oligodendrocytes. *J. Neurosci. Res.*, **43**, 273–81.

Ashman, R. F., Peckham, D. W. and Stunz, L. L. (1996). Fc receptor off-signal in the B cell involves apoptosis. *J. Immunol.*, **157**, 5–11.

Aukrust, P., Müller, F., Nordoy, I. *et al.* (1997a). Modulation of lymphocyte and monocyte activity after intravenous immunoglobulin administration *in vivo*. *Clin. Exp. Immunol.*, **107**, 50–56.

Aukrust, P., Hestdal, K., Lien, E. *et al.* (1997b). Effects of intravenous immunoglobulin *in vivo* on abnormally increased tumor necrosis factor-a activity in human immunodeficiency virus type 1 infection. *J. Infect. Dis.*, 176, 913–923.

Barton, L. L. (1996). Hepatitis C after immunoglobulin administration. *Pediatr. Infect. Dis. J.*, **15**, 558.

Basta, M. and Dalakas, M. C. (1994). High-dose intravenous immunoglobulin exerts its beneficial effect in patients with dermatomyositis by blocking endomysial deposition of activated complement fragments. *J. Clin. Invest.*, **94**, 1729–35.

Blasczyk, R., Westhoff, U. and Grosse-Wilde, H. (1993). Soluble CD4, CD8, and HLA molecules in commercial immunoglobulin preparations. *Lancet*, **341**,

789–90.

Clarkson, S. B., Bussel J. B., Kimberley R. P. *et al.* (1986). Treatment of refractory immune thrombocytopenic purpura with an anti-Fc gamma receptor antibody. *N. Engl. J. Med.*, **314**, 1236–39.

Cook, S., Troiano, R., Rohowsky-Kochan, C. *et al.* (1992). Intravenous gamma globulin in progressive MS. *Acta Neurol. Scand.*, **86**, 171–5.

Cross, A. H. and Antel, J. P. (1998). Antibodies to beta-interferons in multiple sclerosis: can we neutralize the controversy? *Neurology*, **50**, 1206–8.

Dalakas, M. C., Illa, I., Dambrosia, J. M. *et al.* (1993). Efficacy of high-dose intravenous immunoglobulin in the treatment of dermatomyositis: a double-blind, placebo-controlled study. *N. Engl. J. Med.*, **329**, 1993–2000.

Dalakas, M. C. (1994). High-dose intravenous immunoglobulin and serum viscosity: risk of precipitating thromboembolic events. *Neurology*, **44**, 223–6.

Dalakas, M. C. (1997). Intravenous immune globulin therapy for neurologic diseases. *Ann. Intern. Med.*, **126**, 721–30.

Debre, M., Bonnet, M. C., Fridman, W. H. *et al.* (1993). Infusion of Fcg fragments for treatment of children with acute immune thrombocytopenic purpura. *Lancet*, **342**, 945–9.

Deo, Y. M., Graziano, R. F., Repp, R. *et al.* (1997). Clinical significance of Fc receptors and FcgammaR-directed immunotherapies. *Immunol. Today*, **18**, 127–34.

Dietrich, G., Kaveri, S. V. and Kazatchkine, M. D. (1992). Modulation of autoimmunity by intravenous immune globulin through interaction with the function of the immune/idiotypic network. *Clin. Immunol. Immunopathol.*, **62**, S73–S81.

Drews, J. (1986). *Immunpharmakologie*. Springer Verlag.

Dwyer, J. M. (1992). Manipulating the immune system with immune globulin. *N. Engl. J. Med.*, **326**, 107–16.

Fazekas, F., Deisenhammer, F., Strasser-Fuchs, S. *et al.*, for the Austrian Immunoglobulin in Multiple Sclerosis Study Group (1997a). Randomised placebo-controlled trial of monthly intravenous immunoglobulin therapy in relapsing–remitting multiple sclerosis. *Lancet*, **349**, 589–93.

Fazekas, F., Deisenhammer, F., Strasser-Fuchs, S. *et al.*, for the Austrian Immunoglobulin in Multiple Sclerosis Study Group (1997b). Treatment effects of monthly intravenous immunoglobulin on patients with relapsing–remitting multiple sclerosis: Further analysis of the Austrian Immunoglobulin in MS Study. *Multiple Sclerosis*, **3**, 137–42.

Fazekas, F., Strasser-Fuchs, S. and Soelberg-Sørensen, P. (1999). Intravenous immunoglobulin trials in multiple sclerosis. *Intern. MS J.*, **6**, 14–21.

Francis, G. (1999). Intravenous immunoglobulin treatment in multiple sclerosis. *Neurology*, **52**, 214.

Grosse-Wilde, H., Blasczyk, R. and Westhoff, U. (1992). Soluble HLA class I and class II concentrations in commercial immunoglobulin preparations. *Tissue Antigens*, **39**, 74–7.

Hamamoto, Y., Harada, S., Yamamoto, N. *et al.* (1987). Elimination of viruses (human immunodeficiency, hepatitis B, vesicular stomatitis and Sindbis viruses) from an intravenous immunoglobulin preparation. *Vox Sang.*, **53**, 65–9.

Hartung, H. P., Toyka, K. V. and Griffin, J. W. (1998). Guillain-Barré syndrome and chronic inflammatory demyelinating polyneuropathy. In: *Clinical Neuroimmunology* (J. Antel, G. Birnbaum and H. P. Hartung, eds), pp. 294–306. Blackwell Science.

Healey, C. J., Sabharwal, N. K., Daub, J. *et al.* (1996). Outbreak of acute hepatitis C following the use of anti-hepatitis C virus – screened intravenous immunoglobulin therapy. *Gastroenterology*, **110**, 1120–26.

IFNB Multiple Sclerosis Study Group (1993). Interferon beta-1b is effective in relapsing–remitting multiple sclerosis: clinical results of a multicenter, randomized, double-blind, placebo-controlled trial. *Neurology*, **43**, 655–61.

IFNB Multiple Sclerosis Study Group and the University of British Columbia MS/MRI Analysis Group (1995). Interferon beta-1b in the treatment of multiple sclerosis: final outcome of the randomized controlled trial. *Neurology*, **45**, 1277–85.

Imbach, P., Barandun, S., d'Apuzzo, V. *et al.* (1981). High dose intravenous gammaglobulin for idiopathic thrombocytopenic purpura. *Lancet*, **I**, 1228–31.

Imbach, P., Perret, B. A., Babington, R. *et al.* (1991). Safety of intravenous immunoglobulin preparations: a prospective multicenter study to exclude the risk of non-A, non-B hepatitis. *Vox Sang.*, **61**, 240–43.

Jacobs, D. L., Cookfair, D. L., Rudick, R. A. *et al.* (1996). Intramuscular interferon beta-1a for disease progression in relapsing multiple sclerosis. The Multiple Sclerosis Collaborative Research Group (MSCRG). *Ann. Neurol.*, **39**, 6–16.

Johnson, K. P., Brooks, B. R., Cohen, J. A. *et al.* (1995). Copolymer 1 reduces relapse rate and improves disability in relapsing–remitting multiple sclerosis: results of a phase III multicenter, double-blind, placebo-controlled trial. *Neurology*, **45**, 1268–76.

Johnson, K. P., Brooks, B. R., Cohen, J. A. *et al.* (1998). Extended use of glatiramer acetate (Copaxone) is well tolerated and maintains its clinical effect on multiple sclerosis relapse rate and degree of disability. Copolymer 1 Multiple Sclerosis Study Group. *Neurology*, **50**, 701–8.

Kaveri, S., Vassilev, T., Hurez, V. *et al.* (1996). Antibodies to a conserved region of HLA class molecules, capable of modulating CD8 T-cell-mediated function, are present in pooled normal immunoglobulin for therapeutic use. *J. Clin. Invest.*, **97**, 865–9.

Kekow, J., Reinhold, D., Pap, T. *et al.* (1998). Intravenous immunoglobulins and transforming growth factor b. *Lancet*, **351**, 184–5.

Kempf, C., Jentsch, P., Barre-Sinoussi, F. B. *et al.* (1991). Inactivation of human immunodeficiency virus (HIV) by low pH and pepsin (letter). *J. Acq. Immune Def. Syndr.*, **4**, 828–30.

Kimberly, R. P., Salmon, J. E., Bussel, J. B. *et al.* (1984). Modulation of mononuclear phagocyte function by intravenous g-globulin. *J. Immunol.*, **132**, 745–50.

Klaesson, S., Tammik, L., Markling, L. *et al.* (1996). Inhibition of immunoglobulin production *in vitro* by IgG and F(ab')$_2$ fragments, but not by the Fc portion. *Scand. J. Immunol.*, **43**, 574–82.

Klein, J. and Horejsi, V. (1997). *Immunology*. Blackwell Science.

Kondo, N., Ozawa, T., Mushiake, K. *et al.* (1991). Suppression of immunoglobulin production of lymphocytes by intravenous immunoglobulin. *J. Clin. Immunol.*, **11**, 152–8.

Kondo, N., Kasahara, K., Kameyama, T. *et al.* (1994). Intravenous immunoglobulins suppress immunoglobulin productions by suppressing Ca(2+)-dependent signal transduction through Fc gamma receptors in B lymphocytes. *Scand. J. Immunol.*, **40**, 37–42.

Kurlander, R. J. and Hall, J. (1986). Comparison of intravenous gamma globulin and a monoclonal anti-Fc receptor antibody as inhibitors of immune clearance *in vivo* in mice. *J. Clin. Invest.*, **77**, 2010–18.

Lacroix-Desmazes, S., Kaveri, S. V., Mouthon, L. *et al.* (1998). Self-reactive antibodies (natural autoantibodies) in healthy individuals. *J. Immunol. Methods*, **216**, 117–37.

Lam, L., Whitsett, C. F., McNicholl, J. M. *et al.* (1993). Immunologically active proteins in intravenous immunoglobulin. *Lancet*, **342**, 678.

Leung, D. Y. M., Burns, J. C., Newburger, J. W. *et al.* (1987). Reversal of lymphocyte activation in Kawasaki syndrome by intravenous immunoglobulin. *J. Clin. Invest.*, **79**, 468–72.

Lisak, R. P. (1998). Intravenous immunoglobulins in multiple sclerosis. *Neurology*, **51(Suppl. 5)**, S25–S29.

Lutz, H. U., Stammler, P., Jelezarova, E. *et al.* (1996). High doses of immunoglobulin G attenuate immune aggregate-mediated complement activation by enhancing physiologic cleavage of C3b in C3bn-IgG complexes. *J. Immunol.*, **88**, 184–93.

Macey, M. G. and Newland, A. C. (1990). CD4 and CD8 subpopulation changes during high dose intravenous immunoglobulin treatment. *Br. J. Haematol.*, **76**, 513–20.

Marchalonis, J. J., Kaymaz, H., Dedeoglu, F. *et al.* (1992). Human autoantibodies reactive with synthetic autoantigens from T-cell receptor b chain. *Proc. Natl. Acad. Sci. USA*, **89**, 3325–9.

Miller, D. J., Sanborn, K. S., Katzmann, J. A. *et al.* (1994). Monoclonal autoantibodies promote central nervous system repair in an animal model of multiple sclerosis. *J. Neurosci.*, **14**, 6230–38.

Miller, D. J., Bright, J. J., Sriram, S. *et al.* (1997). Successful treatment of established relapsing experimental autoimmune encephalomyelitis in mice with a monoclonal natural autoantibody. *J. Neuroimmunol.*, **75**, 204–9.

Miyagi, F., Horiuchi, H., Nagata, I. *et al.* (1997). Fc portion of intravenous immunoglobulin suppresses the induction of experimental allergic neuritis. *J. Neuroimmunol.*, **78**, 127–31.

Noseworthy, J. H., Weinshenker, B. G., O'Brien, P. G. *et al.* (1997). Intravenous immunoglobulin does not reverse recently acquired, apparently permanent weakness in multiple sclerosis. *Ann. Neurol.*, **42**, 421.

Noseworthy, J. H., O'Brien, P. C., Petterson, T. M. *et al.* (1998). Immunoglobulin administration (IVIg) does not reverse visual acuity loss in long-standing optic neuritis associated with multiple sclerosis. *Neurology*, **A50** (suppl).

Paty, D. W., Li, D. K. B., the UBC MS/MRI Study Group and the IFNB Multiple Sclerosis Study Group (1993). Interferon beta-1b is effective in relapsing–remitting multiple sclerosis: MRI results of a multicenter, randomized, double-blind, placebo-controlled trial. *Neurology*, **43**, 662–7.

Pavelko, K. D., van Engelen, B. G. M. and Rodriguez, M. (1998). Acceleration in the rate of CNS remyelination in lysolecithin-induced demyelination. *J. Neurosci.*, **18**, 2498–2505.

Pozzilli, C., Bastianello, S., Koudriavtseva, T. *et al.* (1996). Magnetic resonance imaging changes with recombinant human interferon b-1a: a short-term study in relapsing-remitting multiple sclerosis. *J. Neurol. Neurosurg. Psychiatr.*, **61**, 251–8.

Prasad, N. K., Papoff, G., Zeuner, A. *et al.* (1998). Therapeutic preparations of normal polyspecific IgG (IVIg) induce apoptosis in human lymphocytes and monocytes: a novel mechanism of action of IVIg involving the Fas apoptotic pathway. *J. Immunol.*, **161**, 3781–90.

PRISMS (Prevention of Relapses and Disability by Interferon b-1a Subcutaneously in Multiple Sclerosis) Study Group (1998). Randomised double-blind placebo-controlled study of interferon b-1a in relapsing/remitting multiple sclerosis. *Lancet*, **352**, 1498–1504.

PSGBS (Plasma Exchange/Sandoglobulin Guillain-Barré Syndrome) Trial Group (1997). Randomised trial of plasma exchange, intravenous immunoglobulin, and combined treatment in Guillain-Barré syndrome. *Lancet*, **349**, 225–30.

Ratko, T. A., Burnett, D. A., Foulke, G. E. *et al.* (1995). Recommendations for off-label use of intravenously administered immunoglobulin preparations. University Hospital Consortium Expert Panel for Off-Label Use of Polyvalent Intravenously Administered Immunoglobulin Preparations. *J. Am. Med. Assoc.*, **273**, 1865–70.

Rodriguez, M. and Lennon, V. A. (1990). Immunoglobulins promote remyelination in the central nervous system. *Ann. Neurol.*, **27**, 12–17.

Rodriguez, M., Miller, D. J. and Lennon, V. A. (1996). Immunoglobulins reactive with myelin basic protein promote CNS remyelination. *Neurology*, **46**, 538–45.

Ross, C., Svenson, M., Hansen, M. B. *et al.* (1995). High avidity IFN-neutralizing antibodies in pharmaceutically prepared human IgG. *J. Clin. Invest.*, **95**, 1974–78.

Rothfelder, U., Neu, I. and Pelka, R. (1982). Therapie der multiplen Sklerose mit Immunglobulin G. *Med. Wochenschr.*, **124**, 74–8.

Roux, K. H. and Tankersley, D. L. (1990). A view of the human idiotypic repertoire. Electron microscopic and immunologic analyses of spontaneous idiotype–anti-idiotype dimers in pooled human IgG. *J. Immunol.*, **144**, 1387–95.

Ruiz de Souza, V., Carreno, M. P., Kaveri, S. V. *et al.* (1995). Selective induction of interleukin-1 receptor antagonist and interleukin-8 in human monocytes by normal polyspecific IgG (intravenous immunoglobulin). *Eur. J. Immunol.*, **25**, 1267–73.

Schiff, R. I. (1994). Transmission of viral infections through intravenous immune globulin. *N. Engl. J. Med.*, **331**, 1649–50.

Schuller, E. and Govaerts, A. (1983). First results of immunotherapy with immunoglobulin G in multiple sclerosis patients. *Eur. Neurol.*, **22**, 205–12.

Schussler, O., Genevaz, D., Latremouille, C. *et al.* (1998). Intravenous immunoglobulins for therapeutic use contain anti-idiotypes against xenophile antibodies and prolong discordant graft survival. *Clin. Immunol. Immunopathol.*, **86**, 183–91.

Schwartz, R. S. (1987). Overview of the biochemistry and safety of a new native intravenous gamma globulin, IGIV, ph 4.25. *Am. J. Med.*, **83(Suppl. 4A)**, 46–51.

Silvestris, F., D'Amore, O., Cafforio, P. *et al.* (1996). Intravenous immune globulin therapy of lupus nephritis: use of pathogenic anti-DNA-reactive IgG. *Clin. Exp. Immunol.*, **104(Suppl. 1)**, 91–7.

Sørensen, P. S. (1994). Treatment of multiple sclerosis with IVIg: potential effects and methodology of clinical trials. *J. Neurol. Neurosurg. Psychiatr.*, **57(Suppl.)**, 62–4.

Sørensen, P. S., Wanscher, B., Jensen, C. V. *et al* (1998). Intravenous immunoglobulin G reduces MRI activity in relapsing multiple sclerosis. *Neurology*, **50**, 1273–81.

Soukop, W. and Tschabitscher, H. (1986). Gamma globulin therapy in multiple sclerosis. Theoretical considerations and initial clinical experience with 7 S immunoglobulin in MS therapy. *Wien Med. Wochenschr.*, **136**, 477–80.

Stangel, M., Hartung, H. P., Marx, P. *et al.* (1997). Side effects of high-dose intravenous immunoglobulins. *Clin. Neuropharmacol.*, **20**, 385–93.

Stangel, M., Hartung, H. P., Marx, P. *et al.* (1998). Intravenous immunoglobulin treatment of neurological autoimmune diseases. *J. Neurol. Sci.*, **153**, 203–14.

Sultan, Y., Kazatchkine, M. D., Maisonneuve, P. *et al.* (1984). Anti-idiotypic suppression of autoantibodies to factor VIII (antihaemophilic factor) by high-dose intravenous gammaglobulin. *Lancet*, **2**, 765–8.

Svenson, M., Hansen, M. B. and Bendtzen, K. (1993). Binding of cytokines to pharmaceutically prepared human immunoglobulin. *J. Clin. Invest.*, **92**, 2533–9.

Takei, S., Arora, Y. K. and Walker, S. M. (1993). Intravenous immunoglobulin contains specific antibodies inhibitory to activation of T-cells by staphylococcal toxin superantigens (see comment). *J. Clin. Invest.*, **91**, 602–7.

Tan, E., Hajinazarian, M., Bay, W. *et al.* (1993). Acute renal failure resulting from intravenous immunoglobulin therapy. *Arch. Neurol.*, **50**, 137–9.

Thornton, C. A. and Ballow, M. (1993). Safety of intravenous immunoglobulin (editorial). *Arch. Neurol.*, **50**, 135–36.

Uemura, Y., Uriyu, K., Hirao, Y. *et al.* (1989). Inactivation and elimination of viruses during the fractionation of an intravenous immunoglobulin preparation: liquid heat treatment and polyethylene glycol fractionation. *Vox Sang.*, **56**, 155–61.

van der Meché, F. G. A. and van Doorn, P. A. (1997). The current place of high-dose immunoglobulins in the treatment of neuromuscular disorders. *Muscle Nerve*, **20**, 136–47.

van Doorn, P. A., Brand, A. and Vermeulen, M. (1988). Anti-neuroblastoma cell line antibodies in inflammatory demyelinating polyneuropathy: inhibition *in vitro* and *in vivo* by IV immunoglobulin. *Neurology*, **38**, 1592–5.

van Engelen, B., Hommes, O., Pinckers, A. *et al.* (1992). Improved vision after intravenous immunoglobulin in stable demyelinating optic neuritis. *Ann. Neurol.*, **32**, 835–6.

Vassilev, T., Gelin, C., Kaveri, S. V. *et al.* (1993). Antibodies to the CD5 molecule in normal human immunoglobulins for therapeutic use (intravenous immunoglobulins, IVIg). *Clin. Exp. Immunol.*, **92**, 369–72.

Voltz, R. and Hohlfeld, R. (1996). The use of intravenous immunoglobulins in the treatment of neuromuscular disorders. *Curr. Opin. Neurol.*, **9**, 360–66.

Voltz, R., Rosen, F. V., Yousry, T. *et al.* (1996). Reversible encephalopathy with cerebral vasospasm in a Guillain-Barré syndrome patient treated with intravenous immunoglobulin. *Neurology*, **46**, 250–51.

Whittam, L. R., Hay, R. J. and Hughes, R. A. C. (1997). Eczematous reactions to human immune globulin. *Br. J. Dermatol.*, **137**, 481–2.

Zavazava, N. and Krönke, M. (1996). Soluble HLA class I molecules induce apoptosis in alloreactive cytotoxic T-lymphocytes. *Nature Med.*, **2**, 1005–10.

7

Azathioprine

Introduction

Azathioprine is an immunosuppressive agent used in combination to prevent rejection during transplantation, and in a variety of immune-mediated diseases including rheumatoid arthritis, ulcerative colitis, myasthenia gravis and multiple sclerosis. It was first given to a 24-year-old man undergoing renal transplantation in 1962, and was initially marketed in Japan in 1965.

Mode of action

Pharmacology (Dollery Therapeutic Drugs, 1999)

Azathioprine, 6-(1-methyl-4-nitroimidanol-5-yl-thio)purine was originally developed as a pro-drug of the cytotoxic agent 6-mercaptopurine (6-MP). It is readily absorbed from the gut, and is rapidly broken down *in vivo* into 6-MP, to which many of its pharmacological effects are attributed. However, the methyl-nitro-imidazole moiety to which it is also cleaved plays an additional role in its biological activity. It is not surprising, therefore, that the determination of the plasma concentration of azathioprine has no prognostic value as regards effectiveness or toxicity (Elion and Hitchings, 1975).

Although it has many effects, the exact mechanism of its immunomodulatory effect is not known. Its action has three major components:

1. Attenuation of B-lymphocyte function, with reduction in IgM and IgG synthesis
2. Inhibition of the cellular component of the inflammatory response
3. Impairment of cell proliferation in general, producing a non-specific depression in the immune response.

In vitro tests suggest that, among lymphocytes, T-cells are the preferential targets (Bach, 1976). This has led to the general idea that azathioprine is mainly a drug for cell-mediated autoimmune diseases. However, extrapolating short-term *in vitro* effects to the long term *in vivo* situation may be misleading, particularly as azathioprine has such a delayed onset of action (see later). In fact, the efficacy of azathioprine in an antibody-mediated disorder such as myasthenia gravis and in some cases of dermatomyositis is also well recognized. The mechanism of action in such diseases may be via suppression of the T-helper B-cell system.

Pharmacokinetics *(Dollery Therapeutic Drugs, 1999)*

Although it is readily absorbed following oral administration, with only 12.6 per cent appearing in the stool over 48 hours, azathioprine can be difficult to detect in the plasma because it is so rapidly broken down. Peak concentration is achieved 1–2 hours after dosing, and the plasma half-life is about 4 hours. It is rapidly distributed throughout the body, although only small amounts enter the brain. Up to 50 per cent of the drug is excreted in urine over the first 24 hours, with only 10 per cent as the unchanged drug.

6-MP readily crosses cell membranes and is converted intracellularly into a number of purine thioanalogues, including the main active nucleotide, thioinosinic acid (Lovatt and Hennings, 1984). This incorporation into DNA may be relevant to its anti-proliferative mode of action. Its elimination via oxidation by xanthine oxidase is inhibited by allopurinol.

Therapeutic effect in multiple sclerosis (MS)

Azathioprine has been used in MS since the 1960s, although the degree of clinical benefit has been difficult to establish. A number of small trials were performed in the 1970s and 1980s, and the results of these were subsequently combined in a meta-analysis (Yudkin *et al.*, 1991). Recently developed clinical treatments have had to be assessed within carefully planned randomized double-blind controlled trials in order to satisfy the regulatory bodies and gain a product licence. The trials have been appropriately powered, have distinguished between relapsing–remitting, primary and secondary progressive multiple sclerosis, and have had narrow and clearly defined entry criteria. Additionally, the advent of MRI as a new surrogate marker has allowed the demonstration of dramatic treatment effects with some of the newer therapeutic agents. Such factors might contribute to the less convincing results of the azathioprine trials when compared to such newer drugs, and makes direct comparison with such products more difficult.

MRI

The effect of the newer agents on MRI change is often used as the primary outcome measure in phase II studies and as a secondary outcome measure in phase III studies. Such data may be influential in the decision-making processes of some of the drug licensing bodies, although MRI measures only correlate weakly with clinical outcome measures. The clinical studies on azathioprine were all performed before MRI was commonly available, and no such studies of aza-thioprine have been performed since; thus its effects on such measures as change in total lesion volume over time and new lesion accumulation rate are unknown.

Relapses

A great deal of importance has been placed on the ability of the newer agents to reduce relapses. Relapse rate has been the primary outcome measure in two (IFNB Multiple Sclerosis Study Group, 1993; PRISMS, 1998) of the three interferon-beta trials (IFNB Multiple Sclerosis Study Group, 1993; Jacobs *et al.*, 1996; PRISMS, 1998) and glatiramer acetate (copolymer 1) study (Johnson *et al.*, 1995, 1998) in relapsing–remitting patients. In contrast, the authors of the azathioprine meta-analysis felt the effect on relapses was not an important clinical outcome (Yudkin *et al.*, 1991*)*. Although most people recognize that long-term disability is the major cause of morbidity in multiple sclerosis, this does not necessarily mean that reducing relapses is not useful.

QALYs and EUROQOLs are measures of quality of life that have been criticized for their usefulness when trying to compare values across different diseases. However, these measures were used in quoting poor cost-effectiveness figures for the newer expensive agents (Development and Evaluation Committee Report, 1997). The quality of life lost in an average relapse is calculated using estimates of the length of time in relapse and the QOL reduction during an attack.

The length of an average relapse has been assumed in some calculations to be 1 month (Paul McNamee and David Parkin, personal communication). However, in the Interferon beta-1a (Rebif®) trial, average relapse length was 47 days (Ares-Serono International SA, Geneva, personal communication). Additionally, a further underestimate of the total QALYs lost in an isolated exacerbation arises from the assumption that there is complete recovery from relapses.

The average decrease in quality of life during an exacerbation has been reported to be 0.5 EUROQOL (Paul McNamee and David Parkin, personal communication) or 0.073–1.03 QOL (Development and Evaluation Committee Report, 1997). One study of stroke patients with residua (Gage *et al.*, 1995) reported a QALY value of 0.75 in patients with mild stroke, and 0.39 in those with moderate to severe strokes. Thus an average MS relapse may produce a reduction in quality of life approximately equal to that of a moderate stroke. Rosser's original matrix (Hopkins, 1992) would suggest that to be disabled to a level of 'work severely limited', 'unable to work' or 'confined to chair', i.e. physical disability greater than that seen in an average MS exacerbation, should only give QALYs of 0.942–0.680 when moderately distressed.

This is surprising, and suggests that factors other than physical disability influence QALYs in MS patients. This suggestion is supported by a study (Rothwell *et al.*, 1997) that showed that the perception of the loss of quality of life that occurs with MS differs between doctors and patients. The authors reported that patients' quality of life assessments are influenced by vitality, general health and mental health scores far more than by physical disability, whilst doctors give the latter most attention and importance. Thus the medical profession is at risk of underestimating the loss of quality of life and distress in MS patients, not only during relapses but generally.

Odds ratio of remaining relapse free

The azathioprine meta-analysis (Yudkin *et al.*, 1991) showed that the chance of remaining relapse free over a 2-year period was significantly reduced. These results are summarized along with those of other treatments in Table 7.1.

Table 7.1 Odds ratio of remaining relapse free

	Odds ratio relapse free	95% CI	Reference
Azathioprine[a]	2.04	1.42–2.93	Yudkin *et al.*, 1991
Interferon β-1b[b]	2.38	1.25–4.25	IFNB Multiple Sclerosis Study Group, 1993
Interferon β-1a (Avonex®)[b]	1.68	0.88–3.16	Jacobs *et al.*, 1996
Interferon β-1a (Rebif®)[b]	2.80	1.68–4.67	PRISMS, 1998
Glatiramer acetate[b]	1.37	0.82–2.34	Johnson *et al.*, 1995
IVIg[b]	2.07	1.07–4.00	Fazekas *et al.*, 1997

[a]included patients with relapsing–remitting and progressive MS
[b]included patients with relapsing–remitting MS
CI, confidence interval.

Relapse rate

Four of the five azathioprine trials used in the meta-analysis showed a reduction in the relapse rate. The results from the largest trial (British and Dutch Multiple Sclerosis Azathioprine Trial Group, 1988) only achieved statistical significance by year four in a group of patients that included some with progressive disease. Two of the three smaller studies were able to identify a statistically significant effect (Ellison *et al.*, 1989; Goodkin *et al.*, 1991). This effect was seen early on in treatment, and despite only progressive (primary and secondary) patients being enrolled in one study (Ellison *et al.*, 1989). One small study (Milanese *et al.*, 1998) included only 13 relapsing–remitting and 10 progressive patients and reported a higher baseline relapse rate in the azathioprine group, which reduced on treatment, whereas the placebo group had a lower baseline rate that increased on treatment to a similar level to the azathioprine group. None of these differences were significant. These results are compared with the effect of other therapeutic agents on relapse rate in Table 7.2.

Two of the azathioprine studies (British and Dutch Multiple Sclerosis Azathioprine Trial Group, 1988; Goodkin *et al.*, 1991) suggested that the effect of azathioprine on relapses is delayed (see Table 7.3). Another demonstrated a greater reduction in relapse rate during year three than in the first 2 years, although the exact rates and statistical analysis for individual years were not given (Ellison *et al.*, 1989). One small study in which there was a non-statistical reduction in relapse rate found a similar effect in years one and two (Swinburn and Liversedge, 1973).

Table 7.2 Effects of therapeutic agents on relapse rate

	% reduction of relapse rate	P value	Study length	Type MS	Reference
Azathioprine[a]	−45	0.08	2 years	RR	Goodkin et al., 1991
Azathioprine	−27	0.025	4 years	RR and P	British and Dutch Multiple Sclerosis Azathioprine Trial Group, 1988
Azathioprine	−50	0.02	3 years	P	Ellison et al., 1989
Azathioprine	[b]Aza 0.92–0.79 Plac 0.6–0.67	ns	3 years	RR and P	Milanese et al., 1988
Azathioprine[c]	−49	ns	2 years	RR	Swinburn and Liversedge, 1973
Interferon β-1b	−34	0.0001	2 years	RR	IFNB Multiple Sclerosis Study Group, 1993
Interferon β-1b	−31	0.0002	2 years	2ry P	European Study Group on Interferon β-1b in Secondary Progressive MS, 1998
Interferon β-1a (Avonex®)	−18[d] −32[e]	0.04 0.002	2 years	RR	Jacobs et al., 1996
Interferon β-1a (Rebif®)	−32	<0.0001	2 years	RR	PRISMS, 1998
Glatiramer acetate	−29[f]	0.007	2 years	RR	Johnson et al., 1995
IVIg	−59	0.0037	2 years	RR	Fazekas et al., 1997
Cyclosporin[g]	−50	0.07	2 years	RR and P	Rudge et al., 1989

[a]year 1, $P = 0.16$; year 2, $P = 0.05$
[b]pre- and post-treatment relapse rate
[c]$n = 19$ azathioprine, $n = 24$ placebo, not intention to treat analysis
[d]if all patient data included
[e]if only data from patients completing 2 years are included
[f]covariate adjusted mean
[g]data from one of two centres (not significant overall).
IVIg, intravenous immunoglobulin therapy; ns, not significant; RR, relapsing–remitting MS, P, progressive (primary and secondary) MS; 2ry P, secondary progressive.

Table 7.3 Percentage reduction in relapse rate

Year 1	Year 2	Year 3	Year 4	Overall	Reference
13 (ns)	19 (ns)	7 (ns)	42 ($P = 0.025$)	27 ($P = 0.025$)	British and Dutch Trial Group, 1988
37 (ns)	62 ($P = 0.05$)			45 ($P = 0.08$)	Goodkin et al., 1991

ns, not significant.

It therefore seems clear that azathioprine does reduce MS relapses, and probably to a similar degree to that seen with the newer therapeutic agents such as interferon beta and glatiramer acetate. The cost of a drug becomes more important if the clinical benefit is only partial and temporary, and thus because azathioprine is so much cheaper it compares favourably when prescribed for its effect on relapses.

Effect on disability

In MS, the effect of treatment on disability is considered more important than the effect on relapse rate. The newer agents are also showing efficacy in this area. Disability at a moment in time (often referred to as unconfirmed disability) can be due to reversible change and/or permanent disability. Temporary disability, as seen during relapses, can also be recorded because of the biological fluctuations (hourly and daily) seen in MS, and falsely charted due to inter- and intra-observer variations in the EDSS score. These latter problems are largely overcome by assuming that only changes of 1 point or more on the EDSS score are relevant, and by excluding changes during fever. Permanent disability is due to incomplete recovery from relapses or progression during the chronic phase of the disease. Reducing permanent disability is recognized by doctors, patients, and hence the pharmaceutical industry, as the ideal aim of MS treatments. The measurement of permanent disability has usually been defined as a sustained change in the EDSS scores on two occasions separated by 3 months. This obviously excludes those relapses that take longer than this to recover, and which may represent up to 24 per cent of all exacerbations (Lui et al., 1998).

Survival analysis of the probability of progressing on the EDSS scale

Sustained disability is the 'gold standard' measure of efficacy in MS drug trials, and this is usually analysed as the probability of progressing by 1 EDSS disability score (stable usually over 3 months). The only azathioprine trial that used survival analysis (Goodkin et al., 1991) reported a significant effect ($P = 0.04$) with azathioprine in patients with relapsing–remitting MS (using a definition of sustained disability at 2 months and a worsening of 0.5 EDSS score when disability was ≥ 5.5 as an endpoint). The Ambulation Index was also statistically significantly affected when analysed in this way ($P = 0.03$). This study found a non-significant reduction in the proportion of relapsing–remitting MS patients who progressed at 2 years. However, this type of analysis has not been reported in the majority of recent trials. These results, together with those from other therapeutic trials in relapsing–remitting MS patients, are summarized in Table 7.4.

Table 7.4 Proportion of patients progressing at 2 years

	Time to progression ($P=$)	Percentage progressed at 2 years[a] ($P=$)	Reference
Azathioprine[b,c]	0.04	ns	Goodkin et al., 1991
Interferon-β 1b[d,e]	ns	ns	IFNB Multiple Sclerosis Study Group, 1993, 1995
Interferon-β 1a[e,f] (Avonex®)	0.02[g] 0.058[h]		Jacobs et al., 1996
Interferon-β 1a[d,e] (Rebif®)	0.040[i] 0.014[j]		PRISMS, 1998
Glatiramer acetate[d,e]		ns	Johnson et al., 1995

[a]not reported in all studies
[b]disability confirmed at 2 months
[c]outcome: EDSS change of 1.0 scores < 5.5, 0.5 at EDSS scores ≥ 5.5
[d]disability confirmed at 3 months
[e]outcome: EDSS change 1.0 for all EDSS scores
[f]disability confirmed at 6 months
[g]all patients analysed
[h]only subgroup of patients completing at least 2 years analysed
[i]22 mcg
[j]44 mcg
ns, not significant.

Mean change in EDSS score

Meta-analysis of the azathioprine trials (Yudkin et al., 1991) revealed a small but just significant effect of azathioprine on the mean change in unconfirmed disability compared to placebo at 2 years (–0.22 EDSS), which lost significance at 3 years. The Rebif® trial (PRISMS, 1998) reported a very similar result, with a just significant effect on the 2-year mean unconfirmed EDSS change, and this measure was also significantly reduced with Glatiramer acetate (Johnson et al., 1995, 1998) and IVIg (Fazekas et al., 1997). The difference in mean EDSS change with Avonex® (Jacobs et al., 1996) in relapsing–remitting patients was significant for unconfirmed and sustained disability (the latter used data from the cohort that completed 130 weeks). In secondary progressive patients, interferon beta-1b produced a significant reduction of unconfirmed mean EDSS change at 2 years of –0.13 EDSS (European Study Group on Interferon beta-1b in Secondary

Progressive MS, 1998) compared to placebo. These results are summarized in Table 7.5. The azathioprine was the only analysis that included patients with all types of MS. There was no significant difference between the azathioprine (Yudkin *et al.*, 1991) and the Avonex® (Jacobs *et al.*, 1996) results when comparing the unconfirmed disability data (Peter Rothwell, personal communication).

Table 7.5 Mean EDSS change compared to placebo

	Mean EDSS change	Type of MS	Reference
Azathioprine	−0.22[a]	RR and P	Yudkin *et al.*, 1991
Interferon β-1b	ns	RR	IFNB Multiple Sclerosis Study Group, 1993
Interferon β-1b	−0.13[b]	2ry P	European Study Group on Interferon β-1b in Secondary Progressive MS, 1998
Interferon β-1a (Avonex®)	−0.49[b,c] −0.59[d]	RR	Jacobs *et al.*, 1996
Interferon β-1a (Rebif®)	−0.25[b]	RR	PRISMS, 1998
Glatiramer acetate	−0.26[b]	RR	Johnson *et al.*, 1995
IVIg	−0.34[b]	RR	Fazekas *et al.*, 1997

[a]mixture of unconfirmed and confirmed/non-relapse disability used in meta-analysis
[b]unconfirmed disability
[c]subgroup completed 104 weeks
[d]sustained disability
ns, not significant; RR, relapsing–remitting; P, progressive (primary and secondary); 2ry P, secondary progressive.

The available data on azathioprine suggest that there may be a positive effect on slowing disability. Lack of sensitivity to an azathioprine effect in the trials performed may be due to a number of factors, such as mixing different types of MS and using less strictly designed protocols. The delayed onset of action of azathioprine is also an important factor. One trial suggested a better effect when corticosteroids (which act more quickly) were added (Ellison *et al.*, 1989). Another showed that the effect on reducing the progression rate increased with time (Milanese *et al.*, 1988). It is not clear at present how such short-term benefits translate into a longer-term reduction in disability, because of the slow natural history of MS and the short-term nature of clinical trials.

Side effects

Although the results of the azathioprine trial (Yudkin *et al.*, 1991) are less robust than those of the newer therapeutic agents, the long-term experience of azathioprine enables the doctor and patient to make a better assessment of the side effect profile. Such knowledge is important when assessing the relative benefits of the treatment against risks in individual patients. Concerns about the long-term risk of cancer may be less for patients with a poor prognosis due to very aggressive MS, and greater for those with a strong family history of cancer or a good long-term prognosis due to mild MS.

Most complications are more likely to occur at higher doses (3–5 mg/kg), especially with renal insufficiency (Penn, 1971). Most side effects can be reversed by stopping the drug (Harris *et al.*, 1971).

Haematological and hepatic *(McGrath et al., 1975)*

Azathioprine is associated with an increase in mean corpuscular volume with normal B_{12} and folate levels. This seems to be a dose-related phenomenon. Significant anaemia is rare. Azathioprine commonly reduces the lymphocyte count, but this is rarely of clinical concern. Neutropenia is rarer, but is an indication for dose reduction or drug withdrawal. Haematological abnormalities (excluding macrocytosis) were found in 18 per cent of myasthenia gravis (MG) patients in one study (Hohlfeld *et al.*, 1988), and either reversed spontaneously or reversed with reduction or temporary cessation of the drug. Such side effects were dose-dependent. Abnormal liver function tests were reported in 6 per cent of cases, and all resolved spontaneously without drug dose alteration. The authors' experience is of a lower incidence of haematological side effects. The incidence of azathioprine-induced haematological or hepatic abnormalities sufficient to necessitate permanent drug withdrawal was found to be 0–5.5 per cent and 0–3 per cent, respectively, in the azathioprine MS trials (Swinburn and Liversedge, 1973; British and Dutch Multiple Sclerosis Azathioprine Trial Group, 1988; Milanese *et al.*, 1988; Ellison *et al.*, 1989; Goodkin *et al.*, 1991).

Infections

When azathioprine is used for indications other than for organ transplantation, infections have not generally been reported to be frequent or severe (Lovatt and Hennings, 1984). Patients on doses of 2 mg/kg or more might be at greater risk (Hohlfeld *et al.*, 1988), although coincidental treatment with corticosteroid treatment in this study may have contributed. No significant increase was seen in MS patients treated with azathioprine compared to placebo (Swinburn and Liversedge, 1973; British and Dutch Multiple Sclerosis Azathioprine Trial Group, 1988; Milanese *et al.*, 1988; Ellison *et al.*, 1989; Goodkin *et al.*, 1991).

Gastrointestinal (GI) disturbance

GI disturbance tends to occur during initiation of azathioprine, and usually results in permanent withdrawal of the drug. It was reported in 13 per cent of MG patients (Hohlfeld *et al.*, 1988), some of whom were also treated with corticosteroids. In the MS trials, a frequency of 0–21 per cent was reported (Swinburn and Liversedge, 1973; British and Dutch Multiple Sclerosis Azathioprine Trial Group, 1988; Milanese *et al.*, 1988; Ellison *et al.*, 1989; Goodkin *et al.*, 1991); the higher incidence was seen in a study that initiated treatment at the full dose of 2.5 mg/kg taken as a single daily dose (Swinburn and Liversedge, 1973). These authors advised patients who developed such side effects to divide the dose or take it nocté to relieve such symptoms. Discontinuation of the drug due to such side effects is less likely if started at doses of 25–50 mg per day (Vallalba and Adams, 1996); therefore, azathioprine should be initiated in a graded fashion.

Allergic skin reactions

These are rare, and were seen in none of the 104 patients with myasthenia gravis (Hohlfeld *et al.*, 1988). Rashes or fever leading to withdrawal of azathioprine were reported in 0–3 per cent of patients in four studies of MS patients (Swinburn and Liversedge, 1973; British and Dutch Multiple Sclerosis Azathioprine Trial Group, 1988; Milanese *et al.*, 1988; Ellison *et al.*, 1989). One study, which set the highest target dose (3 mg/kg), had a higher incidence of 17 per cent (Goodkin *et al.*, 1991). However, this maintenance dose was reached over months and allergic reactions generally occur early on, although the timing of such problems was not stated in this study. Interestingly, the number of patients discontinuing treatment was similar in the azathioprine and the placebo groups.

Pregnancy

Teratogenicity has been seen in a number of animal species (*Dollery Therapeutic Drugs, 1999*), and azathioprine and its metabolites have been found in low concentrations in amniotic fluid and foetal blood (Saarikoski and Seppala, 1976). However, epidemiological evidence indicates that the frequency of congenital abnormalities is similar in the offspring of maternal transplant patients to that of the general population (Lovatt and Hennings, 1984). A recent report of azathioprine in inflammatory bowel disease confirmed that there is no increase in the malformation rate of foetuses, the rate of abortion or of prematurity, even when used in early pregnancy at therapeutic doses (Alstead *et al.*, 1990).

Cancer risk

The evidence suggesting an increased risk of cancer with azathioprine treatment is inconclusive. Initial reports of an increased risk of malignancy were in transplant patients who were additionally immunosuppressed because of their underlying disease process as well as multiple drug therapy. Additionally, immunologically-mediated diseases may have an increased risk of cancer. A 10-fold background risk has been reported in rheumatoid arthritis (Silman *et al.*, 1988), and a relative risk of 1.29 was seen in MS (Moller *et al.*, 1991) although this latter excess was mainly in cancers most likely to be detected by increased medical surveillance. Conflicting reports exist as to whether azathioprine or other cytotoxic treatments further increase the background risk (Kirsner *et al.*, 1982;

Kinlen, 1985; Silman et al., 1988; Matteson et al., 1991; Hazleman, 1982) in rheumatoid arthritis. In MS, concern was raised when 10 out of 131 patients developed epitheliomas (Lhermitte et al., 1984) when treated with azathioprine for a mean duration of 73 months. However, none of the randomized studies have found a statistically significant increase in malignancy in MS patients on azathioprine (Swinburn and Liversedge, 1973; British and Dutch Multiple Sclerosis Azathioprine Trial Group, 1988; Milanese et al., 1988; Ellison et al., 1989; Goodkin et al., 1991), although only small numbers of patients were included in some of them. The reported increased risk of non-Hodgkin's lymphoma seen in association with immunosuppression is thought to be due to an increased expression of viral associated tumours. This sort of malignancy has not been reported in excess in MS patients, even those on immunosuppressive treatment. A case control study (Confavreux et al., 1996) that included 23 MS cancer patients suggested that the relative risk of developing cancer with azathioprine treatments was 1.3 with less than 5 years use, 2.0 with 5–10 years use, and 4.4 with more than 10 years use. These results were not significant, but analysis of linear trend was.

A similar pattern was seen when analysing for cumulative dose. In addition, a statistically significant relative risk of 6.7 at doses greater than 600 g was found. The types of cancer were those commonly found in the general population, and non-Hodgkin's lymphoma was not increased. The only case (out of a total of 23) that developed non-Hodgkin's lymphoma was a patient who had not received azathioprine. The major flaw of case-control studies is that the patients are not randomized to treatment. It is possible that those patients with more aberrant immune systems are at greater risk of developing malignancies, and also at greater risk of having aggressive MS. This group of patients would be more likely to receive treatments such as azathioprine, and thus the increased cancer risk reported could be related to the underlying immune defect rather than the treatment itself. Against this is the dose and time response seen (Confavreux et al., 1996), which favours a causal effect of azathioprine. Overall, it is likely that any increased risk is low and related to long-term treatment.

Azathioprine regimen

Dosage

The variability of MS makes it difficult to monitor the effectiveness of treatment in individual patients. Various azathioprine regimens have been used in studies, with maintenance doses of between 2.0–3.0 mg/kg (Swinburn and Liversedge, 1973; British and Dutch Multiple Sclerosis Azathioprine Trial Group, 1988; Milanese et al., 1988; Ellison et al., 1989; Goodkin et al., 1991). These trials generally had a high incidence of azathioprine side effects, and drug withdrawals were often related to early GI upset or rashes. It should be noted that most studies did not have a slow initiation regimen, and one that did (Goodkin et al., 1991) started on 150 mg daily with subsequent increases. Only one study (Goodkin et al., 1991) had a regimen for altering the azathioprine dose if the blood count or liver function tests became abnormal. Such adjustments can usually allow the drug to be continued, since these abnormalities are not usually associated with symptoms. Although side effects were greater in those on azathioprine than on placebo, there was no difference in the number of patients discontinuing treatment between the groups in the three large trials (British and Dutch Multiple Sclerosis Azathioprine Trial Group, 1988; Ellison *et al.*, 1989; Goodkin *et al.*, 1991).

It would be logical to use a regimen that works in other more easily monitored diseases, such as myasthenia gravis (Palace *et al.*, 1998). A slow initiation regimen, such as starting with 25 mg and increasing by 25 mg daily, or increasing by 50 mg daily per week, may reduce early GI upset. The optimal dose is probably around 2.5 mg/kg per day, and should be taken in divided doses. The onset of action is delayed in myasthenia gravis by 12–21 months (Palace *et al.*, 1998), and by more than 6 months in inflammatory myopathies (Bunch, 1981). It is common practice to allow only 3 months for azathioprine to start working in rheumatoid disease, and up to 6–7 months for the full effect (Swinson and Swinburn, 1980; Butler, 1990). Whether azathioprine has a similar time of onset of action and a similar dose response across all immunologically mediated diseases is not known. Randomized studies of azathioprine in myositis have not distinguished between polymyositis (cell-mediated) and dermatomyositis (antibody-mediated) (Bunch, 1981). Because of the delay in onset of action and the suggestion that the addition of corticosteroids to azathioprine may improve efficacy (Ellison *et al.*, 1989), it may be useful to cover with prednisolone early on. It has also been reported that the macrocytosis, which often results from azathioprine treatment, is a prognostic marker for a beneficial treatment effect in myasthenia gravis (Witte *et al.*, 1986), and it was suggested that a lack of a macrocytosis associated with a poor therapeutic response may indicate under-dosage. However, this observation was not supported in a trial of MS patients (British and Dutch Multiple Sclerosis Azathioprine Trial Group, 1988). Despite the controversy, it seems reasonable to consider an increase in azathioprine dose to 3 mg/kg in those MS patients without a macrocytosis who continue to deteriorate rapidly despite azathioprine treatment for at least 18 months. After 2–3 years of treatment on full dosage, if it is felt that the MS is responding and there are plans to continue treatment indefinitely the azathioprine can be slowly reduced to a lower maintenance dose. However, judging the individual response to such treatment is not easy because of the partial therapeutic effect and the biological variability of MS.

Monitoring blood tests

Most abnormalities arise early in the course of the treatment. Blood should initially be taken weekly for full blood count (to include differential white cell count) and liver function tests until the maintenance dose has been reached for 8 weeks. After this, the blood can be checked 3-monthly.

Progressive anaemia, total WBC $< 3.0 \times 10^9/l$, neutrophil count $< 1.5 \times 10^9/l$, platelets $< 100 \times 10^9/l$ and progressive liver function abnormalities can be managed by stopping the azathioprine until blood tests return to normal and restarting with a dose 50 mg lower than previously. A repeat abnormality on the reduced dose (an infrequent occurrence) is an indication to withdraw azathioprine permanently.

Which patients should receive treatment

At present the evidence for the effectiveness of azathioprine is weak, although it may be as good as the newer treatments. Because of the side effect profile, it is usually reserved for patients with moderately aggressive disease. Subgroup analysis of one study (British and Dutch Multiple Sclerosis Azathioprine Trial Group, 1988) suggested a greater effect in women and those aged over 40 years, although statistical significance is lost if the Bonferroni correction is made. In patients with frequent significant relapses or rapid progression for whom the newer therapeutic agents cannot be prescribed (for example due to inadequate funding, contraindications or needle phobia), azathioprine is a reasonable alternative. The treatment effect has also been seen in studies that have included primary progressive patients, and thus treatment in this group can be considered against the individuals' background cancer risk (in view of the older age of onset in many such patients). Because of the delayed onset of action, any attempt to assess whether azathioprine is effective in an individual patient should be delayed until the second year of therapy. Any increase in the risk of developing cancer is likely to be well after this time, i.e. at least 5 years later (Confavreux et al., 1996).

Combination therapy

Azathioprine, interferon beta and Glatiramer acetate all partially reduce the relapse rate. However, their mechanisms of action probably differ. Combinations of azathioprine with the newer agents might increase the efficacy and reduce the side effect profiles of the individual drugs by reducing the doses used. Additionally, it has been suggested that the addition of azathioprine to interferon beta might suppress the development of anti-interferon beta antibodies (Kappos, 1996). There is no theoretical reason to predict adverse interactions between these drugs, and indeed combinations of azathioprine and interferon beta are being used in clinical practice and have been reported in small studies (Kappos, 1996; Moreau et al., 1997). However, leucopenia necessitated reduction or discontinuation of azathioprine in two out of six patients in one of these studies (Kappos, 1996). Combinations with the more established agents such as cyclosporin (Gold, 1990) and alternating regimens with chloramphenicol have also been used (Chofflon et al., 1992). Combination treatments with azathioprine generally appear to be well tolerated. A study to compare azathioprine with interferon beta (EZAZIMUS) was proposed by EDMUS (Witte et al., 1986); however, combination therapy using both these agents versus interferon beta alone is now felt to be a more feasible study (C. Confavreux, personal communication). This is partly because of the ethical and compliance issues raised in withholding interferon beta treatment from appropriate patients, but also because only an add-on trial will attract funding from the pharmaceutical industry.

Future trials

Many new MS treatments will appear within the next decade, and they are all likely to be expensive because of the large costs involved in the pre-marketing stage of drug development. It would seem logical, therefore, to have more data on the effectiveness of the established drugs and how they directly compare with the newer treatments, and some factors for consideration appear below.

Advantages of Azathioprine	Disadvantages of Azathioprine
Cheap	Side effect profile, especially allergic reactions such as rashes and GI disturbance
Reduces relapses, probable equal effect to newer agents	Possible increase risk of cancer with long-term treatment
Probable effect on reducing disability	Delay in onset of action
Long-term experience available allows better assessment of rarer long-term side effects	Lack of data from equivalently well designed clinical trials with MRI data, when compared to newer agents

References

Alstead, E. M., Ritchie, J. K., Lennard-Jones, J. E. *et al.* (1990). Safety of azathioprine in pregnancy in inflammatory bowel disease. *Gastroenterology*, **99**, 443–6.

Bach, J. F. (1976). The pharmacological and immunological basis for the use of immunosuppressive drugs. *Drugs*, **11**, 1–13.

British and Dutch Multiple Sclerosis Azathioprine Trial Group (1988). Double-masked trial of Azathioprine Trial Group. *Lancet*, **ii**, 179–83.

Bunch, T. W. (1981). Prednisone and azathioprine for polymyositis: long-term follow-up. *Arthr. Rheum.*, **24(1)**, 45–8.

Butler, R. (1990). Monitoring drug therapy in rheumatoid arthritis: efficacy. *A.R.C.* **July, No. 15**.

Chofflon, M., Juillard, C., Juillard, P. *et al.* (1992). Tumor necrosis factor a production as a possible predictor of relapse in patients with multiple sclerosis. *Eur. Cytokine Net.*, **3(6)**, 523–31.

Confavreux, C., Saddier, P., Grimaud, J. *et al.* (1996). Risk of cancer from azathioprine therapy in multiple sclerosis: a case-control study. *Neurology*, **46**, 1607–12.

Development and Evaluation Committee (1997). *Interferon Beta-1a in*

Relapsing–Remitting Multiple Sclerosis. Report No 77, The Wessex Institute for Health Research and Development.

Dollery Therapeutic Drugs (1999). *Azathioprine*. Colin Dollery, Ed. Churchill Livingstone, pp. A181–5.

Elion, G. B. and Hitchings, G. H. (1975). *Handbook of Experimental Pharmacology*, Vol. 38. Springer-Verlag.

Ellison, G. W., Myers, L. W., Mickey, M. R. *et al.* (1989). A placebo-controlled, randomised, double-masked, variable dosage, clinical trial of azathioprine with and without methylprednisolone in multiple sclerosis. *Neurology*, **39**, 1018–26.

European Study Group on Interferon β-1b in Secondary Progressive MS (1998). Placebo-controlled multicentre randomised trial of interferon b-1b in treatment of secondary progressive multiple sclerosis. *Lancet*, **352**, 1491–7.

Fazekas, F., Deisenhammer, F., Strasser-Fuchs, S. *et al.* for the Austrian Immunoglobulin in Multiple Sclerosis Study Group (1997). Randomised placebo-controlled trial of monthly intravenous immunoglobulin therapy in relapsing–remitting multiple sclerosis. *Lancet*, **349**, 589–93.

Gage, B. F., Cardinalli, A. B., Albers, G. W. and Owens, D. K. (1995). Cost-effectiveness of warfarin and aspirin for prophylaxis of stroke in patients with non-valvular atrial fibrillation. *J. Am. Med. Assoc.*, **274**, 1839–45.

Gold, R. (1990). Combined immunosuppression with azathioprine and cyclosporin: results of an open MRI pilot study. *J. Neurol.*, **237(Suppl. 1)**, 20.

Goodkin, D. E., Bailey, R. C., Teetzen, M. L. *et al.* (1991). The efficacy of azathioprine in relapsing–remitting multiple sclerosis. *Neurology*, **41**, 20–25.

Harris, J., Jessop, J. D. and Chaput de Saintonge, D. M. (1971). Further experience with azathioprine in rheumatoid arthritis. *Br. Med. J.*, **iv**, 463–4.

Hazleman, B. L. (1982). The comparative incidence of malignant disease in rheumatoid arthritis exposed to different treatment regimes. *Ann. Rheum. Dis.*, **41(Suppl. 1)**, 12–17.

Hohlfeld, R., Michels, M., Heininger, K. *et al.* (1988). Azathioprine toxicity during long-term immunosuppression of generalised myasthenia gravis. *Neurology*, **38**, 258–61.

Hopkins, A. (1992). *Measures of the Quality of Life and the Uses to which Such Measures may be put*. RCP Publications.

IFNB Multiple Sclerosis Study Group (1993). Interferon beta-1b is effective in relapsing–remitting multiple sclerosis. 1. Clinical results of a multicenter, randomized, double-blind, placebo-controlled trial. *Neurology*, **43**, 655–61.

IFNB Multiple Sclerosis Study Group and the University of British Columbia MS/MRI Analysis Group (1995). Interferon beta-1b in the treatment of multiple sclerosis: Final outcome of the randomized controlled trial. *Neurology*, **45**, 1277–85.

Jacobs, L. D., Cookfair, D. L., Rudick, R. A. *et al.* (1996). Intramuscular interferon beta-1a for disease progression in relapsing multiple sclerosis. *Ann. Neurol.*, **39**, 285–94.

Johnson, K. P., Brooks, B. R., Cohen, J. A. (1995). Copolymer 1 reduces relapse rate and improves disability in relapsing remitting multiple sclerosis: Results of a phase 111 multicenter, double-blind, placebo-controlled trial. *Neurology*, **45**, 1268–76.

Johnson, K. P., Brooks, B. R., Cohen, J. A. *et al.* (1998). Extended use of glatiramer acetate (Copaxone) is well tolerated and maintains its clinical effect on multiple sclerosis relapse rate and degree of disability. *Neurology*, **50**, 701-8.

Kappos, L. (1996). Combinations of drugs. *Multiple Sclerosis*, **1**, 400–403.

Kinlen, L. J. (1985). Incidence of cancer in rheumatoid arthritis and other disorders after immunosuppressive treatment. *Am. J. Med.*, **78(1a)**, 44–9.

Kirsner, A. B., Farber, S. J., Sheon, R. P. *et al.* (1982). The incidence of malignant disease in patients receiving cytotoxic therapy for rheumatoid disease. *Ann. Rheum. Dis.*, **41(Suppl. 1)**, 32–3.

Lhermitte, F., Marteau, R., Roullet, E. *et al.* (1984). Prolonged treatment of Multiple sclerosis with average doses of Azathioprine. An evolution of 15 years experience. *Rev. Neurol. (Paris)*, **140**, 553–8.

Lovatt, G. E. and Hennings, R. C. (1984). *Imuran Adverse Reactions*. Wellcome Group Research and Development, The Wellcome Foundation.

Lui, C., Wan Po, A. L. and Blumhardt, L. D. (1998). 'Summary measure' statistic for assessing the outcome of treatment trials in relapsing–remitting multiple sclerosis. *J. Neurol. Neurosurg. Psychiatr.*, **64**, 726–9.

Matteson, E. L., Hickey, A. R., Maguire, L. *et al.* (1991). Occurrence of neoplasia in patients with rheumatoid arthritis enrolled in a DMARD registry. Rheumatoid Arthritis Azathioprine Registry Steering Committee. *J. Rheumatol.*, **18(6)**, 809–14.

McGrath, E. P., Ibels, L. S., Raik, E. *et al.* (1975). Erythroid toxicity of azathioprine. *Q. J. Med.*, **XLIV/173**, 57–63.

Milanese, C., La Manta, L., Salmaggi, A. *et al.* (1988). Double-blind controlled randomized study on azathioprine efficacy in multiple sclerosis. Preliminary results. *Ital. J. Neurol. Sci.*, **9**, 53–7.

Moller, H., Kneller, R. W., Boice, J. D. and Olsen, J. H. (1991). Cancer incidence following hospitalisation for multiple sclerosis in Denmark. *Acta Neurol. Scand.*, **84**, 214–20.

Moreau, T., Blanc, S., Grimaud, J. *et al.* (1997). EZAZIMUS: early azathioprine versus interferon in multiple sclerosis. *Multiple Sclerosis*, **3**, 339.

Palace, J., Newsom-Davis, J., Lecky, B. and the Myasthenia Gravis Study Group (1998). *Neurology*, **50**, 1778–83.

Penn, I. (1971). Complications of immunosuppression. *Minerva Chir.*, **26**, 718–20.

PRISMS (Prevention of Relapses and Disability by Interferon β-1a Subcutaneously in Multiple Sclerosis) Study Group (1998). Randomized double-blind placebo-controlled study of interferon beta-1a in relapsing/remitting multiple sclerosis. *Lancet*, **352**, 1498–1504.

Rothwell, P. M., McDowell, Z., Wong, C. K. and Dorman, P. J. (1997). Doctors and patients don't agree: cross-sectional study of patients' and doctors' perceptions and assessment of disability in multiple sclerosis. *Br. Med. J.*, **314,** 1580–83.

Rudge, P., Koetsuer, J. C., Mertin, J. *et al.* (1989). Randomised double-blind controlled trial of cyclosporin in multiple sclerosis. *J. Neurol. Neurosurg. Psychiatr.*, **52,** 559–65.

Saarikoski, S. and Seppala, M. (1976). Immunosuppression during pregnancy: transmission of azathioprine and its metabolites from the mother to the fetus. *Int. J. Pharmacol. Biopharm.*, **14/4,** 298–302.

Silman, A. J., Petrie, J., Hazelman, B. and Evans, S. J. (1988). Lymphoproliferative cancer and other malignancies in patients with rheumatoid arthritis treated with azathioprine: a 20-year follow-up study. *Ann. Rheum. Dis.*, **47(12),** 988–92.

Swinburn, W. R., Liversedge, L. A. (1973). Long-term treatment of multiple sclerosis with azathioprine. *J. Neurol. Neurosurg. Psychiatr.*, **36,** 123–6.

Swinson, D. R. and Swinburn, W. R. (1980). Rheumatoid arthritis. In: *Rheumatology* (D. R. Swinson and W. R. Swinburn, eds), p. 51. Hodder and Stoughton.

Villalba, L. and Adams, E. M. (1996). Update on therapy for refractory dermatomyositis and polymyositis. *Curr. Opin. Rheumatol.*, **8,** 544–51.

Witte, A. S., Cornblath, D. R., Schatz, N. J. and Lisak, R. P. (1986). Monitoring azathioprine therapy in myasthenia gravis. *Neurology*, **36,** 1533–4.

Yudkin, P. B., Ellison, G. W., Ghezzi, A. *et al.* (1991*).* Overview of azathioprine treatment in multiple sclerosis. *Lancet*, **338,** 1051–5.

8

Mitoxantrone

Introduction

The molecule mitoxantrone (Mx) was discovered in the 1970s, and is a member of the anthracenedione family. Originally developed as an antineoplastic drug, Mx has a proven immunosuppressive activity, and is also thought to have some antiviral and antibacterial activity. In the USA it is approved for the treatment of acute myeloid leukaemia in adults (since 1989) and advanced hormone-refractory prostate cancer (since 1996), and in Europe for the treatment of breast cancer, lymphoma and hepatoma. The dose given in cancer patients is usually higher and given more frequently than in MS patients ($12 \, mg/m^2$ per day every 3 days for two to three courses in acute myeloid leukaemia, $12 \, mg/m^2$ every 3 weeks for 6–10 courses for advanced hormone-refractory prostate cancer, $12–14 \, mg/m^2$ every 3–4 weeks in Europe). In the USA, there are several thousand cancer patients treated each year with Mx, usually in combination with other chemotherapeutic drugs, and the range of a single administered dose is $12–90 \, mg/m^2$.

The molecular weight of Mx is 517 daltons (interferon beta: 20 kda), its long terminal half-life ranges from 23–215 hours, and it has an extensive distribution to diverse tissues. Interestingly, research in monkeys has shown that its distribution to brain, spinal cord and cerebrospinal fluid (CSF) is low, suggesting that it does not cross the intact blood–brain barrier (BBB) or blood–CSF barrier (Lenk et al., 1987).

In principle, Mx has a dual molecular mechanism of action (Rosenberg et al., 1986); on one hand it exerts a direct effect on nucleic acids by intercalating with the DNA and RNA, causing inter- and intra-band crosslinks and band scissions, and on the other hand it has more recently been discovered that it inhibits DNA repair via inhibition of topoisomerase II.

The basic immune mechanism of action is also two-fold. Mx exerts an immunosuppressive effect on CD4-helper and cytotoxic T-cells, on B-lymphocytes and macrophages. Its immunomodulatory effect is by augmenting the suppressor T-cell activity (Fidler et al., 1986a). More recently, it was shown in animal models that Mx enhances apoptosis in tumour cells. A recent study looking at human B-chronic lymphocytic leukaemia cells suggests that the cytotoxic effect of Mx is due to induction of apoptosis via DNA fragmentation and caspase activation (Bellosillo et al., 1998).

Mx in the animal model of multiple sclerosis

Over the last 15 years, Mx has been tested in experimental allergic encephalomyelitis (EAE), an animal model of MS. Both acute and chronic EAE have been investigated, and with regard to acute EAE, studies have been performed in both active and passive EAE models – the main difference being that in the latter there is no induction phase. In Lewis rats, both in active EAE and passively transferred T-cell EAE, Mx showed a significant suppression of clinical symptoms and a strong reduction of inflammatory infiltrates. It appears to be 10 times more potent than cyclophosphamide (Ridge *et al.*, 1985; Lublin *et al.*, 1987). In chronic relapsing SJL/J EAE mice, Mx inhibited the disease development over a 3-month treatment period but not thereafter (Levine and Saltzman, 1986). Mx was also effective when given between two relapses in chronic relapsing mice, in preventing the expected next relapse as compared to untreated EAE mice. In addition, there is a suggestion from *in vitro* data that Mx can suppress demyelination (Watson *et al.*, 1991). These positive *in vivo* and *in vitro* pre-clinical studies stimulated the clinical investigations of Mx in MS patients.

Phase I, II and III studies in multiple sclerosis

Single-arm open-label trials

Since 1990 there have been a number of single-arm studies of MS patients treated with Mx (Gonsette and Demonty, 1990; Kappos *et al.*, 1990; Mauch *et al.*, 1992; Noseworthy *et al.*, 1993; Ruggero and Marciano, 1993; Mesaros *et al.*, 1998; Reeß *et al.*, 1998).

Gonsette and Demonty (1990) used Mx to treat 22 MS patients (16 with relapsing–remitting (RR) and six with secondary progressive (SP) MS). The dose was 14 mg/m^2 Mx every 3 weeks, and the aim was to reduce the lymphocyte count to 1000/mm^2 or less. The EDSS was stable after a mean follow-up of 1 year, and in six patients the EDSS had increased. Twelve patients had a high relapse rate prior to treatment, and the relapse rate was reduced in eight of these patients at follow-up, and unchanged in four.

Kappos *et al.* (1990) treated 14 SP patients with rapidly progressing MS. The treatment schedule was 10 mg/m^2 every 3 weeks for three to five courses, the number of courses depending on the leucocyte count and/or disease activity. Eight patients were studied beyond 3 months: three of these eight patients improved on the DSS, and five remained stable.

Mauch *et al.* (1992) treated 10 MS patients (six RR, four SP) with evidence of rapid deterioration of at least 1 point on the EDSS within the preceding 12 months, using 12 mg/m^2 Mx every 3 months. Eight of the nine patients were followed for 1 year and showed an improvement compared to their enrolment DSS and standard neurological status (SNS).

Noseworthy *et al.* (1993) treated 13 patients with progressive MS (8 mg/m^2 every 8 weeks, total of seven infusions). Only three of 13 patients showed an increase in the EDSS of more than 0.5 after 18 months, but the authors felt that the EDSS changes were consistent with the natural history of the disease.

Ruggero and Marciano (1993) treated 14 SPMS patients with 6–10 mg/m^2 Mx every 3 months. Six patients received 6 mg/m^2 Mx due to pre-study treatment with other chemotherapeutics. After a follow-up of between five and 21 months, EDSS was 6.3 as compared to 6.4 at baseline.

Reeß et al. (1998) treated 52 RR and 23 SPMS patients with 12 mg/m^2 Mx; mean cumulative dose 101 mg, mean treatment period 21 months, mean time between two courses 4.4 months. The authors concluded that the progression of the disease could be stopped both in RR and SPMS patients, and that the side effects were well tolerated.

Mesaros et al. (1998) treated 23 (seven RR and 16 SPMS) patients using 20 mg Mx and 1 g methylprednisolone every month for 6 months. To enter the trial, the patients had to have suffered at least two relapses and/or at least a 2-point deterioration on the EDSS in the preceding 24 months. At the end of the trial, 13 patients had improved by at least 0.5 point on the EDSS, nine were stable and one had deteriorated. The authors observed no serious side effects, including cardiotoxicity.

Gd-DTPA-enhanced MRI and single-arm Mx trials

In the early 1990s, three single-arm Mx studies of MS patients included Gd-enhanced MRI and observed a remarkable treatment effect of Mx on the blood–brain barrier.

Krapf et al., 1995 (see also Mauch et al., 1992) studied 10 patients with a total of 169 Gd-enhancing lesions at month 0 (M0), and found 40 Gd-enhancing lesions at M3, five at M6, one at M9, ten at M12, and five at M24.

Kappos et al. (1991) studied 14 SPMS patients with a total of 139 Gd-enhancing lesions at M0, and at M6, after three to five courses of Mx (10 mg/m^2 every 3 weeks), there were four Gd-enhancing lesions.

Noseworthy et al. (1993) observed 43 Gd-enhancing lesions in 13 SPMS patients at M0. After 6 months of Mx 8 mg/m^2 every 3 weeks, only a single Gd-enhancing lesion remained in these 13 patients; at M18 there were six Gd-enhancing lesions.

The indication of clinical efficacy in single-armed Mx trials in MS, although unblinded, and the striking effect of Mx in protecting the impaired blood–brain barrier as evidenced by Gd-enhanced MRI, prompted phase II and phase III MX trials

The French and British multicentre controlled trial
(Edan et al., 1997)

This randomized, MRI-controlled (but clinically unblinded and not placebo-controlled) trial evaluated the efficacy of Mx over 6 months in a group of 42 patients with aggressively active clinical and radiological disease. All patients received monthly IV injections of methylprednisolone (Tables 8.1, 8.2). The patients had either suffered two relapses with sequelae or progression of 2 points on the EDSS during the 12 months previously, and on MRI there had to be at least one new active lesion on monthly Gd-enhanced MRI scans during a 2-month baseline period. Patients fulfilling these clinical and MRI criteria were randomized to 6 months' treatment with intravenous mitoxantrone (20 mg/month) and methylprednisolone (1 g methylprednisolone/month), or 1 g methylprednisolone/month alone. Six patients in the control group and four patients in the mitoxantrone group had secondary progressive MS, whereas the others had the relapsing–remitting form of MS. The patients were evaluated with monthly Gd-enhanced and T2-weighted scans, and blinded analysis was performed by two experienced readers. Monthly clinically unblinded examinations of the patients were performed by neurologists in five French centres. In the control group, five patients dropped out due to severe exacerbations and EDSS progression. All drop-outs were extremely active on MRI; 33 of their 34 MR scans showed new Gd-enhancing lesions, with a mean number of 8.7 per patient scan. There were no drop-outs in the Mx group.

The primary endpoint of the study was the percentage of patients without new

Table 8.1 Treatment schedules

	French study	MIMS
Indication		
Diagnosis	Clinically definite multiple sclerosis	
EDSS	EDSS ≤ 6	EDSS 3–6
Disease activity	Two or more relapses in	Relapsing remitting or
Clinical activity	prior 12 months or two or more points EDSS increase in prior 12 months	secondary progressive forms of multiple sclerosis in an active stage of the disease (i.e. deterioration of at least 1 point on the EDSS within the previous 18 months)
MRI activity	At least one active lesion on gadolinium-enhanced MRI during the 2-month baseline period with monthly MRI scan	No MRI activity requested
Treatment protocol	Every month for 6 months; a single intravenous infusion of 20 mg Mx, 1 g IV methylprednisolone	Every 3 months for 2 years: 12 mg/m^2 body surface (as IV infusion)
Maximum cumulative dose	120 mg/patient	96 mg/m^2/patient

Table 8.2 Mitoxantrone and multiple sclerosis – reduction of clinical and MRI activity in the controlled trials

	French study	Italian study	MIMS
Clinical form of MS	Very active MS; RP or SP	RR	RR or SP
Treatment	20 mg/month for 6 months	8 mg/m^2 per month for 12 months	12 mg/m^2 per 3 months for 24 months
Duration of follow-up (months)	6	24	24
Reduction in relapses (%)	77	60	60
Reduction of clinical progression (% of patients with ≥ 1 point EDSS increase)	84	79	64
Reduction in the number of new MRI lesions (%)	84	52	88
Reduction of active MRI lesions (%)	86	–	86

active MRI lesions. At entry (month 0), this was 4.8 per cent in the non-Mx group and 10 per cent in the Mx group. This percentage increased during the treatment period in the Mx group, starting from month 2, and reached 90 per cent by month 6. In contrast, the increase in the control group was 31 per cent ($P < 0.001$).

With regard to secondary endpoints, during the baseline period the mean monthly number of new enhancing lesions varied between 4.6 and 9.1. During the treatment period the mean monthly number of new enhancing lesions varied between 2.9 and 13.2 in the non-Mx group, and between 0.1 and 2.6 in the Mx group. Thus, the numbers were less for the Mx group at all time points (Figure 8.1), and the differences were significant from months 1–6. Over the whole 6-month period, there was an 85 per cent reduction in new enhancing lesions in the Mx group. Comparing the T2-weighted images at exit with those at month 0, there was also an 80 per cent reduction in new T2-weighted lesions in the Mx group (5.5 vs 1.1).

Clinical assessment of the patients, though unblinded, showed a clear clinical benefit for the Mx group. The change in the EDSS with respect to month 0 was significant: From months 2–6, the Mx group continuously improved at all time points, reaching a final mean EDSS improvement of about 1 point compared to month 0. By contrast, the non-Mx group deteriorated from months 0–4, and apparent improvement at months 5 and 6 was seen after five patients had dropped out due to severe deterioration. Furthermore, the distribution of the confirmed variation of 1 point in EDSS between month 0 and the end of the study was clearly different, showing that in the Mx group 12 out of 21 patients improved by 1 point or more on the EDSS, and only one patient deteriorated. By contrast, in the non-Mx group six patients deteriorated and only three improved. During the 2-month baseline period, the Mx and non-Mx groups had 12 and nine exacerba-

Mean cumulative no of new enhancing lesions/scan

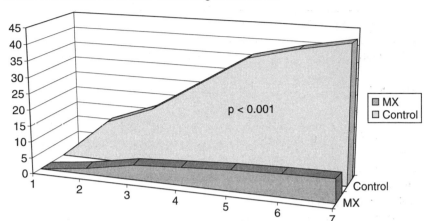

Figure 8.1 French and British Mx trial: monthly MRI data.

tions respectively, giving extrapolated annual rates of 3.4 and 2.6, similar to those of the 12 preceding months (3.1 and 2.4). However, during the treatment period there were fewer relapses in the Mx group as compared to the non-Mx group (7 vs 31 relapses). This effect was even more pronounced during the last 4 months of the treatment (1 vs 18 relapses). During the treatment period, 14 out of 21 patients were free of exacerbations in the Mx group, and 7 out of 21 in the control group.

More adverse events were recorded in the Mx group than in the control group (18 vs 6 patients). There was no evidence of serious side effects, and in particular no cardiotoxicity was detected. Minor and transient alopecia occurred in seven patients. Eight of 15 women developed amenorrhea, beginning between months 2 and 6; this was transient in seven women and persistent in one (aged 44 years). All patients in the Mx group had an expected pronounced neutropenia, starting about 2 weeks after injection, which resolved within a few days. At the next monthly injection, leucopenia was minor in four patients, and there was no need to adjust the dose. In nine patients, concomitant treatment for nausea became necessary.

The Italian multicentre controlled trial *(Millefiorini et al., 1997)*

This placebo-controlled trial evaluated the efficacy of mitoxantrone over 2 years in a group of 51 relapsing–remitting multiple sclerosis patients (Table 8.2). The patients were clinically selected as having a disability rated 2–5 on the Kurtzke EDSS at entry, with at least two exacerbations in the previous 2 years. They were randomized to 1 year of mitoxantrone treatment (27 patients received IV infusion of 8 mg/m² per month) or to the placebo group (24 patients received IV infusion of saline every month for 1 year). The patients were examined by four blinded EDSS physicians (especially trained in applying the EDSS, during a joint session) and evaluated prior to the start of the therapy, and 12 and 24 months later. Monitoring and recording of exacerbations and other medical events were documented by an unblinded treating physician in each of the eight Italian clinical centres. MRI studies without contrast, using T2-weighted spin echo sequence, were performed at 0, 12 and 24 months.

The primary endpoint of the study was the proportion of patients with a 1-point EDSS progression. During the total period of the study (0–2 years), nine of 24 (37 per cent) placebo patients deteriorated by at least 1 point on the EDSS as compared with two of 27 (7 per cent) patients receiving Mx ($P = 0.02$).

With regard to the secondary endpoints, a significant decrease in the mean annual number of exacerbations was observed in the Mx group compared with the placebo group (0.4 vs 1.3, $P < 0,001$). Furthermore, there was a significant increase in the number of exacerbation-free patients in the Mx group compared to the placebo group (17 vs 5, $P < 0.01$). A significant worsening in EDSS was also observed in the placebo group between the baseline and the end of the study (placebo: 3.5, SD 1.2 vs 4.2, SD 1.6, $P < 0.01$; Mx: 3.6, SD 0.9 vs 3.5, SD 1.4, $P = NS$). Forty-two of 51 patients completed the annual MRI for 2 years, and a comparison between the 23 Mx-treated patients and the 19 patients of the placebo group showed a 52 per cent reduction of new T2 lesions in the Mx group (7.3 vs 3.5, $P = 0.05$) although there was no difference in the number of enlarging lesions.

Several adverse events were recorded, but there were no signs of cardiotoxicity on electrocardiogram and echocardiography, no serious infections, no moderate or severe alopecia and no haematological adverse reactions. The most common side effect was nausea, which was generally mild and easily controlled with antiemetics. Five women out of 17 developed amenorrhea, beginning between months 4 and 8 after starting Mx, although this resolved rapidly after cessation of therapy.

The controlled phase III MIMS trial *(Hartung et al., 1998, Krapf et al., 1998)*

This randomized, placebo-controlled, observer-blind study was presented in September 1998 at the 14th Congress of ECTRIMS (MIMS, Tables 8.1, 8.2). One hundred and ninety-nine patients with relapsing–remitting or secondary progressive MS (EDSS at entry 3–6, age 18–55 years) were randomized to 12 mg/m^2 IV Mx, 5 mg/m^2 IV Mx or placebo (IV methylene blue). The regimen was given every 3 months for 2 years, and there were 188 clinically evaluable patients. In predetermined centres, a subgroup of 110 patients was examined with Gd-enhanced and T2-weighted MRI at months 0, 12 and 24, and centrally analysed by two experienced MR readers blinded to the clinical status of the patients.

There were five primary endpoints of the study: change from baseline of EDSS, Ambulation index (AI) and standard neurological status (SNS), the number of treated relapses, and the time to the first treated relapse. After 24 months, all five primary endpoints in the two Mx groups were significantly different from the placebo group. The changes were as follows:

	$12\,mg/m^2$ group	$5\,mg/m^2$ group	Placebo group
Change in EDSS	-0.13	-0.23	$+0.23$
Change in AI	0.3	0.4	0.8
Number of treated relapses in 2 years	0.4	0.7	1.2
Time to first relapse requiring steroids	Not reached within 24 months	Not reached within 24 months	15 months

The positive clinical impact of Mx in MS was seen as early as 6 months after initiation of the treatment in the $12\,mg/m^2$ Mx group as compared to 12 months in the $5\,mg/m^2$ group.

The secondary outcome criteria were confirmed EDSS progression of 1 point, and MRI evaluation. In the $12\,mg/m^2$ Mx group 7 per cent had a 3-month confirmed 1-point EDSS progression, compared with 19 per cent in the placebo group ($P = 0.03$). On MRI, there was a significant reduction in the percentage of active scans at months 12 and 24 from baseline with both doses (about 86 per cent and 75 per cent in the $12\,mg/m^2$ and the $5\,mg/m^2$ Mx groups, respectively), whereas the percentage of active scans remained stable in the placebo group. There was almost no progression detectable in both treatment groups in regard to the lesion load, whereas in the placebo group a continuous increase was found at months 12 and 24 ($P < 0.05$).

Mx – toxicity profile

Its potential for toxicity clearly limits the use of Mx, and this therefore needs to be considered in detail (Posner *et al.*, 1985; Table 8.3).

Table 8.3 Exclusion criteria for Mx treatment in MS

1 Evidence of previous treatment with Mx, **and** maximum cumulative dose $\geq 120\,mg/m^2$
2 Evidence of previous treatment with anthracenediones or anthracyclines
3 Mediastinal radiotherapy
4 Cardiac risk factors (e.g. congestive heart failure, myocardial infarction, uncontrolled ischaemic heart disease, uncontrolled arterial hypertension, LVEF ≤ 50 per cent)
5 Association with other drugs that are potentially cardiotoxic (e.g. neuroleptics, antidepressive drugs such as lithium)
6 Pregnant or nursing MS patients

Bone marrow depression

This is the principal dose-limiting toxic side effect of mitoxantrone, requiring careful clinical management tailored to each individual patient. It is predominantly granulocytopenia, which develops 10 days after a single large dose and persists for 4–7 days. Full recovery usually occurs by days 18–21 after drug administration (Crossley, 1984). A haemoglobin level, WBC and platelet count must be performed before each course of Mx. The absolute neutrophil count (ANC) has to be above 1500/mm^2 and the platelet count more than 150 000/mm^2 before a course of Mx is started. In cases of haematological toxicity, the next dose must be reduced (Table 8.4).

Table 8.4 MIMS – 12 mg/m^2 treatment arm: dose reduction in case of toxicity

Leukocytes ($\times 10^9$/l)	Platelets ($\times 10^9$/l)	Next dosage (mg/m^2)
Severe infection after Mx infusion		
<2000	< 50 000	10
<1000	< 25 000	8
7 days preceding next Mx infusion		
<4000	<100 000	9
<3000	< 75 000	6
<2000	< 50 000	STOP

Cardiotoxicity *(Table 8.5)*

Table 8.5 Cardiac monitoring in Mx-treated MS patients

1 No relevant past history of cardiac disease
2 No relevant ECG abnormalities:
   • perform ECG before starting Mx
3 Echocardiogram:
   • perform baseline echocardiograph to assess LVEF
   • ensure that LVEF is > 50 per cent
   • ensure that the same method is always used to assess the LVEF for the same patient
     (and if possible, performed by the same cardiologist)
     Stop Mx treatment, and continue cardiac monitoring:
   • if LVEF drops by ≥ 10 per cent
   • if LVEF is below 50 per cent
4 If clinical evidence of heart disease:
   • stop Mx treatment immediately
   • continue cardiac monitoring
   • seek cardiologist's advice
5 No relevant history of cardiotoxic drugs

Mx-related cardiotoxicity is characterized by reduction of the left ventricular ejection fraction (LVEF) and congestive heart failure. The risk of cardiac damage increases as the total dose increases. Histologically, there is ultrastructural myofibrillar damage and the development of vacuoles. In spontaneous hypertensive rats, Mx induces apoptosis in renal tubular and intestinal epithelium cells but not in myocytes. It was hypothesized that cardiotoxicity of Mx may be due to reactive oxygen intermediates, which are produced as a result of the formation of an Fe-III-Mx-complex. However, the formation of reactive oxygen intermediates occurred in Mx-treated animals at much higher doses than with doxorubicin, accounting for the comparatively reduced cardiotoxicity of the former (Herman et al., 1997). Apart from the cumulative dose, the risk of cardiac damage increases significantly with increasing patient age and pre-existing cardiac disease. Previous studies have suggested that the risk of Mx cardiac effects is low when it is given to patients with no previous cardiotoxic therapies or pre-existing heart disease and at a cumulative dose lower than $160\,mg/m^2$ (De Forni and Armand, 1994). In order to prevent cardiotoxicity, it is mandatory to monitor the LVEF by performing either an echocardiogram or a radionuclide ventriculogram. The recommendation is to obtain a baseline echocardiogram before treatment, and to repeat the examination once the cumulative dose exceeds half the nominal limit (i.e. $80\ mg/m^2$) prior to each alternate dose. The administration of Mx should be discontinued if the LVEF is reduced by more than 10 per cent between two readings, or if the LVEF is less than 50 per cent at any time. Respecting these guidelines, no symptomatic cardiotoxicity was seen in the three controlled trials using Mx in MS at a cumulative dose of between 70 and $96\,mg/m^2$ (De Castro et al., 1995; see also Millefiorini et al., 1997; Edan et al., 1997; Hartung et al., 1998). Although the dose used in these studies seemed safe, the possibility cannot be dismissed that subclinical, permanent and minor cardiac injury induced by the drug may later become clinically symptomatic as patients age and develop the common form of heart disease. If Mx is used to treat a non-life-threatening disease such as MS, it is the responsibility of the treating physician to continue to follow the cardiac status of the patients for up to 10 years after completing Mx therapy (Steinherz et al., 1991). In a pilot study performed by Gonsette (personal communication), 52 patients with active MS disease were treated with Mx ($14\,mg/m^2$ of Mx every 3 weeks). Three cases of congestive heart failure were encountered; two were reversible, and the cumulative doses were $106\,mg/m^2$ and $176\,mg/m^2$, respectively. One patient, who was concomitantly treated with lithium 250 t.i.d. and prothipendyl hydrochloride, died at a cumulative dose of $207\,mg/m^2$ (total dose 336 mg Mx).

Gonadal function

Fertility problems can be a delayed side effect of chemotherapy, and this must be discussed with young patients because it is such an important issue of quality of life. In women, the risk of gonadal dysfunction is related to the age of the patients. Experience with women treated with Mx for breast cancer (Bines et al., 1996) showed that few of those less than 36 years of age became amenorrheic, and amenorrhea was usually transitory. Older women are more likely to develop permanent amenorrhea. The increased rate of gonadal failure in older women might be explained by the lower number of remaining follicles. In young men treated for Hodgkin's disease, mitoxantrone in combination with other chemotherapy (vincristine, vinblastine, prednisone) caused significant decreases in sperm count and mobility; however, recovery occurred within 3–4 months of the end of the chemotherapy (Meistrich *et al.*, 1997). In contrast to other regimens with alkylating agents (for example, cyclophosphamide), it is known that after cessation of Mx there is a complete recovery of the sperm production without morphological changes *in vitro* or genotoxic effects on germinal cells *in vivo*.

Other acute side effects (Table 8.6)

Nausea or vomiting occurs in about 60 per cent of patients on any course of mitoxantrone, and is usually mild or moderate. Alopecia, if present, is usually minimal and does not require a wig.

Table 8.6 Common adverse events (usually transient)

1 Nausea (give IV antiemetics before IV Mx infusion)
2 Alopecia
3 Urinary tract infection
4 Menstrual disorders
5 Leukocytopenia/thrombocytopenia
6 Liver enzymes elevation

Discussion

There is now a growing body of evidence indicating that Mx has a proven clinical benefit in multiple sclerosis (Table 8.2). Mx is able to reduce the annual relapse rate and improve or stabilize clinically RR and/or SPMS patients as assessed by a number of clinical scores (EDSS, Ambulation Index and Standard Neurological Status). The clinical benefit of the drug has been shown in a number of phase I trials, a couple of phase II trials and, more recently, in a European phase III trial (MIMS). The clinical findings of Mx in MS patients are corroborated by MRI results, especially Gd-enhanced MRI, where a striking reduction in the number of Gd-enhancing lesions has been a constant finding after Mx treatment (Kappos *et al.*, 1990; Noseworthy *et al.*, 1993; Krapf *et al.*, 1995, 1998; Edan *et al.*, 1997). In line with the clinical benefits of Mx in MS patients are the clinical and histological findings in several EAE studies, where Mx has been shown to reduce the relapse rate, improve or prevent clinical deterioration and, histologically, reduce the number of inflammatory infiltrates.

Despite its clear clinically positive impact on MS patients and on the animal model of MS there are a number of important questions to be addressed before considering its routine use in MS patients, and these are discussed below.

What is the role of Mx in progressive MS?

Given its unknown potential for long-term toxicity, especially cardiotoxicity, Mx should today be considered as a second-line drug for the treatment of secondary progressive MS patients. Interferon beta-1b has recently been approved by European regulatory agencies as the only approved drug for this important group of MS patients. However, given the fact that in an interferon beta-1b phase III trial about 40 per cent of SPMS patients failed to respond to the drug in terms of delaying confirmed disease progression, it is obvious that a substantial number of non-responders will continue to progress. In this population of non-responders, Mx deserves to be considered as an alternative therapy. However, even if the 3-month interval between two infusions allows a long period of treatment (about 2 years for 12 mg/m^2 dosage and 5 years for 5 mg/m^2 dosage), the potential toxicity of the drug will ultimately limit its use.

Is there a role for Mx in very active MS patients?

The important issue of treating rapidly deteriorating MS patients ('malignant' MS) with Mx was addressed by Edan *et al.* (1997). In previous trials, such a group of patients represented only a small percentage of the whole cohort (e.g. 22 out of 354 in the British and Dutch Multiple Sclerosis Azathioprine Trial, 1988). The strong and rapid reduction in the number of Gd-enhancing lesions, along with its clinical benefit as observed in the monthly combination of Mx and methylprednisolone, suggests a potential role for this Mx regimen as rescue therapy in very active cases of multiple sclerosis. Furthermore, Mx is an attractive but temporary option in RRMS patients who do not respond to interferon beta-1a or -1b, or glatiramer acetate.

What is the short- versus long-term clinical efficacy of Mx in MS?

As discussed above, Mx has shown impressive clinical efficacy in MS patients, usually during treatment or shortly after stopping it. However, to date there are no substantial data concerning the long-term efficacy of Mx after cessation of treatment. In this regard, it should be noted that European approval by regulatory agencies of interferon beta-1b in progressive MS was given based on data from a 24-month trial. In a 2-year follow-up of the French study (De Marco *et al.*, 1996), it was found that most of the patients remained stable for 18 months after cessation of Mx. Regarding the MIMS patients, clinical data collection for the 3-year period will be available soon (Wyeth Lederle, Germany, personal communication). As for the duration of its effect in markedly reducing inflammatory activity as assessed by Gd-enhancement, again no substantial data are available today. There is, however, some evidence from single-arm Mx trials that the reduction of

Gd-enhancement is observed for as long as 12–18 months after stopping the drug. However, more data are clearly warranted to determine the long-term clinical benefits of Mx, and more MRI follow-up is needed to determine the effect of Mx on the blood–brain barrier and the T2-weighted MRI lesions.

What is known about mitoxantrone's mechanism of action in MS?

There is an increasing amount of evidence from *in vivo* and *in vitro* studies, both in EAE and MS patients, that Mx is an immunosuppressive and modulating agent that acts non-selectively on a number of pivotal immune responses (T-cells, B-cells and macrophages). With regard to the white cell count, the relative and earlier decrease in the number of B-cells as compared to T-cells is suggestive of a strong effect on the humoral arm (G. Edan, unpublished data). Clinically, it would be of interest if the response in MS patients with and without evidence of Gd-enhancement was different, and similarly, if its impact was different in relapsing–remitting MS as compared to progressive patients without relapses. Furthermore, there are no data available looking at its role in primary progressive MS, where increasing evidence suggests that a primary attack on the oligodendrocytes, and not inflammation, is the initial step of the disease (Bruck *et al.*, 1994; Ozawa *et al.*, 1994; Lucchinetti *et al.*, 1996). Interestingly, an Mx trial in primary progressive MS is planned in the USA (D. Goodkin, personal communication, 1999).

How do the short- and long-term toxic effects of Mx affect its use?

In Europe, there seems to be a consensus among MS specialists with long-term experience of Mx in MS that the short-term adverse effects are usually transient and negligible. This also holds true for cardiotoxicity, where it is mandatory to perform cardiac monitoring (essentially ECG and echocardiography) before, during and after stopping treatment. This experience is corroborated by the recent major clinical trials in MS patients. In this regard, Mauch *et al.* (1992) are currently reviewing their Mx MS patients ($n = 450$) in order to assess the long-term toxicity profile of mitoxantrone. It is of note that in none of these patients was there clinical evidence of heart failure (Mauch, personal communication). Similarly, Edan *et al.* (1997) are re-evaluating the Rennes cohort of Mx-treated MS patients ($n = 150$), including a follow-up with LVEF. Regarding the German experience (Mauch *et al.*, 1992), in the French centre there was no evidence of clinical heart failure. However, in two patients there was a drop in the LVEF noted at follow-up, which led to stopping the medication.

What is the management in patients who worsen after having received the maximal cumulative dose of Mx?

There are no substantial data available to answer this question. In practice, this implies that it is left to the discretion of the treating MS specialist to decide which treatment, usually one with minor side effects, will be added after Mx.

Is there a rationale for sequential treatment?

The concept of induction treatment followed by long-term treatment combining several drugs has been proven effective in infectious diseases and in oncology, but has not been investigated in MS. Since both interferon beta (Hall *et al.*, 1997) and mitoxantrone have proven efficacy, sequential administration offers a good opportunity to test this therapeutic concept in MS. The specific and complementary effects of these two compounds in terms of immunosuppressive activity (global action for mitoxantrone versus selective action for interferon beta), rapid action (strong and immediate action for mitoxantrone versus progressive immuno-modulation for interferon beta) and treatment duration (prescription limited to a few years for mitoxantrone, 3-monthly infusions versus several years for interferon beta) suggest that they might, when combined in a sequential schedule, exhibit synergic action in MS. In this regard, Edan and colleagues are starting a new trial aiming to determine whether a treatment strategy combining induction treatment by mitoxantrone followed by interferon beta-1b (as compared with interferon beta alone) can delay disease progression in patients having a very active relapsing course of the disease that threatens to lead rapidly to severe disability.

References

Bellosillo, B., Colomer, D., Pons, G. and Gil, J. (1998). Mitoxantrone, a topoisomerase II inhibitor, induces apoptosis of B-chronic lymphocytic leukaemia cells. *Br. J. Haematol.*, **100(1)**, 142–6.

Bines, J., Oleske, D. M. and Cobleigh, M. A. (1996). Ovarian function in premenopausal women treated with adjuvant chemotherapy for breast cancer. *J. Clin. Oncol.*, **14**, 1718–29.

British and Dutch Multiple Sclerosis Azathioprine Trial Group (1988). Double masked trial of aziathioprine in multiple sclerosis. *Lancet*, **ii**, 179–83.

Bruck, W., Schmied, M., Suchanek, G. *et al.* (1994). Oligodendrocytes in the early course of multiple sclerosis. *Ann. Neurol.*, **35**, 65–73.

Crossley, R. J. (1984). Clinical safety and tolerance of mitoxantrone. *Sem. Oncol.*, **11(Suppl. 1)**, 54–9.

De Castro, S., Cartoni D., Millefiorini E. *et al.* (1995). Non-invasive assessment of mitoxantrone cardiotoxicity in relapsing–remitting multiple sclerosis. *J. Clin. Pharmacol.*, **35**, 627–32.

De Forni, M. and Armand, J. P. (1994). Cardiotoxicity of chemotherapy. *Curr. Opin. Oncol.*, **6**, 340–44.

De Marco, O., Cortinovis, P., Clanet, M. *et al.* (1996) In MS patients with very active disease, the benefit of the association mitoxantrone/methylprednisolone lasts at least 18 months. The 12th Congress of the European

Committee for Treatment and Research in Multiple Sclerosis. *Eur. J. Neurol.*, **3(Suppl. 4),** 59.

Edan, G., Miller, D., Clanet, M. *et al.* (1997). Therapeutic effect of mitoxantrone combined with methylprednisolone in multiple sclerosis: a randomized multicenter study of active disease using MRI and clinical criteria. *J. Neurol. Neurosurg. Psychiatr.*, **62,** 112–18.

Fidler, J. M., Dejoy, S. Q., Smith, F. R. *et al.* (1986a). Selective immunomodulation by the antineoplastic agent mitoxantrone. II. Non-specific adherent suppressor cells derived from mitoxantrone-treated mice. *J. Immunol.*, **136,** 2747–54.

Fidler, J. M., Dejoy, S. Q. and Gibbons, J. R. (1986b). Selective immunomodulation by the antineoplastic agent mitoxantrone. I. Suppression of B lymphocyte function. *J. Immunol.*, **137,** 727–32.

Gonsette, R. E. and Demonty, L. (1990). Immunosuppression with mitoxantrone in multiple sclerosis: a pilot study for 2 years in 22 patients. *Neurology*, **40(Suppl. 1),** 261.

Hall, G., Compston, D. A. S. and Scolding, N. J. (1997). Beta-interferon and multiple sclerosis. *Trends Neurosci.*, **20,** 63–7.

Hartung, H. P., Gonsette, R. E. and the MIMS Study Group (1998). Mitoxantrone in progressive multiple sclerosis: a placebo-controlled, randomized, observer-blind European phase III multicentre study. Clinical data. 14th Congress of the European Committee for Treatment and Research in Multiple Sclerosis. *Multiple Sclerosis*, **4,** 325.

Herman, E. H., Zhang, J., Hasinoff, B. B. *et al.* (1997). Comparison of the structural changes induced by doxorubicin and mitoxantrone in the heart, kidney and intestine, and characterization of the Fe(III)-mitoxantrone complex. *J. Mol. Cell Cardiol.*, **29(9),** 2415–30.

Kappos, L., Gold, R., Künstler, E. *et al.* (1990). Mitoxantrone in the treatment of rapidly progressive multiple sclerosis: a pilot study with serial gadolinium-enhanced MRI. *Neurology*, **40(Suppl. 1),** 261.

Krapf, H., Mauch, E., Fetzer, U. *et al.* (1995). Serial gadolinium-enhanced magnetic resonance imaging in patients with multiple sclerosis treated with mitoxantrone. *Neuroradiology*, **37,** 113–19.

Krapf, H., Morrissey, S., Zenker, O. *et al.* (1998). Mitoxantrone in progressive multiple sclerosis: a placebo-controlled, randomized, observer-blind European phase III multicentre study. MRI data. 14th Congress of the European Committee for Treatment and Research in Multiple Sclerosis. *Multiple Sclerosis*, **4,** 380.

Lenk, H., Müller, U. and Tanneberger, S. (1987). Mitoxantrone: mechanism of action, antitumor activity, pharmakokinetics, efficacy in the treatment of solid tumors and lymphomas, and toxicity. *Anticancer* Res., **7,** 1257–64.

Levine, S. and Saltzman, A. (1986). Regional suppression therapy after onset and prevention of relapses in experimental allergic encephalomyelitis with mitoxantrone. *J. Neuroimmunol.*, **13,** 175–81.

Lublin, F. D., Lasava, M., Viti, C. and Knobler, R. L. (1987) Suppression of acute and relapsing experimental allergic encephalomyelitis with mitoxantrone. *Clin. Immunol. Immunopathol.*, **45**, 122–8.

Lucchinetti, C. F., Bruck, W., Rodriquez, M. and Lassmann, H. (1996). Distinct patterns of multiple sclerosis pathology indicates heterogeneity in the pathogenesis. *Brain Pathol.*, **6**, 259–74.

Mauch, E., Kornhuber, M. H., Krapf, H. *et al.* (1992). Treatment of multiple sclerosis with mitoxantrone. *Eur. Arch. Psychiatr. Clin. Neurosci.*, **242**, 96–102.

Meistrich, M. L., Wilson, G., Mathur, K. *et al.* (1997). Rapid recovery of spermatogenesis after mitoxantrone, vincristine, vinblastine, and prednisone chemotherapy for Hodgkin's disease. *J. Clin. Oncol.*, **15**, 3488–95.

Mesaros, S., Levic, Z., Drulovic, J. *et al.* (1998). Treatment of multiple sclerosis with mitoxantrone. 14th Congress of the European Committee for Treatment and Research in Multiple Sclerosis. *Multiple Sclerosis*, **4**, 387.

Millefiorini, E., Gasperini, C., Pozzilli, C. *et al.* (1997). Randomized placebo-controlled trial of mitoxantrone in relapsing–remitting multiple sclerosis: 24-month clinical and MRI outcome. *J. Neurol.*, **244**, 153–9.

Noseworthy, J. H., Hopkins M. B., Vandervoort, M. K. *et al.* (1993). An open-trial evaluation of mitoxantrone in the treatment of progressive MS. *Neurology*, **43**, 1401–6.

Ozawa, K., Suchanck, G., Breitschopf, H. *et al.* (1994). Patterns of oligodendroglia pathology in multiple sclerosis. *Brain*, **117**, 1311–22.

Posner, L. E., Dukart, G., Goldberg, J. *et al.* (1985). Mitoxantrone: an overview of safety and toxicity. *Invest. New Drugs*, **3**, 123–32.

Reeß, J., Eisenmann, S., Mauch, E. *et al.* (1998). Results of an open study with 75 MS patients treated with mitoxantrone. 14th Congress of the European Committee for Treatment and Research in Multiple Sclerosis. *Multiple Sclerosis*, **4**, 382.

Ridge, S. C., Sloboda, A. E., McReynolds R. A. *et al.* (1985). Suppression of experimental allergic encephalomyelitis by mitoxantrone. *Clin. Immunol. Immunopathol.*, **35**, 35–42.

Rosenberg, L. S., Carvlin, M. J. and Krugh, T. R. (1986). The antitumor agent mitoxantrone binds cooperatively to DNA: evidence for heterogeneity in DNA conformation. *Biochemistry*, **25**, 1002–8.

Ruggero, C. and Marciano, N. (1993). Mitoxantrone therapy of secondary progressive multiple sclerosis: pilot study. *Neurology*, **43(4)(Suppl. 2)**, 494S.

Steinherz, L. J., Steinherz, P. G., Charlotte, T. C. *et al.* (1991). Cardiac toxicity 4 to 20 years after completing anthracycline therapy. *J. Am. Med. Assoc.*, **266**, 1672–7.

Watson, C. M., Davison, A. N., Baker, D. *et al.* (1991). Suppression of demyelination by mitoxantrone. *Int. J. Immunopharmacol.*, **13(7)**, 923–30.

Disease modifying drugs – progressive disease

9

Treatments for progressive forms of MS

Introduction

In recent years, multiple sclerosis has emerged as a treatable disease. Approximately 85 per cent of patients with MS initially experience an acute attack of symptoms, and almost 50 per cent of these patients experience recurrent exacerbations with or without complete recovery. This clinical pattern is called relapsing–remitting MS if patients are clinically stable between attacks, and treatment options for patients with this form of MS are reviewed in Chapters 3–8.

Nearly 50 per cent of relapsing–remitting patients later experience gradual progression of disability, with or without clinical exacerbations. This clinical pattern is called secondary progressive MS (SPMS). There remain 10–15 per cent of patients who experience a progressive course from onset, and this is called primary progressive MS (PPMS). In 1998 and 1999, interferon beta-1b was approved in Europe and Canada for the treatment of SPMS. Applications for approval of interferon beta-1b and mitoxantrone for SPMS are pending in the USA. This chapter reviews the various therapeutic options, supported by published clinical trails, for progressive forms of MS: interferon beta-1b, methotrexate, cyclical pulses of intravenous methylprednisolone, and cyclophosphamide. Reported results from trials of promising treatment options in SPMS are also reviewed: mitoxantrone and 2-chlorodeoxyadenosine.

Published phase III and II trials of disease modifying therapies for SPMS

Interferon beta-1b

Interferon beta-1b is an approved treatment for relapsing–remitting MS in the USA, Canada and Europe, and in this context it has been addressed elsewhere in this book (see Chapter 3). In February 1998, a multicentre (32 MS centres in 12 European countries) Phase III clinical trial of interferon beta-1b in secondary progressive MS was terminated early because of 'overwhelming efficacy'. The results of this study, which were published in November 1998 in *The Lancet*

(ESG, 1998), provided convincing evidence of a clinically significant treatment effect in SPMS patients. In this collaborative study, 718 patients met the entry criteria of ages 18–55 years, baseline EDSS (Kurtzke, 1983) scores of 3.0–6.5, and a history of two or more relapses or a 1 or more point increase in EDSS over the previous 2 years. Secondary progression was defined as a period of deterioration, independent of relapses, sustained for at least 6 months and following a period of RRMS. Patients were randomized to receive subcutaneous injections of 8 Miu interferon beta-1b every other day ($n = 360$), or placebo ($n = 358$). The primary outcome measure was time to confirmed progression of disability sustained for 3 or more months. Confirmed progression of disability was defined as a 1-point increase on the EDSS for baseline EDSS scores of 3.0–5.5, and a 0.5-point increase for baseline EDSS scores of 6.0–6.5. The average disease duration was 13 years, and 70 per cent of enrolled patients experienced SPMS with superimposed relapses.

After 2 years of study, there was a significant difference in time to onset of sustained progression of disability favouring interferon beta-1b ($P = 0.0008$). The treatment effect was notable at 9 months ($P = 0.058$) and significant after 12 months ($P = 0.003$), and sustained progression was delayed by 9–12 months. Of the placebo group, 49.7 per cent experienced sustained progression of disability; this compared to 38.9 per cent in the treated group ($P = 0.0048$), a reduction of approximately 22 per cent in the proportion of patients experiencing progression. This effect was independent of the level of disability at baseline, or the presence of clinical exacerbations during the 2 years preceding enrolment or during the treatment period. Treatment also had a favourable effect on delaying the time to wheelchair requirement (EDSS 7.0), reducing the relapse rate, decreasing the number of new MRI lesions, and reducing steroid treatment and hospital admissions. Overall, interferon beta-1b was very well tolerated in SPMS patients, with a similar incidence of flu-like symptoms and injection-site reactions to those in previous trials.

As a result of this trial, interferon beta-1b was approved for treatment of patients with SPMS in Europe and Canada. The North American trial of interferon beta-1b in SPMS has been terminated prematurely, and the results of this trial are awaited. Table 9.1 outlines the differences in the designs of the European (EUSPMS) and North American SPMS (NASPMS) trials, and Table 9.2 summarizes the baseline clinical and demographic data of the patients enrolled in both trials. On average, patients in the NASPMS trial were older at baseline (46.8 years compared to 41 years) and had longer mean disease duration (14.7 years compared to 13.1 years). The treatment effect reported in the EUSPMS trial was independent of baseline EDSS, but the relationship between treatment effect and disease duration has not been previously explicitly considered. A *post hoc* analysis of the relationship between treatment effect, age and disease duration may be of interest in the analysis of the results of the NASPMS trial. Also, the proportion of patients who did not experience relapses during the 2 years prior to enrolment was significantly greater in the NASPMS trial. Although the treatment effect reported in the EUSPMS trial was independent of relapses during the 2 years before enrolment, a *post hoc* analysis to investigate the relationship between

Table 9.1 Differences in the designs of the EUSPMS and NASPMS trials

	EUSPMS	NASPMS
Number of subjects	718 (EDSS 3.0–6.5)	939 (EDSS 3.0–6.5)
Treatment groups	Interferon beta-1b 8.0 Miu sub-cutaneous, alternate days, vs placebo for 3 years	Interferon beta-1b 8.0 Miu vs 5.0 Miu subcutaneous, alternate days, vs placebo for 3 years
Dose escalation period (weeks)	2	4
Drug-related AEs	NSAIDs recommended	Ibuprofen required for 7 weeks
Entry age (years)	18–55	18–65
Disease duration (years)	1 or more	2 or more
Clinical course entry requirement	RR onset followed by gradual progression of disability for 6 or more months independent of relapses, and either two or more relapses **OR** an increase of 1 or more EDSS points during 24 months preceding study entry	RR onset followed by gradual progression of disability for 6 or more months independent of relapses **AND** an increase of 1 or more EDSS points during 24 months preceding study entry
Rx for relapses	IV methylprednisolone 1 g for 3 days with or without tapering doses of oral prednisone up to a maximum of three courses in 1 year	IV methylprednisolone 1 g for 5 days without tapering doses of oral prednisone
Primary outcome	Worsening EDSS without relapse sustained for 3 or more months	Worsening EDSS with or without relapse sustained for 6 or more months
Other planned outcomes	1. Time to reach EDSS 7.0 2. Severity of exacerbation graded subjectively by investigator 3. QOL measured by SIP 4. Rao cognitive tests at selective sites 5. Montgomery Asberg Depression Rating Scale (physician-recorded) 6. Frequent MRI cohort ($n = 125$) monthly Gd+ MRI scans months 0–6 and 18–24 7. No pharmacokinetics study	1. Not planned outcome 2. Severity of exacerbation graded by Scripps Scale 3. QOL measured by MSQLI 4. Rao cognitive tests plus Perdue pegboard and Trials A and B tests at all sites 5. Beck Depression Inventory (self-recorded) 6. Frequent MRI cohort ($n = 164$) monthly Gd+ MRI for 3 years 7. Pharmacokinetics substudy
Analysis of results	Pre-planned interim analysis at 2 years*	6-monthly pre-planned interim analysis*

*EUSPMS: $P = 0.013$ (Lan–Demets adaptation of O'Brien–Fleming procedure). NASPMS: $P = 0.0007, 0.0008, 0.0010. 0.0012, 0.0016, 0.0016, 0.048$ (Fleming, Harrington, O'Brien procedure).

treatment effect and relapses during those 2 years may also be of interest in the NASPMS trial.

Although interferon beta-1b is not approved for treatment of patients with SPMS in the USA, interferon beta-1b (Betaseron®) and interferon beta-1a (Avonex®) are widely prescribed for patients with SPMS who experience super-imposed relapses, a practice reflecting a general opinion that relapsing forms of MS, with or without progression, are difficult to distinguish and probably share a similar biology. With convincing evidence of efficacy in SPMS without relapses, interferon beta-1b may be prescribed off-label for patients with SPMS without superimposed relapses. It is anticipated that interferon beta-1b will be the most widely prescribed treatment for patients with SPMS, with or without superim-posed relapses, if approved by the United States Food and Drug Administration (FDA) for this indication.

Table 9.2 Comparison of baseline data for EUSPMS and NASPMS trials

Measures of interest	EUSPMS ($n=718$)	NASPMS ($n=939$)
Women	439 (61%)	588 (63%)
Mean age (SD, years)	41.0 (7.8)*	46.8 (8.3)*
Mean disease duration (SD, years)	13.1 (7.1)*	14.7 (8.3)*
Mean time since onset of gradual progression (SD, years)	3.8 (3.1)	4.0 (3.4)
Mean EDSS at baseline (SD)	5.2 (1.1)	5.1 (1.2)
EDSS by category:		
<4.0	114 (16%)	99 (11%)
4.0–5.5	282 (39%)	394 (42%)
>5.5	322 (45%)	446 (48%)
Patients without relapses 2 years prior to study	216 (30%)*	422 (45%)*
Mean annual relapse rate in 2 years prior to study (SD)	0.85 (0.8)*	0.41 (0.65)*

*Differences between study populations: $P < 0.001$.

Methotrexate

Methotrexate, N-10-methyl-aminopterin, is a competitive inhibitor of dihydrofo-late reductase, interfering with the production of reduced cofactors necessary for the synthesis of DNA and RNA (Grosflam and Weinblatt, 1991). Low-dose weekly oral methotrexate (MTX) is a standard, effective and relatively safe regimen in the treatment of rheumatoid arthritis (RA) (Weinblatt et al., 1992). The exact mechanism of action in RA is unclear (Cronstien, 1997), but low-dose MTX has immunosuppressive activity (Calabrese et al 1988; Alarcon et al., 1990; Hine et al., 1990), anti-inflammatory activity (Weinblatt et al., 1985; Segal et al.,

1990; Sperling *et al.*, 1992; Tak *et al.*, 1997; Dolhain *et al.*, 1998) and immunoregulatory effects (Neilson *et al.*, 1991; Nielsen and Hammer, 1992). Although no major toxicity has yet been observed in patients with multiple sclerosis treated with methotrexate, instances of major toxicity may be expected with more widespread use of this drug. The RA population has provided reliable information regarding tolerability of oral MTX at the same dosage (Goodman and Polisson, 1994). Major toxicity observed in patients with rheumatoid arthritis consists principally of interstitial pulmonary fibrosis, liver cirrhosis and bone marrow suppression.

The results from the first double-blind, placebo-controlled Phase II trial of low-dose, weekly oral methotrexate (MTX) in 60 chronic progressive MS patients (42 with SPMS, 18 with PPMS) were reported in 1995 (Goodkin *et al.*, 1995). Patients enrolled in the study met the entry criteria of age 21–60 years, disease duration greater than 1 year, and an EDSS score of 3.0–6.5. Participants were stratified by their ability to walk without (EDSS < 6.0) or with (EDSS > 6.0) assistance, and then randomized to receive 7.5 mg oral MTX or placebo one day per week. The primary outcome measure for the study was the proportion of patients experiencing 'treatment failure' on methotrexate versus placebo, using a composite outcome measure of disability. Patients met the requirements for sustained treatment failure by experiencing any of the following changes sustained for a minimum of 2 months:

- Worsening of the entry EDSS by ≥ 1.0 point for patients with an entry score of 3.0–5.0 or by ≥ 0.5 point for those patients with an entry score of 5.5–6.5
- Worsening of the entry Ambulation Index (AI) (Hauser *et al.* 1983) score of 2–6 by ≥ 1.0 point
- Worsening of ≥ 20 per cent from baseline value on best performance of two consecutive performances of box and block test (BBT) (Goodkin *et al.*, 1988); scores obtained with either hand
- Worsening of ≥ 20 per cent from baseline value on best performance of two consecutive performances of 9-hole peg test (9HPT) (Goodkin *et al.*, 1988); scores obtained with either hand.

The relationship between sustained progression and the treatment group favoured methotrexate as follows: MTX = 51.6 per cent and placebo = 82.8 per cent ($P = 0.011$). Analysis of each of the components of the composite showed that the effect was strongest for 9HPT ($P = 0.007$) and was seen to a lesser extent in the BBT ($P = 0.068$) and the EDSS ($P = 0.205$). Sustained treatment failure as defined by change in AI did not differ between the groups. The time before 50 per cent of patients achieved sustained treatment failure was 74.4 weeks in the MTX-treated group and 23.4 weeks in the placebo. The difference between overall sustained treatment failure distributions for these groups was highly significant ($P < 0.001$).

Forty-two of the 60 patients entered into this study had secondary progressive MS. A statistically significant MTX treatment effect on the rates of sustained treatment failure measured with the composite outcome variable was found for secondary progressive patients ($P = 0.005$), but not for primary progressive patients ($P = 0.630$). The power to detect differences between groups in the primary disease group was limited due to the small sample size ($n = 18$).

In addition to the clinical neurological evaluations, a standardized neuropsychological testing battery was administered to all patients at study entry and then annually for 2 years. A significant treatment effect favouring MTX was seen on measures of information-processing speed ($P < 0.025$), confrontational naming ($P < 0.05$) and prose recall ($P < 0.05$) (Fischer et al., 1994). Additionally, 35 consecutively enrolled patients were scheduled for gadolinium-enhanced MRI scans at 6-week intervals for the first 6 months of treatment. The results of exploratory analyses demonstrated a treatment effect favouring MTX on absolute change in T2-weighted total lesion area (Goodkin et al., 1996), and the change in T2-weighted total lesion area was significantly related to sustained progression of disability as measured by tests of manual dexterity but not the EDSS.

This study demonstrated a statistically significant treatment effect favouring MTX that was most evident on validated tests of upper extremity function (Goodkin et al., 1988). The difference in outcome between treatment groups was apparent within 6 months of initiating therapy, and was sustained for 2 years without evidence of significant toxicity. No patient discontinued therapy because of drug toxicity. The therapeutic benefit was not sufficiently robust to be statistically significant when measured solely by the EDSS. It is possible that the therapeutic benefits observed with MTX in the context of this Phase II study may be restricted to patients with secondary rather than primary progressive MS, although this conclusion is supported only by preliminary data and may be premature.

Low-dose weekly oral methotrexate is not approved for use in patients with multiple sclerosis. Nonetheless, the observed treatment effect, modest toxicity, ready availability and limited cost make it an attractive therapeutic option for some patients with progressive MS, and it is widely used off-label in the treatment of SPMS. Treatment decisions made under these circumstances should be individualized, and optimally should follow consultation with a physician who is experienced in the care of patients with MS and is thoroughly familiar with the administration procedures, pharmacokinetics, potential drug interactions and adverse effects known to occur with this drug.

Cyclical pulses of intravenous methylprednisolone

Intravenous pulse glucocorticoids shorten the duration of acute MS exacerbations and remain the treatment of choice for relapses in MS (Kupersmith et al., 1994; Olivieri et al., 1998). This has prompted study of the use of steroids as disease modifying agents in progressive MS. Two previous studies (Rinne et al., 1968; Milligan et al., 1987) examining the use of glucocorticoids in chronic progressive MS have suggested a treatment effect, but because of design limitations the results were difficult to interpret. In 1998, results from the Phase II dose comparison trial of cyclical pulses of intravenous methylprednisolone in SPMS patients demonstrated a modest treatment effect in favour of the high-dose treatment option (Goodkin et al., 1998).

In this Phase II study, 108 patients with secondary progressive MS met the entry criteria of age 21–60 years, disease duration longer than 1 year, and baseline EDSS 4.0–6.5. SPMS was defined as progression of > 0.5 EDSS points over 5 months in patients who had experienced one or more exacerbations, with or without recovery to baseline EDSS, during the 2 years preceding entry. Participants were randomized to receive either high-dose (500 mg, $n = 54$) or low-dose (10 mg, $n = 54$) methylprednisolone every 8 weeks for 2 years. Each bimonthly pulse was administered intravenously once a day for 3 days, followed by a tapering course of oral methylprednisolone starting on day 4 and concluding on day 14. High-dose recipients initiated their tapering dose at 64 mg and took the following doses on days 2–11 respectively: 64 mg, 48 mg, 48 mg, 32 mg, 32 mg, 24 mg, 24 mg, 8 mg, 8 mg and 8 mg. Low-dose recipients initiated their tapering dose at 10 mg and took the following doses on days 2–11 respectively: 10 mg, 8 mg, 8 mg, 6 mg, 6 mg, 4 mg, 4 mg, 2 mg, 2 mg and 2 mg.

The primary outcome measure was a comparison of the proportion of patients experiencing treatment failure in each treatment arm. Treatment failure was defined as sustained worsening for 5 or more months on any component of a composite outcome measure, or by relapse rate (three exacerbations treated with unscheduled methylprednisolone during 12 successive months). Components of the composite outcome measure included EDSS (> 1 point increase for baseline EDSS 4.0–5.0 or > 0.5 point increase for baseline EDSS 5.5–6.5), timed ambulation (> 1 point increase from baseline) and standardized tests of manual dexterity (20 per cent or more increase from baseline time on the best of two consecutive performances of BBT or 9HPT in either hand).

At the end of the 2 years, 53.7 per cent of the low-dose group and 38.9 per cent of the high-dose group met the criteria for treatment failure. This difference was not statistically significant ($P = 0.18$). However, a significant treatment effect was seen with the pre-planned secondary outcome, a log rank comparison of the survival curves of the low- and high-dose groups. The time to onset of sustained treatment failure was found to be delayed in the high-dose group ($P = 0.04$). Because the high-dose treatment failure rate did not reach 50 per cent, an estimated median time to onset of sustained treatment failure could not be compared across treatment groups. More high-dose than low-dose recipients experienced drug-related adverse events, but serious drug-related adverse events were uncommon. High-dose treatment was discontinued in only one patient, who experienced a transient psychotic reaction.

The results of this preliminary study demonstrate that cyclical pulses of steroids are safe and well-tolerated, appear to be efficacious in delaying progression of disability in SPMS patients, and may provide an additional alternative disease modifying treatment for SPMS patients with or without superimposed relapses. While widely used off-label, the optimal dose, route of administration and frequency of administration of this promising treatment for SPMS remains unknown.

Cyclophosphamide (Cytoxan®)

Cyclophosphamide is an alkylating agent widely used in the treatment of neoplastic and autoimmune disorders because of its potent cytotoxic and immunosuppressive effects. Although several unblinded trials of cyclophosphamide in chronic progressive MS have suggested a positive treatment effect (Hommes *et al.*, 1980; Hauser *et al.*, 1983; Goodkin *et al.*, 1987; Weiner *et al.*, 1993), these benefits have not been confirmed in placebo-controlled trials (Likosky *et al.*, 1991; TCCMSG, 1991). The variable results have been attributed to differences in patient selection, drug doses and criteria used to define clinical progression (Noseworthy *et al.*, 1991; Weiner *et al.*, 1991).

The toxicity of cyclophosphamide has been well characterized, and side effects include alopecia, haemorrhagic cystitis, leucopenia, myocarditis, pulmonary interstitial fibrosis, infertility and malignancy. In the light of these problems and the conflicting evidence for efficacy, the role of cyclophosphamide as a disease modifying therapy in SPMS is unclear. Cyclophosphamide is most frequently used for selected patients with SPMS who have not responded to other, less toxic, alternatives.

Reported results from phase III trials of disease modifying therapies for SPMS

The following section reviews the results of two phase III trials of disease modifying therapies in SPMS; 2-chlorodeoxyadenosine (Cladribine®) and mitoxantrone (Novantrone®). The results of these trials have been presented at international meetings, but full manuscripts have not yet been published and are not available for review.

2-chlorodeoxyadenosine (Cladribine®)

Cladribine® is a purine nucleoside which is resistant to adenosine deaminase and selectively targets lymphoid cells, both dividing and at rest. It was originally developed to mimic the immunodeficient state of hereditary adenosine deaminase deficiency (Carson *et al.*, 1983, 1984). It has been approved for the treatment of hairy cell leukaemia, but has also been shown to be effective in the treatment of autoimmune haemolytic anaemia and immune thrombocytopenia (Beutler, 1992).

In 1990 Sipe and colleagues conducted a phase II pilot study, treating four patients with chronic progressive MS with a 7-day infusion of six doses of IV Cladribine 0.087 mg/kg per day. The results of this pilot study suggested a positive treatment effect as measured by sustained improvement on the Scripps Neurologic Rating Scale (SNRS) (Sipe *et al.*, 1984), prompting further study of this therapy in a larger population. In 1994, the results of a 2-year double-blind, placebo-controlled, crossover study of Cladribine in 51 chronic progressive MS patients were published (Sipe *et al.*, 1994), and suggested a positive treatment effect on neurological rating scales.

In 1999, the results of the phase III study of Cladribine® in 159 patients with chronic progressive MS were reported (Rice *et al.*, 2000). EDSS scores of participants ranged from 3.0–6.5; 48 of the 159 patients had PPMS and 111 patients SPMS. Participants were randomly assigned to receive 2-chlorodeoxyadenosine 0.07 mg/kg per day for 5 consecutive days every 4 weeks for either two low-dose ($n = 53$) or six high-dose ($n = 52$) cycles, or placebo ($n = 54$). All participants completed eight treatment cycles; those completing active therapy cycles were switched to placebo for their remaining cycles to give a total of eight treatment cycles, and placebo recipients also received eight treatment cycles. Patients underwent neurological evaluations (EDSS) bimonthly and MRI scanning session every 6 months for 12 months.

No clinical treatment effects were seen across groups, as measured by mean changes in disability scores (EDSS and Scripps Neurological Rating Scale), proportion of patients experiencing a sustained increase on the EDSS scale (>1 point on the EDSS scale for baseline EDSS 3.0–5.0 or > 0.5 point for baseline EDSS 5.5–6.5), or time to onset of confirmed progression of disability. However, the placebo-controlled phase of this study lasted only 12 months, a time-frame that may be too brief to detect a significant effect on sustained progression of disability. Subgroup analyses demonstrated no significant difference in treatment effect between PPMS and SPMS patients. Analysis of MRI data, however, demonstrated a positive treatment effect favouring Cladribine®. Both low-dose and high-dose recipients with SPMS experienced fewer numbers of gadolinium-enhanced T1-weighted lesions ($P = 0.007$, $P = 0.001$ respectively), and the proportion of SPMS patients having gadolinium-enhanced T1-weighted lesions was significantly lower in Cladribine® recipients (low dose, $P = 0.013$; high-dose, $P = 0.002$). None of these treatment effects were observed in the PPMS recipients.

Cladribine® was well tolerated, with the exception of a dose-dependent lymphocytopenia and thrombocytopenia. There is significant potential for unwanted long-term marrow suppression and possible complications of bleeding, anaemia or opportunistic infection. In the absence of a convincing effect on sustained progression of disability, it is unlikely that Cladribine will be widely accepted or used as an alternative disease modifying therapy for patients with SPMS.

Mitoxantrone (Novantrone®)

Mitoxantrone is a cytotoxic anthracenedione that is currently approved as a first-line agent in the combination therapy of acute non-lymphocytic leukaemia and as initial chemotherapeutic in conjunction with corticosteroids for pain related to advanced hormone-refractory prostate cancer. It has also been successfully used to treat breast cancer, non-Hodgkin's lymphoma and hepatoma. Its mechanism of action has not been fully elucidated, but it is a DNA-intercalating agent with cytocidal activity on both proliferating and non-proliferating cultured human cells. It has also been shown to have potent immunosuppressive actions on B- and T-lymphocyte activity (Wang *et al.*, 1984, 1986; Fidler *et al.*, 1986). Because of these immunosuppressive actions, mitoxantrone has been studied in animal models of

MS as well as in phase II and phase III trials for the treatment of RRMS and SPMS. The use of mitoxantrone in RRMS is addressed in Chapter 8.

In 1998, the results of the European multicentre placebo-controlled phase III trial of mitoxantrone in progressive MS demonstrated a beneficial effect favouring treatment (Hartung and Gonsette, 1998). In this study, 194 patients with SPMS (with or without relapses) and aged 18–55 years with EDSS scores of 3.0–6.0 were randomized to receive mitoxantrone every 3 months for up to 24 months at a dose of 5 mg/m^2 ($n = 66$) or 12 mg/m^2 ($n = 63$), or placebo ($n = 65$). Participants underwent neurological evaluations every 3 months, and in a subgroup of 110 patients, brain MRI sessions were performed annually for 2 years. The primary outcome measure was mean change in EDSS. Additional clinical outcomes included mean change in Ambulation Index, number of relapses requiring steroid therapy, time to first relapse requiring steroid therapy, proportion of patients experiencing sustained worsening of EDSS, percentage of patients without relapses requiring treatment, mean number of relapses, and time to first relapse.

There were significant treatment effects measured by the primary outcome measure ($P = 0.038$) and most of the secondary clinical outcomes. In general, high-dose recipients experienced a more robust treatment effect. In the subgroup who completed annual MRI scanning sessions, there was a significant reduction in the number of new T2-weighted lesions in both low-dose and high-dose groups ($P < 0.05$) compared to placebo at the end of 2 years. A significant decrease in the number of new gadolinium-enhanced T1-weighted lesions was seen in the high-dose group only, at the end of 1 year ($P = 0.016$), and this effect was sustained at the end of 2 years ($P = 0.004$).

Overall, mitoxantrone was well tolerated during this study. Common side effects included a predictable and reversible leucopenia, mild alopecia, nausea and menstrual disorders. The left ventricular ejection fraction decreased by 10 per cent in 19 patients on mitoxantrone (19.2 per cent) and nine patients on placebo (13.8 per cent). An irreversible cardiomyopathy is reported to occur at cumulative doses of mitoxantrone over 140 mg/m^2 in cancer patients, but no evidence of clinically significant cardiac dysfunction was observed in this or other studies involving MS patients. Mitoxantrone is not currently widely used for the treatment of patients with SPMS, but its use will increase if approved by the FDA. Concern remains regarding cardiac toxicity with long-term usage of mitoxantrone, and careful attention should be directed at monitoring cardiac status with serial transthoracic echoes, particularly as patients approach or exceed cumulative doses of 140 mg/m^2.

Choosing disease modifying therapy for SPMS patients

It is often difficult to apply the results of controlled phase II and III clinical trials to clinical practice. Ideally, treatment decisions are data driven, but ultimately the choice of therapy for patients with progressive forms of MS reflects a clinician's clinical judgement and breadth of experience with various agents, as well as patient expectations. Table 9.3 outlines the authors' treatment algorithm for the available off-label therapies for secondary progressive MS.

Table 9.3 The authors' algorithm for treatment of secondary progressive MS

Population	Treatment considerations
Gradual progression of disability accompanied by frequent exacerbations **OR** accompanied by new Gd+ lesions	Interferon beta-1a or -1b (preferred); glatiramer acetate; methotrexate; cyclical pulses of IV methylprednisolone
Gradual progression of disability without frequent relapses and unaccompanied by new Gd+ lesions	Interferon beta-1b (preferred); oral weekly methotrexate; cyclical pulses of IV methylprednisolone; mitoxantrone; cyclophosphamide in selected patients with aggressive disease (women under 40 years of age may benefit more)

For patients with SPMS who experience frequent relapses, interferon beta therapy is a most appealing disease modifying treatment. If the suspicion of relapses is difficult to confirm clinically, an MRI scan may provide evidence of recent disease activity. Both interferon beta-1a and -1b products have been shown to decrease the relapse rate, reduce MRI activity and delay the time to onset of sustained progression of disability. If, however, interferon beta is poorly tolerated, or patients exhibit an inadequate response to therapy (either by relapse rate or progression of disability), glatiramer acetate, methotrexate, cyclical pulses of intravenous methylprednisolone, or mitoxantrone present alternative treatment options. The relative efficacies of these monotherapies, or combinations thereof, is unknown.

For SPMS patients who do not experience superimposed relapses, interferon beta-1b is approved for use in Europe and Canada, and is used off-label in the USA. For patients who continue to experience gradual progression of disability while taking interferon beta, treatment with methotrexate, cyclical pulses of intravenous methylprednisolone, or mitoxantrone should be considered. Cyclophosphamide is used by some investigators, especially in young patients who have an aggressive course. Some investigators believe that interferon beta may be an attractive treatment option for SPMS patients who experience new MRI lesions in the absence of clinical exacerbations, and the authors subscribe to this view.

There are currently no approved therapies for PPMS patients. In the absence of a rigorous controlled clinical trial for patients with primary progressive MS, it remains unclear how to treat this form of the disease. The results of on-going controlled clinical trials of interferon beta-1a, mitoxantrone and glatiramer acetate in primary progressive MS are awaited with interest.

References

Alarcon, G. S., Schrohenloher, R. E., Bartolucci, A. A. *et al.* (1990). Suppression of rheumatoid factor production by methotrexate in patients with rheumatoid arthritis. Evidence for differential influences of therapy and clinical status on IgM and IgA rheumatoid factor expression. *Arthr. Rheum.*, **33**, 1156–61.

Beutler, E. (1992). Cladribine (2-chlorodeoxyadenosine). *Lancet*, **340**, 952–6.

Calabrese, L. H., Taylor, J .V., Wilke, W. S. *et al.* (1988). Methotrexate (MTX) immunoregulatory T-cell subsets and rheumatoid arthritis: is MTX an immunomodulator? *Arthr. Rheum.*, **31(Suppl. 1)**, C20.

Carson, D. A., Wasson, D. B., Taetle, R. and Yu, A. (1983). Specific toxicity of 2-chloro-deoxyadenosine towards resting and proliferating human lymphocytes. *Blood*, **62**, 737–43.

Carson, D. A., Wasson, D. B. and Beutler, E. (1984). Antileukemic and immunosuppressive activity of 2-chloro-2′-deoxyadenosine. *Proc. Natl. Acad. Sci. USA*, **81**, 2232–6.

Cronstein, B. N. (1997). The mechanism of action of methotrexate. *Rheum. Dis. Clin. North. Am.*, **23(4)**, 739–55.

Dolhain, R. J. E. M., Tak, P. P., Dijkmans, B. A. C. *et al.* (1998). Methotrexate reduces inflammatory cell numbers, expression of monokines and of adhesion molecules in synovial tissue of patients with rheumatoid arthritis. *Br. J. Rheum.*, **37**, 502–8.

ESG (1998). European Study Group on interferon beta-1b in secondary progressive MS. Placebo-controlled multicentre randomised trial of interferon beta-1b in treatment of secondary progressive multiple sclerosis. European Study Group on interferon beta-1b in secondary progressive MS. *Lancet*, **352**, 1491–7.

Fidler, J. M., DeJoy, S. Q., Smith, F. R. III and Gibbon, J. J. (1986). Selective immunomodulation by the antineoplastic agent MTXN: suppression of B lymphocyte function. *J. Immunol.*, **137**, 727–32.

Fischer, J. S., Goodkin, D. E., Rudick, R. A. *et al.* (1994). Low-dose (7.5 mg) oral MTX improves neuropsychological function in patients with chronic progressive multiple sclerosis. *Ann. Neurol.*, **36**, 289.

Goodkin, D. E., Plencner, S., Palmer-Saxerud, K. *et al.* (1987). Cyclophosphamide in chronic progressive multiple sclerosis: maintenance vs non-maintenance therapy. *Arch. Neurol.*, **44**, 823–32.

Goodkin, D. E., Hertzgaard, D. and Seminary, J. (1988). Upper extremity function in multiple sclerosis: improving assessment sensitivity with box-and-block and nine-hole peg tests. *Arch. Phys. Med. Rehabil.*, **69**, 850–54.

Goodkin, D. E., Rudick, R. A., VanderBrug Medendorp, S. *et al.* Low-dose (7.5 mg) oral methotrexate reduces the rate of progression in chronic progressive multiple sclerosis. *Ann. Neurol.*, **37**, 30–40.

Goodkin, D. E., Rudick, R. A., VanderBrug Medendorp, S. *et al.* (1996). Low-dose oral methotrexate in chronic progressive multiple sclerosis: analyses of serial MRIs. *Neurology*, **47**, 1153–7.

Goodkin, D. E., Kinkel, R. P., Weinstock-Guttman, B. *et al.* (1998). A phase II study of IV methylprednisolone in secondary progressive multiple sclerosis. *Neurology*, **51**, 239–45.

Goodman, T. A. and Polisson, R. P. (1994). Methotrexate: adverse reactions and major toxicities. *Rheum. Dis. Clin. North. Am.*, **20(2)**, 513–28.

Grosflam, J. and Weinblatt, M. E. (1991). Methotrexate: mechanism of action, pharmacokinetics, clinical indications, and toxicity. *Curr. Opin. Rheumatol.*, **3**, 363–8.

Hartung, H. P. and Gonsette, R. (1998). MTX in progressive multiple sclerosis (MS): a PLC-controlled, randomized, observer-blind European phase III multi-center study-clinical results. *Multiple Sclerosis*, **4**, 325.

Hauser, S. L., Dawson, D. M., Lehrich, J. R. *et al.* (1983). Intensive immunosuppression with high dose cyclophosphamide, plasma exchange, and ACTH. *N. Engl. J. Med.*, **308**, 173–80.

Hine, R. J., Everson, M. P., Hardon, J. M. *et al.* (1990). Methotrexate therapy in rheumatoid arthritis patients diminishes lectin-induced mono-nuclear cell proliferation. *Rheumatol. Int.*, **10**, 165–9.

Hommes, O. R., Lamers, K. J. B. and Reekers, P. (1980). Effect of intensive immunosuppression on the course of chronic progressive multiple sclerosis. *J. Neurol.*, **223**, 177–90.

Kupersmith, M. J., Kaufman, D., Paty, D. *et al.* (1994). Megadose corticosteroids in MS. *Neurology*, **44**, 1–4.

Kurtzke, J. F. (1983). Rating neurological impairment in multiple sclerosis: an expanded disability scale (EDSS). *Neurology*, **33**, 1444–52.

Likosky, W. H., Fireman, B., Elmore, R. *et al.* (1991). Intense immunosuppression in chronic progressive multiple sclerosis: the Kaiser study. *J. Neurol. Neurosurg. Psychiatr.*, **54**, 1055–60.

Milligan, N. M., Newcombe, R. and Compston, D. A. S. (1987). A double-blind controlled trial of high dose methylprednisolone in patients with multiple sclerosis: 1. Clinical effects. *J. Neurol. Neurosurg. Psychiatr.*, **50**, 511–16.

Nielsen, H. J. and Hammer, J. H. (1992). Possible role of histamine in pathogenesis of autoimmune diseases: implications for immunotherapy with histamine-2 receptor antagonists. *Med. Hypoth.*, **39**, 349–55.

Nielsen, H. J., Nielsen, H. and Georgsen, J. (1991). Ranitidine for improvement of treatment resistant psoriasis. *Arch. Dermatol.*, **127**, 270.

Noseworthy, J. A., Vandervoort, M. K. and Penman, M. *et al.* (1991). CTX and plasma exchange in multiple sclerosis (letter). *Lancet*, **337**, 1540–41.

Olivieri, R. L., Valentino, P., Russo, C. *et al.* (1998). Randomized trial comparing two different high doses of methylprednisolone in MS: a clinical and MRI study. *Neurology*, **50**, 1833–6.

Rice, G. P. A., Filippi, M., and Comi, G. (2000). Cladribine and progressive MS: clinical and MRI outcomes of a multicenter controlled trial. Cladribine MRI Study Group. *Neurology* **54(5)**, 1145–55.

Rinne, U. K., Sonninen, V. and Tuovinen, T. (1968). Corticotrophin treatment in multiple sclerosis. *Acta Neurol. Scand.*, **44**, 207–18.

Segal, R., Yaron, M. and Tartakovsky, B. (1990). Methotrexate: mechanism of action in rheumatoid arthritis. *Sem. Arthr. Rheum.*, **20**, 190–200.

Sipe, J. C., Knobler, R. L., Braheny, S. L. *et al.* (1984). A neurologic rating scale (NRS) for use in multiple sclerosis. *Neurology*, **34**, 1368–72.

Sipe, J. C., Romine, J. S., Koziol, J. A. *et al.* (1994). Cladribine in the treatment of chronic progressive multiple sclerosis. *Lancet*, **344**, 9–13.

Sperling, R. I., Benincaso, A. I., Anderson, R. J. *et al.* (1992). Acute and chronic suppression of leukotriene B_4 synthesis ex vivo in neutrophils from patients with rheumatoid arthritis beginning treatment with methotrexate. *Arthr. Rheum.*, **35**, 376–84.

TCCMSG, The Canadian Cooperative Multiple Sclerosis Group (1991). The Canadian cooperative trial of cyclophosphamide and plasma exchange in progressive multiple sclerosis. *Lancet*, **337**, 441–6.

Tak, P. P., Smeets, T. J. M., Daha, M. R. *et al.* (1997). Analysis of the synovial cell infiltrate in early rheumatoid synovial tissue in relation to local disease activity. *Arthr. Rheum.*, **40**, 217–25.

Wang, B. S., Lumanglas, A. L., Ruzalla-Mellon, V. M. *et al.* (1984). Induction of alloreactive immunosuppression by 1,4-bis[(2-aminoethyl)amino]-5,8-dihydroxy-9,10-anthracenedione dihydrochloride. *Int. J. Immunopharmacol.*, **6**, 475.

Wang, B. S., Lumanglas, A. L., Silva, J. *et al.* (1986). Inhibition of induction of alloreactivty with MTXN. *Int. J. Immunopharmacol.*, **8(8)**, 967–73.

Weinblatt, M. E., Coblyn, J. S., Fox, D. A. *et al.* (1985). Efficacy of low-dose methotrexate in rheumatoid arthritis. *N. Engl. J. Med.*, **312**, 818–22.

Weinblatt, M. E., Weissman, B. N., Holdsworth, D. E. *et al.* (1992). Long-term prospective study of methotrexate in the treatment of rheumatoid arthritis. 84-month update. *Arthr. Rheum.*, **35**, 129–37.

Weiner, H. L., Hauser, S. L., Dawson, D. M. *et al.* (1991). CTX and plasma exchange in multiple sclerosis (letter). *Lancet*, **337**, 1033–4.

Weiner, H. L., Mackin, G. A., Orav, E. J. *et al.* (1993). Intermittent cyclophosphamide pulse therapy in progressive multiple sclerosis: final report of the Northeast Cooperative Multiple Sclerosis Treatment Group. *Neurology*, **43**, 910–18.

Disease modifying drugs – emerging therapies

10

Emerging therapies

This chapter will assess how emerging therapies may be able to target possible molecular mechanisms involved in the pathogenesis of MS. The detailed immunological control and mechanisms of dysregulation in MS are complex and outside the scope of this work; the reader is therefore referred to a comprehensive review on this subject (Hohlfeld, 1997). However, on the basis of current understanding several lines of disease modification could be or have been targeted, including:

1. Blockade of T-cell activation by the trimolecular complex; anti-T-cell receptor therapies
2. Neutralization of T-cell activation markers
3. Oral tolerance to autoantigens
4. Inhibition of adhesion and migration of inflammatory cells through the blood–brain barrier (BBB)
5. Anti-inflammatory agents
6. Agents promoting remyelination
7. Agents preventing axon loss.

A number of newer agents have already undergone preliminary trials in MS. Others are still in the very early stages of assessment, but will be discussed on the merits of their potential benefit.

T-cell receptor immunotherapy

There has been much interest in the possibility of developing a therapy that targets the trimolecular complex; T-cell receptor (TCR), major histocompatability complex molecules and antigenic peptides. This hypothesis has developed from experiments performed in the early 1980s, in which rats immunized to myelin basic protein (MBP) were resistant to developing experimental allergic encephalomyelitis (EAE) if they had been first exposed to inactivated encephalitogenic T-cells (Ben-Nun et al., 1981).

After determining the amino acid sequence of the TCR, synthetic peptides were used to show that anti-TCR peptide immunity suppressed responses to myelin basic protein and the development of EAE (Vandenbark *et al.*, 1989).

However, it is not clear whether the principles of immunotherapy for EAE are applicable to human disease. In MS, the spreading and diversification of the autoimmune response to additional myelin antigens, such as proteolipid protein and myelin oligodendrocyte protein, during the course of the disease raises questions regarding the applicability of specific anti-TCR therapy. Nevertheless, the work in EAE has led to preliminary trials using TCR immunotherapy in MS patients.

A double-blind, placebo-controlled study using a TCR peptide vaccine from the Vβ5.2 sequence expressed in MS lesions and on MBP-specific boosted peptide-reactive T-cells has been performed in patients with progressive MS (Vandenbark *et al.*, 1996). Vaccination with Vβ5.2 peptides, but not placebo, induced strong T-cell recognition of the TCR Vβ5.2 sequences. Significant boosting of T-cell responses to Vβ5.2-38-58 peptides occurred only in patients who received peptides. The authors were unable to detect any statistically significant differences in clinical outcome between the TCR peptide responders and the placebo-treated patients. However, a clinical benefit was reported in patients who responded to TCR peptide vaccination (none of six were clinically worse) versus non-responders receiving either peptide or placebo (10 of 17 were clinically worse). There was no evidence of drug toxicity or any apparent effects of immunosuppression.

Interpretation of this study has to be cautious given the small sample size, the short duration of follow-up, the absence of MRI data and the difficulty in detecting disability over time using the current measurement systems. However, it is promising that this study has shown the potential for immunological manipulation in MS without significant side effects.

One difficulty with this approach is the diversification of the immune response to additional myelin (and possibly even non-myelin) antigens during the course and progression of the disease. Such heterogeneity indicates that several TCR peptides may be required to suppress ongoing disease activity in MS. A study by Zipp *et al.* (1998) has shown a marked diversity of the anti-T-cell receptor immune response. It has therefore been suggested that candidate TCR peptides should be screened *in vitro* in functional experiments before they are clinically applied for TCR vaccination therapy (Hawke, 1998).

Another strategy is to use altered peptide ligands (APLs). These peptides, which differ from the original by one or two amino acids, have been shown to alter the pattern of cytokine production from T-cells and to produce T-cell anergy. A double-blind, randomized, placebo-controlled study took this approach in 30 MS patients, using an altered myelin basic protein peptide administered subcutaneously. This was well tolerated in the short term (Lindsey *et al.*, 1998), although the effect on clinical outcome is still unknown. A number of trials using T-cell receptor peptides or T-cell vaccination are now ongoing.

Neutralization of T-cell activation markers

Chimeric and humanized monoclonal antibodies

The premise of this therapy is to deplete specific subsets of T-lymphocytes in the systemic circulation, thus preventing cell migration and inflammation within the central nervous system (CNS).

Myelin-specific T-cells of the $CD4^+$ phenotype are known to exist in man, and are suspected to play an important role in the development of inflammation. Following activation and migration into the CNS, $CD4^+$ T-cells initiate a cascade of events, including release of pro-inflammatory cytokines. Using anti-CD4 antibody, a double-blind placebo-controlled randomized study was performed in 71 patients with clinically active relapsing–remitting or secondary progressive MS, using MRI and clinical outcome measures (van Oosten et al., 1997). Although there was an effective reduction in the circulating CD4 count in the treated group, no effect was observed in the frequency of new enhancing MRI lesions. The number of clinical exacerbations was lower by 41 per cent in the treatment group compared to placebo group.

A humanized monoclonal antibody has also been tested against CD52 T-cells in the form of CAMPATH-1H (Moreau et al., 1994). This treatment gave rise to a profound and prolonged lymphopenia, and was also associated with acute transient worsening of current symptoms or a recurrence of symptoms from previous clinical episodes. These episodes were associated with a marked increase in circulating levels of TNFα, IL-6 and interferon gamma. In addition, about 40 per cent of the patients on treatment developed autoimmune thyroid disease in the second year of treatment.

In 28 secondary progressive MS patients receiving a 5-day pulse of CAMPATH-1H, there was a virtual cessation of inflammatory activity for at least 18 months as detected by gadolinium-enhanced MR imaging. Despite this, approximately half the patients on treatment became progressively more disabled over time. Magnetic resonance studies showed progressive cerebral atrophy in these patients, which correlated with axon loss measured by proton magnetic resonance spectroscopy (Coles et al., 1999; Paolillo et al., 1999).

It is clearly disappointing that axonal degeneration seems to continue despite the absence of ongoing inflammation. It may be that the processes contributing to axon loss are already 'primed' in patients with longstanding progressive disease.

Cytokine based treatments

T-cells differentiate into distinct populations defined by the pattern of cytokines that they secrete. Th1 cells mainly secrete pro-inflammatory cytokines such as tumour necrosis factor (TNFα), IL-2 and interferon gamma, while Th2 cells predominantly secrete IL-4 and IL-10, which provide help for antibody-producing B-cells and can ameliorate autoimmune disease. A number of therapies have been advocated that attempt to downregulate the expression of Th1 cells and upregulate Th2 expression, but a major difficulty with this approach is that the precise role of Th1 and Th2 cells is not fully understood, and their effect may vary in different situations. Manipulation of the T-cell response can lead to clinical worsening rather than improvement. An example of this difficulty in predicting response occurred with preliminary treatment studies using TNFα antagonists. A study using an anti-TNF monoclonal antibody (cA2) showed an increase in MRI activity and worsening of CSF parameters (van Oosten et al., 1996a). A recent study using Lenercept (Lenercept Multiple Sclerosis Study Group et al., 1999), a recombinant TNF-receptor p55 immunoglobulin fusion protein, was stopped early. This agent neutralizes the effect of TNF, and patients receiving the active agent had an increased number of relapses with greater attack severity compared to the placebo group. There was also a trend towards greater MRI activity in the treatment groups, although this was not statistically significant. There is some evidence, however, that TNFα can have a potent anti-inflammatory effect, and it may be important for signalling in the elimination of inflammatory infiltrates (Eugster et al., 1999). A number of pharmacological inhibitors of TNFα synthesis, including thalidomide and pentoxifylline, are being assessed in trials. Regarding pentoxifylline, the preliminary results to date have been conflicting. Myers et al. (1995) failed to demonstrate an immunological effect at any dose, with continuing clinical and MRI evidence of deterioration in most of the 14 patients. Similarly, van Oosten et al. (1996b) failed to show an immunological effect in 20 patients. However, one study showed suppression of TNFα and IL-12 and enhanced production of IL-10 and IL-4 after oral administration of pentoxifylline (Rieckmann et al., 1998).

There is little information on attempts to increase expression of Th2-secreted cytokines, which may be expected to suppress inflammation. A study using transforming growth factor (TGFβ) showed no clinical or MRI effect over the course of a phase I trial in 11 patients (Calabresi et al., 1998). Five of the patients developed reversible nephrotoxicity. The use of IL-10 awaits evaluation.

Bone marrow transplantation

A less specific form of immune therapy is autologous or allogenic bone marrow transplantation (BMT). Autologous BMT has less significant morbidity, since there is no graft versus host response. Fassas et al. (1997) reported on 15 patients with progressive MS who underwent peripheral blood stem-cell transplantation after ablative treatment with bis carbo nitroso urea (BCNU), etoposide, cytosine arabinoside and melphelan, with antilymphocyte globulin given after transplantation. There was significant toxicity associated with the immediate procedure, although all patients survived. At a 6-month follow-up, seven patients were felt to have improved, one was worse and seven unchanged. However, by 1 year 12 of the 15 patients were dead.

Preliminary data have been presented by Samijn et al. (1999) regarding three patients who underwent T-cell depleted autologous BMT. The patients received total body irradiation and cyclophosphamide. Antithymocytic immunoglobulins were administered for in vivo T-cell depletion, and this was followed by CD34 selected autologous BMT. All patients suffered general malaise and two patients developed liver function disturbances and moderately severe skin problems, with two patients requiring parenteral feeding because of severe mucosal involvement. The follow-up reported to date is only 4 months, with no change in clinical outcome measures.

This form of treatment does not appear to stop clinical relapses, as evidenced by the patient who developed optic neuritis 2 months after allogenic BMT with ongoing evidence of activity on enhanced MRI (Jeffery and Alshami, 1998). Nevertheless, there are moves afoot for larger bone marrow transplant studies in MS.

Oral tolerance to autoantigens

Oral administration of an antigen can lead to immunological tolerance by two mechanisms; active cellular suppression and clonal anergy. Low doses of oral antigen mediate active suppression by the induction of regulatory T-cells in the gut-associated lymphoid tissue (GALT). These cells then migrate to the systemic immune system. Higher doses of oral antigen produce clonal anergy and deletion. It has been demonstrated that exposure to a specific oral autoantigen can produce widespread or bystander suppression to several antigens. This has the advantage in MS that there is no need to know the specific antigen that produces an autoimmune response. A phase III randomized, double-blind, placebo-controlled study of oral bovine myelin in 516 relapsing–remitting patients has been completed and published in abstract form (Francis *et al.*, 1997; Panitch *et al.*, 1997), and no improvement in MRI indices were observed. There was no significant difference in relapse rate between the treatment group and control group. Further studies using the principle of oral tolerance are in progress.

Inhibition of adhesion and migration of inflammatory cells through the blood–brain barrier

In order to target brain and spinal cord, activated T-cells must penetrate the blood–brain barrier. The process of homing and transmigration of activated T-lymphocytes is regulated by numerous adhesion molecules, which are reciprocally expressed on endothelial cells and leucocytes. There appear to be three important steps in the migration of activated T-cells across the BBB. First, leucocytes under shear stress attach to the vessel wall; the selectin group of adhesion molecules are of importance at this stage of tethering. Next, rolling leucocytes are stopped at the vascular lining under the influence of chemo-attractants such as C5a, chemokines and platelet-activating factor. Finally, the interaction of integrins such as ICAM-1 and VCAM-1 promotes strong adhesion to endothelium before transmigration through the endothelium occurs. The activated T-cells, having gained entry into the CNS, migrate along a path determined by chemotactic molecules released at the site of inflammation. It can therefore be concluded that adhesion molecules are critically important in leucocyte migration through endothelial barriers.

Adhesion molecules

Integrins are among the most versatile of the adhesion molecule families. They are thought to be essential for the interaction of endothelial cells with extracellular matrix components such as basement membranes. One such integrin is alpha-4 beta-1 ($\alpha4\beta1$) integrin (also called very late antigen-4, VLA-4). The interaction of $\alpha4\beta1$ integrin on T-lymphocytes with its counter receptor, vascular adhesion molecule-1 (VCAM-1) on endothelial cells, is an important mechanism in the trafficking of leucocytes across the endothelium and into the central nervous system.

Following a number of promising studies in experimental allergic encephalomyelitis models (Yednock *et al.*, 1992), it was proposed that antibodies against $\alpha4\beta1$ integrin might have therapeutic value in MS, both as a potential treatment of acute exacerbation and to inhibit the occurrence of subsequent attacks.

A preliminary multicentre randomized, double-blind, placebo-controlled trial has now been performed by Tubridy *et al.* (1999) in 70 patients with clinically definite, active, relapsing–remitting and secondary progressive MS. Two treatment doses were given 1 month apart. In total, 37 patients received anti-$\alpha4\beta1$ antibody and 33 received placebo. The active treatment group exhibited significantly fewer new active and new enhancing MRI lesions than the placebo group over the first 12 weeks, but there was no significant difference in the number of new active or new enhancing lesions in the second 12 weeks of the study. The number of patients with acute MS exacerbations was not significantly different in the two groups during the first 12 weeks, but was significantly higher in the treatment group in the second 12 weeks. The treatment group developed a significant lymphocytosis between weeks 1 and 12. The only statistically significant adverse effect was fatigue, which was reported by 12 patients in the treatment group and four in the placebo group.

In terms of clinical outcome, at week 12 there was a significant difference in the number of patients with an improved (from baseline) EDSS score in favour of the treated group. By the end of the study (week 24) the placebo group had returned to baseline mean EDSS score, and there was no significant difference between the two groups.

This was the first study to use a humanized monoclonal antibody to anti-$\alpha4\beta1$ integrin in patients with MS. The finding of a significant difference in the number of new active lesions between treatment group and placebo in the first 12 weeks of the study suggests that new lesion formation was suppressed, presumably by preventing the migration of T-lymphocytes and monocytes across the BBB. There was no effect on already established inflammatory lesions. This is not particularly surprising, since the $\alpha4\beta1$ integrin/VCAM interaction is a relatively early step in the process of cell trafficking and BBB breakdown in the formation of new MS lesions, with additional mechanisms likely to perpetuate the inflammatory process.

No treatment effect was observed in the second half of the study, in keeping with the return to normal levels of the lymphocyte count in this period and the very low levels of detectable anti-$\alpha4\beta1$ integrin levels. However, the relapse rate was significantly higher during this period in the treated group. This difference was partly related to a low relapse rate in the placebo group in this period. The authors noted that the number of MS relapse exacerbations was a secondary end-point, and that the study was therefore not powered to detect an effect on relapse rate; nevertheless, it remains quite possible that a rebound effect on exacerbation rate was associated with stopping treatment. This could perhaps be due to upregulation of VCAM-1 expression. There was no persistent effect on the clinical status scores.

In summary, this very short-term treatment did appear to have a short-lived effect on disease activity. Whether such an effect can be extended by repeated infusions at monthly intervals remains to be proven. However, no data exist for long-term safety and tolerance of the treatment with repeated administration. Finally, the treatment has yet to be shown to have a positive effect on the frequency or severity of clinical relapses. Further studies of longer duration and larger patient groups will need to concentrate not simply on MRI findings but also on clinical outcome as a primary endpoint.

Anti-inflammatory agents

Metalloproteinases

Matrix metalloproteinases (MMPs) are a large group of proteolytic enzymes that are involved in restructuring the extracellular matrix in response to a number of stimuli. An elevated expression of MMP contributes to tissue destruction and passage of cells across the BBB in MS. MMPs also seem to be involved in the regulation of a number of pro-inflammatory cytokines, such as tumour necrosis factor (TNFa). In a recent study, Lee *et al.* (1999) demonstrated an increase in a particular MMP, gelatinase B, and of the tissue inhibitors of matrix metalloproteinases (TIMP) TIMP-1 and TIMP-2 in a group of 21 patients with relapsing–remitting MS. Furthermore, gelatinase B levels were significantly higher during a clinical relapse compared with periods in which the patient was clinically quiescent. This study also showed a significant positive correlation between increased levels of gelatinase B and number of T1-weighted enhancing MRI lesions. It may seem unlikely that treatment with TIMP will have a disease modifying effect, given that large quantities of metalloproteinase inhibitor are already expressed *in vivo* in patients undergoing active relapse, but treatment at a very early stage in the inflammatory process may prevent upregulation of MMP expression and the activation of other proteases. There has been some success with matrix metalloproteinase inhibitors in the treatment of EAE (Liedtke *et al.*, 1998), and it seems quite likely that this form of treatment will be tried in the near future in MS patients.

Promotion of remyelination

There is good evidence that remyelination can and does occur in MS lesions (Prineas *et al.*, 1993). However, the degree to which remyelination can be enhanced in a manner that provides restoration of function in patients with the disease is still unknown. The issue of promoting remyelination is clearly a complex one. This form of treatment depends on being able simultaneously to switch off the inflammatory and demyelinating components of the disease, and it is almost certain that any remyelinating strategies would have to be combined with other agents that could fulfil this role. In this respect, intravenous immunoglobulin treatment is of interest. As discussed in Chapter 6, immunoglobulins have been shown to have a potential role in the inflammatory phase of the illness. Evidence that IVIg may have a potential role in remyelination comes from an observation of enhanced remyelination in animals with Theiler's murine encephalomyelitis virus (Rodriguez *et al.*, 1987) treated with immune serum raised by immunization with spinal cord homogenate. The remyelination effects were shown to be associated with the immunoglobulin fraction. However, use of IVIg in the human disease has not shown an improvement in either the vision or the visual evoked potential latency in patients with fixed deficit following an attack of optic neuritis (Noseworthy *et al.*, 1998). Similarly, no effect has been demonstrated after administration in patients with recently acquired and apparently permanent weakness (Noseworthy *et al.*, 1997).

Although mature oligodendrocytes are unable to divide and remyelinate, it has been shown that oligodendrocyte progenitor cells (which are capable of migration and remyelination) are present in the human adult nervous system (Scolding *et al.*, 1995) and, more specifically, in the MS lesion (Scolding *et al.*, 1998). A number of factors have been identified that, at least *in vitro*, can enhance oligodendrocyte cell division, migration and survival. One strategy that has been suggested is the harvesting of oligodendrocyte precursors from a patient, growing up this cell line *in vitro* using appropriate growth factors and then implanting these cell lines into lesions that have produced a well defined persistent clinical deficit. A clinical situation where this may be promising is selective remyelination of the superior cerebellar peduncle in patients with severe rubral tremor (Compston, 1998).

Agents preventing axon loss

Although recognized since the time of Charcot, it is only recently that axon loss has been considered an important pathological event in the evolution of the MS lesion. A number of new immunohistochemical techniques, including amyloid precursor protein staining (Ferguson *et al.*, 1997) and staining with the monoclonal antibody SMI-32 (Trapp *et al.*, 1998), have revealed transections of axons in human *post mortem* tissue, particularly in acute inflammatory lesions. Further evidence for axon loss and dysfunction comes from a number of studies using proton magnetic resonance spectroscopy (MRS). By measuring changes in N-acetyl aspartate (NAA), an amino acid localized to neurones and their axon processes, a number of groups have shown a correlation between axon loss and fixed clinical disability in MS patients (Davie *et al.*, 1995; de Stefano *et al.*, 1997). MRS has also shown reduced NAA (indicating axon loss or dysfunction) in normal-appearing white matter (Davie *et al.*, 1997; Fu *et al.*, 1998). The mechanisms that lead to axon loss are still not clear. It is of interest that matrix metalloproteinase expression is most conspicuous in areas of active inflammation, with a distribution coincident with amyloid protein precursor staining (Anthony *et al.*, 1997). Furthermore, an animal model based on a delayed hypersensitivity reaction to BCG, which produces early axonal damage, has shown that matrix metalloproteinase inhibitors can reduce both blood–brain barrier damage and the area of axonal and myelin damage (Matyszak and Perry, 1996).

It has also been hypothesized that axon loss in MS may occur as a form of programmed cell death. If this is initiated by some component of the inflammatory cascade, then there may be potential for therapies that enhance axon survival.

Conclusion

Future therapeutic progress will be based on, and refined by, a more detailed understanding of the mechanisms that trigger and mediate tissue damage in MS. The clinical course of the disease and the evolving pathology as detected using a range of MRI techniques (Miller *et al.*, 1998) should clarify which of these strategies is most likely to succeed in a particular patient, and also influence the timing of intervention.

One crucial aim in the next few years is to identify what is likely to be a number of genes responsible for the pathophysiological events occurring in the disease process. This should provide a greater focus in deciding which therapies should go forward for more intensive study. Given the diverse natural history of the disease, the constraints of phase II and III trials and the limitations of surrogate markers, such focus is needed. The number of patients unexposed to previous treatments and the resources of independent researchers are finite, and it is therefore fundamentally important that the continuing efforts to find a cure are driven by good science.

Table 10.1 Emerging therapies in the treatment of MS

Therapy	Putative mode of action	Type of MS (No. treated)	Outcome measure	Reference
TCR peptide vaccine Vβ5.2	Blockade of T cell activation	PP, SP (23)	Immunogenicity, clinical outcome	Vandenbark et al. (1996)
Altered peptide ligand	T cell anergy	RR, SP (30)	Tolerability, pharmacokinetics	Lindsey et al. (1998)
Anti CD4 antibody	Neutralization of T cell activation markers	RR (71)	MRI, clinical outcome	van Oosten et al. (1997)
Anti CD52 antibody	Neutralization of T cell activation markers	SP, PP (14)	MRI, MRS, clinical outcome, cytokine profile	Moreau et al. (1994), Coles et al. (1999)
Anti TNF-α antibody	Anti-cytokine effect	RR (2)	MRI, clinical outcome	van Oosten et al. (1996a)
TNFr fusion protein	Anti-TNF effect	RR (168)	MRI, clinical outcome	Lenercept Multiple Sclerosis Study Group et al. (1999)
Pentoxifylline	Inhibits TNF-α synthesis	RR, SP (>35)	MRI, clinical outcome, immunogenicity	Myers et al. (1995), van Oosten et al. (1996b), Rieckmann et al. (1996)
TGF-β	Suppresses inflammatory activity; inhibition of pro-inflammatory cytokines	SP (11)	MRI, clinical outcome	Calabresi et al. (1998)
Autologous bone marrow transplantation	Immune inactivation and reconstitution	SP (15)	Clinical outcome	Fassas et al., 1997
Oral bovine myelin	Immunological tolerance, bystander suppression	RR (516)	Clinical outcome, MRI	Francis et al. (1997), Panitch et al. (1997)
Anti-α4β1 integrin antibody	Blocks leucocyte transport across blood–brain barrier	RR, SP (70)	MRI, clinical outcome	Tubridy et al. (1999)

References

Anthony, D. C., Miller, K. M., Fearn, S. *et al.* (1997). Differential matrix metalloproteinase expression in cases of multiple sclerosis and stroke. *Neuropathol. Appl. Neurobiol.*, **23**, 406–15.

Ben-Nun, A., Wekerle, H. and Cohen, I. R. (1981). Vaccination against autoimmune encephalomyelitis with T-lymphocyte line cells reactive against myelin basic protein. *Nature*, **292**, 60–61.

Calabresi, P. A., Fields, N. S., Maloni, H. W. *et al.* (1998). Phase I trial of transforming growth factor beta 2 in chronic progressive MS. *Neurology*, **51**, 289–92.

Coles, A. J., Wing, M. G., Molyneux, P. *et al.* (1999). Monoclonal antibody treatment exposes three mechanisms underlying the clinical course of multiple sclerosis. *Ann. Neurol.*, **46**, 296–304.

Compston, A. (1998). Future options for therapies to limit damage and enhance recovery. *Sem. Neurol.*, **18**, 405–11.

Davie, C. A., Barker, G. J., Webb, S. *et al.* (1995). Persistent functional deficit in multiple sclerosis and autosomal dominant cerebellar ataxia. *Brain*, **118**, 1583–92.

Davie, C. A., Barker, G. J., Thompson, A. J. *et al.* (1997). 1H magnetic resonance spectroscopy of chronic cerebral white matter lesions and normal appearing white matter in multiple sclerosis. *J. Neurol. Neurosurg. Psychiatr.*, **63**, 736–42.

de Stefano, N., Matthews, P. M., Narayanan, S. *et al.* (1997). Axonal dysfunction and disability in a relapse of multiple sclerosis: longitudinal study of a patient. *Neurology*, **49**, 1138–41.

Eugster, H. P., Frei, K., Bachmann, R. *et al.* (1999). Severity of symptoms and demyelination in MOG-induced EAE depends on TNFR1. *Eur. J. Immunol.*, **29**, 626–32.

Fassas, A., Anagnstopolous, A., Kassis, A. *et al.* (1997). Peripheral blood stem cell transplantation in the treatment of progressive multiple sclerosis: first results of a pilot study. *Bone Marrow Trans.*, **20**, 631–8.

Ferguson, B., Matyszak, M. K., Esiri, M. M. and Perry, V. H. (1997). Axonal damage in acute multiple sclerosis lesions. *Brain*, **120**, 393–9.

Francis, G., Evans, A. and Panitch, H. (1997). MRI reults of a phase III trial of oral myelin in relapsing–remitting MS (abstract). *Ann. Neurol.*, **42**, 467.

Fu, L., Matthews, P. M., de Stefano, N. *et al.* Imaging axonal damage in normal appearing white matter. *Brain*, **121**, 103–13.

Hawke, S. (1998). T-cell receptor immunotherapy in multiple sclerosis (editorial). *Brain*, **121**, 1391–3.

Hohlfeld, R. (1997). Biotechnical agents for the immunotherapy of multiple sclerosis. Principles, problems and perspectives. *Brain*, **120**, 865–916.

Jeffery, R. and Alshami, E. (1998). Allogenic bone marrow transplantation in multiple sclerosis (abstract). *Neurology*, **50**, A147.

Lee, A. M., Palace, J., Stabler, G. *et al.* (1999). Serum gelatinase B, TIMP-1 and

TIMP-2 levels in multiple sclerosis. A longitudinal clinical and MRI study. *Brain*, **122**, 191–7.

Lenercept Multiple Sclerosis Study Group and University of British Columbia MS/MRI Analysis Group (1999). TNF neutralization in MS: results of a randomized, placebo-controlled multicenter study. *Neurology*, **53**, 457–65.

Liedtke, W., Cannella, B., Mazzaccaro, R. J. *et al.* (1998). Effective treatments of models of multiple sclerosis by matrix metalloproteinase inhibitors. *Ann. Neurol.*, **44**, 35–46.

Lindsey, J. W., Lublin, F. D., Stark, S. R. *et al.* (1998). Double-blind, randomized, placebo-controlled evaluation of the safety, tolerability, and pharmacokinetics of CGP 77116 in patients with multiple sclerosis (abstract). *Neurology*, **50**, A139.

Matyszak, M. K. and Perry, V. H. (1996). Delayed-type hypersensitivity lesions in the CNS are prevented by inhibitors of matrix metalloproteinases. *J. Neuroimmunol.*, **69**, 141–9.

Miller, D. H., Grossman, R. I., Reingold, S. C. and McFarland, H. F. (1998). The role of magnetic resonance techniques in understanding and managing multiple sclerosis. *Brain*, **121**, 3–24.

Moreau, T., Thorpe, J., Miller, D. *et al.* (1994). Reduction in new lesion formation in multiple sclerosis following lymphocyte depletion with CAMPATH-1H. *Lancet*, **344**, 298–301.

Myers, L. W., Ellison, G. W., Merrill, J. E. *et al.* (1995). Pentoxifylline: not a promising treatment for multiple sclerosis. *Neurology*, **459(Suppl. 4)**, A419.

Noseworthy, J. H., Weinshenker, B. G., O'Brien, P. C. *et al.* (1997). Intravenous immunoglobulin (IVIg) does not reverse recently acquired, apparently permanent weakness in multiple sclerosis. American Neurological Association, San Diego. *Ann. Neurol.*, **42**, 42.

Noseworthy, J. H., O'Brien, P. C., Petterson, T. M. *et al.* (1998). Immunoglobulin administration (IVIG) does not reverse visual acuity loss in long-standing optic neuritis associated with multiple sclerosis. American Neurological Association, Minneapolis. *Neurology*, **50A**.

Panitch, H., Francis, G. and the Oral Myelin Study Group (1997). Clinical results of a phase III trial of oral myelin in relapsing-remitting multiple sclerosis (abstract). *Ann. Neurol.*, **42**, 459.

Paolillo, A., Coles, A., Molyneux, P. *et al.* (1999). Quantitative MRI in patients with secondary progressive MS treated with monoclonal antibody, CAMPATH-1H. *Neurology*, **53**, 751–7.

Prineas, J. W., Barnard, R. O., Kwon, E. E. *et al.* (1993). Multiple sclerosis: remyelination of nascent lesions. *Ann. Neurol.*, **33**, 137–51.

Rieckmann, P., Weber, F., Gunther, A. *et al.* (1996). Pentoxifylline, a phosphodiesterase inhibitor, induces immune deviation in patients with multiple sclerosis. *J. Neuroimmunol.*, **64**, 193–200.

Rodriguez, M., Lennon, V. A., Benviste, E. N. and Merrill, J. E. (1987). Remyelination by oligodendrocytes stimulated by antiserum to spinal cord. *J. Neuropathol. Exp. Neurol.*, **46**, 84–95.

Samijn, J. P. A., Schipperus, M. R., van Doorn, P. A. *et al.* (1999). T-cell depleted autologous bone marrow transplantation for multiple sclerosis: transplantation toxicity and early results in three patients (abstract). *J. Neurol.*, **246**, 1/36–1/37.

Scolding, N. J., Rayner, P. J., Sussman, J. *et al.* (1995). A proliferative adult human oligodendrocyte progenitor. *Neuroreport*, **6**, 441–5.

Scolding, N., Franklin, R., Stevens, S. *et al.* (1998). Oligodendrocyte progenitors are present in the normal adult human CNS and in the lesions of multiple sclerosis. *Brain*, **121**, 2221–8.

Trapp, B. D., Peterson, J., Ransohoff, R. M. *et al.* (1998). Axonal transection in the lesions of multiple sclerosis. *N. Engl. J. Med.*, **338**, 278–85.

Tubridy, N., Behan, P. O., Capildeo, R. *et al.* (1999). The effect of anti-alpha 4 integrin antibody on brain lesion activity in MS. *Neurology*, **53**, 466–72.

Vandenbark, A. A., Hashim, G. and Offner, H. (1989). Immunization with synthetic T-cell receptor V-region peptide protects against experimental autoimmune encephalomyelitis. *Nature*, **341**, 541–4.

Vandenbark, A. A., Chou, Y. K., Whitham, R. *et al.* (1996). Treatment of multiple sclerosis with T-cell receptor peptides: Results of a double-blind pilot trial. *Nat. Med.*, **2**, 1109–15.

van Oosten, B., Barkhof, F., Truyen, L. *et al.* (1996a). Increased MRI activity and immune activation in two multiple sclerosis patients treated with the monoclonal anti-tumour necrosis factor antibody cA2. *Neurology*, **47**, 1531–4.

van Oosten, E. W., Rep, M. H. G., van Lier, R. A. W. *et al.* (1996b). A pilot study investigating the effects of orally administered pentoxifylline on selected immune variables in patients with multiple sclerosis. *J. Neuroimmunol.*, **66**, 49–55.

van Oosten, B. W., Lai, M., Hodgkinson, S. *et al.* (1997). Treatment of multiple sclerosis with the monoclonal anti-CD4 antibody cM-T412; results of a randomised, double-blind placebo-controlled, MR monitored phase 11 trial. *Neurology*, **49**, 351–7.

Yednock, T. A., Cannon, C., Fritz, L. C. *et al.* (1992). Prevention of experimental autoimmune encephalomyelitis by antibodies against alpha4-beta1. *Nature*, **356**, 63–6.

Zipp, F., Kerschensteiner, M., Dornmair, K. *et al.* (1998). Diversity of the anti-T-cell receptor immune response and its implications for T-cell vaccination therapy of multiple sclerosis. *Brain*, **121**, 1395–1407.

Disease modifying drugs – overview

Overview of treatment strategies for relapsing and progressive disease

Introduction

With the development of new treatments in multiple sclerosis, it will be necessary to adopt treatment strategies for the practising clinician in order to decide on the most appropriate regimen to use in an individual patient at a particular point in time. Information about a drug's benefit and side effects will necessarily reflect an evolving database of knowledge. However, it is now a convenient time to consider a rational approach to treatment, with many of the larger clinical trials completed and reported on and new putative treatments being considered as a result.

Relapsing–remitting disease with minor or no cumulative disability (EDSS 0–3)

On the basis of data currently available from clinical trials, it would be appropriate to consider treating a patient who has had two relapses in a 3-year period. However, an individual clinician may decide to commence therapy in patients with less frequent relapses if clinical presentation or MRI lesion load suggest that this would be appropriate. Should the patient's relapses be of a generally mild type, without having a significant effect on daily life and without causing a major residual or accumulating deficit, then interferon beta or glatiramer acetate would be expected to reduce relapse rate by about one-third (see Chapters 3–5). Glatiramer acetate is a suitable drug for those patients who would like to minimize side effects, although it needs to be injected subcutaneously on a daily basis. However, interferon beta is an equally suitable option, and although generally has more side effects in the first 6 months, it requires less frequent injections. Interferon beta-1b or -1a could be used, and interferon beta-1a can be administered by thrice weekly subcutaneous or weekly intramuscular injections. The relative merits of a treatment in slowing down the progress of the condition will not be such an important issue in patients with a minor cumulative deficit. Immunoglobulin could also be considered for such patients, although whether benefit continues in the long term is unknown, and the theoretical but unlikely possibility of viral transmission must be taken into account (see Chapter 6).

Relative advantages and disadvantages of available treatments are given in Table 11.1.

Table 11.1 Relapsing–remitting disease with minor or no cumulative disability (EDSS 0–3)

	Advantages	Disadvantages
Glatiramer acetate	Reduction in relapse rate similar to interferon beta, minimal side effects	Daily injection, occasional systemic reactions
Interferon beta-1b	Sustained reduction in relapse rate (3 years)	Initial systemic side effects (initial frequent neutralizing antibodies)
Interferon beta-1a (Rebif®)	Reduced relapse rate (with delayed progression in short term)	Subcutaneous injection reactions, thrice weekly injection
Interferon beta-1a (Avonex®)	Reduced relapse rate (with delayed progression in short term)	Intramuscular injection not always tolerated, initial systemic side effects
Immunoglobulin	Apparent effect on relapse rate (and progression in short term), theoretical remyelination potential	Infrequent hypersensitivity reactions (theoretical viral transmission)

Relapsing–remitting disease with moderate cumulative disability (EDSS ≥ 3.5)

In patients who have more aggressive relapsing–remitting disease, with relapses affecting the activities of daily life and incomplete recovery leading to cumulative neurological deficit over a short time period, a different therapeutic strategy might be adopted. In general, patients in this group will have had at least two relapses in the previous 2 years, at least one of which has been a severe relapse without complete recovery. Interferon beta-1a has been shown to be of benefit in delaying the progression of the condition in the short term, as well as reducing relapse rate (see Chapter 4). Avonex® has not been formally studied in this group of patients. Subgroup analysis of the Rebif® trial has suggested that patients who have a Kurtzke EDSS > 3.5 would benefit from the higher dose of 12 Miu rather than the standard 6 Miu thrice weekly (see Chapter 4). Retrospective analysis of the pivotal interferon beta-1b trial suggested delayed progression for patients with EDSS ≥ 4 (see Chapter 3). Glatiramer acetate has also been shown to delay progression in the short term (see Chapter 5), and immunoglobulin may be considered although further studies are required to confirm its effect on progression of disability (see Chapter 6). Alternative possibilities would include azathioprine, particularly in those patients who cannot tolerate injection, although its therapeutic effect is often delayed and the long-term risks of immunosuppression and possibly malignancy need to be considered (see Chapter 7). Mitoxantrone could be contemplated in patients with particularly aggressive disease, although the total dose of the drug given will be limited by potential cardiotoxicity (see Chapter 8).

Medications are compared and contrasted in Table 11.2.

Table 11.2 Relapsing–remitting disease with moderate cumulative disability (EDSS ≥ 3.5)

	Advantages	Disadvantages
Immunomodulation		
Interferon beta-1a (Rebif®)	Reduced relapse rate with delayed progression in short term	Subcutaneous injection reactions, thrice weekly injection
Interferon beta-1b	Reduced relapse rate (and delayed progression in short term, EDSS ≥ 4)	Initial systemic side-effects (initial frequent neutralizing antibodies)
Glatiramer acetate	Reduction in relapse rate and delayed progression in short term, similar to interferon beta, minimal side effects	Daily injection, occasional systemic reactions
Immunoglobulin	Apparent effect on relapse rate and progression in short term, theoretical remyelination potential	Infrequent hypersensitivity reactions (theoretical viral transmission)
Immunosuppression		
Azathioprine	Similar effect on relapse rate to interferon beta/glatiramer acetate	Delayed treatment effect, immunosuppression, possible malignancy
Mitoxantrone	Marked effect on relapse rate (in patients with frequent relapses)	Potential toxicity (including cardiotoxicity)

Secondary progressive disease

Most patients will enter a slowly progressive phase of their condition after a variable period of time. Such progression is a gradual phenomenon, usually affecting motor and cerebellar function, and although relapses may continue to occur, progression is not clearly dependent on clinically defined relapses or neurological deficit resulting from them. The usual type of progressive disease is secondary progression following an initial relapsing–remitting course. Interferon beta-1b has been shown to be of modest benefit in slowing progression in the early stages of secondary progressive disease; however, whether this benefit continues after a 2-year period is uncertain, and follow-up data may clarify matters (see Chapters 3 and 9). Interferon beta-1a (Rebif®) was found to have a less convincing effect on progression over a 3-year period in patients with established progressive disease (see Chapter 4). Immunoglobulin is currently being studied in this group of patients (see Chapter 6). Azathioprine is not thought to have a major effect on secondary progression (see Chapter 7). The results of mitoxantrone in secondary progressive disease are encouraging, and long-term toxicity studies are awaited with interest (see Chapters 8 and 9). There are currently no effective therapies for patients whose progressive disease begins in the absence of well-defined relapses; therapy for the primary progressive forms of MS remains under investigation.

The term 'chronic progression' has been used to describe patients who have a slowly progressive course without accompanying relapses, and many will have secondary progressive disease although a proportion will be primary progressive. Methotrexate appears to be of modest benefit in this group of patients in slowing the progression of upper limb dysfunction (see Chapter 9).

A concluding table of the relative merits of possible treatments is given in Table 11.3.

Table 11.3 Secondary progressive disease

	Advantages	Disadvantages
Interferon beta-1b	Delayed progression in short term, and reduced relapse rate	Subcutaneous injection reactions, initial systemic side effects
Interferon beta-1a (Rebif®)	Reduced relapse rate with suggested delayed progression in females only (in short term)	Subcutaneous injection reactions, initial systemic side effects
Mitoxantrone	Reduced relapse rate with delayed progression in short term	Potential toxicity (including cardiotoxicity)
Methotrexate	Modest effect on upper limb function (for example, in patients increasingly dependent on wheelchair)	Potential immunosuppression, possible hepatic or respiratory complications

Clearly a rational approach to treatment will depend on an individual patient's needs. In certain circumstances it may be inappropriate to consider disease modifying treatments, or a compromise may be chosen to modify the disease but minimize side effects and concentrate on the important aspects of symptomatic therapy and neurological rehabilitation (in relatively disabled patients). These matters will be addressed in the remaining chapters of this book.

Symptomatic management

Management of spasticity – pharmacological agents

Introduction

Spasticity in multiple sclerosis is common and often disabling, but its management can be successful and highly rewarding. The main purpose of this chapter is to describe the pharmacological management of spasticity, and Chapter 13 will describe the management of focal spasticity, particularly by the use of botulinum toxin. However, it is important to emphasize that although spasticity can often be managed by the use of systemic or focal pharmacological agents, the overall treatment strategy should remain multidisciplinary. The physiotherapist and orthotist are important contributors to the overall management.

What is spasticity?

Spasticity is basically an increase in muscle tone, which on examination is characterized by hyperactive stretch reflexes. Spasticity is velocity dependent; in other words, it increases the faster the muscle is stretched. This initial increase in resistance to passive stretch is often followed by a loss of tone – the clasp-knife phenomenon. However, spasticity is usually seen in association with other features of the upper motor neurone (UMN) syndrome, which encompasses an array of positive and negative phenomena that will often influence the overall treatment strategy. Positive phenomena are characterized by excessive motor activity, and include such phenomena as clonus, rigidity, and flexor and extensor spasms. These features can themselves contribute to functional disability, and are often responsible for problems in hygiene and self-care, and for some of the more distressing features of spasticity, such as pain. However, the UMN syndrome also encompasses a number of negative phenomena characterized by a reduction in motor activity, such as weakness, fatigue, slow initiation and consequent loss of dexterity. These are features that can also be associated with significant disability. Thus, it is the whole UMN syndrome that should be taken into account when treatment goals and strategies are being designed. Such an assessment should include the management of other complications of hypertonia, including muscle and soft tissue contracture.

This chapter does not allow for a detailed discussion of the pathophysiology of spasticity. However, it does seem that very little of the clinical UMN syndrome arises because of interruption of the pyramidal tracts (Brown, 1994). Isolated lesions of the pyramidal tracts usually only produce some mild loss of manual dexterity, perhaps an extensor plantar response with mild hypertonia and hyper-reflexia. Most of the features of the UMN syndrome result from involvement of the para-pyramidal tracts, particularly the dorsal reticulo-spinal, medial reticulo-spinal and vestibulo-spinal tracts. These three tracts (the first inhibitory and the latter excitatory) provide control over the interneuronal networks in the spinal cord, which in turn are the main neural influence upon the lower motor neurones. If the neuronal balance between inhibitory and excitatory influences is disturbed in favour of an overall excitation of the system, then spasticity and other features of the UMN syndrome will result. Most of the pharmacological agents used in spasticity seem to have an effect on this inhibitory/excitatory balance.

Treatment goals

The first step in management strategy for spasticity is identification of treatment goals. Spasticity may be abnormal, but is not necessarily harmful and increased muscle tone can be helpful to promote standing and transfers in an otherwise weak muscle. Flexor or extensor spasms can sometimes be utilized to assist in standing or dressing. Occasionally spasticity, whilst unhelpful, is relatively mild, and the minimal resulting disability needs to be balanced against the potentially disabling side effects of treatment. This balance is usually most difficult to achieve in mild spasticity, and, as a generalization, the more severe the spasticity, the more likely the need for therapeutic intervention. There are many potential goals for treatment, all of which need proper discussion primarily with the patient but also with the carer or family and the rehabilitation team. The commonest goals are likely to be:

• Reduction in pain
• Improvement in mobility
• Improved seating position
• Easier fitting of orthoses or easier physiotherapy exercises
• Reduction in risk of complications from contractures and/or pressure sores
• Ease of nursing care during such procedures as washing, transferring and changing a catheter.

Naturally, an individual may have more than one treatment goal; nevertheless, each one should be agreed and carefully recorded so that the effect of any intervention can be monitored and the treatment adjusted accordingly.

Outcome measures

The treatment goal should determine an appropriate outcome measure. If, for example, reduction of pain is the desired goal, then a pain scale is an appropriate outcome measure. If ease of nursing care or improvement of hygiene are the desired outcomes, then the nurse or carer should attend (or provide a report for) each outpatient or treatment session. The actual measurement of spasticity is rarely necessary in a clinical setting, and there are very few simple valid and reliable measures of spasticity that can be applied in a busy outpatient clinic. There are various biomechanical measures of resistance to passive stretch, including the Wartenburg pendulum test (Bajd and Bowmand, 1982), and a variety of torque generators that can be fixed to the limb and measure the amount of force induced by moving a limb over a certain angle. However, biomechanical equipment tends to be expensive and not readily applicable in a clinical setting. Quantitative neurophysiological measurements of spasticity have largely been developed as research tools, and measurements mainly focus on characteristics of the H reflex, particularly suppression of the reflex by vibration and reciprocal inhibition. These techniques are well reviewed by Shahani and Cross (1990).

However, these measures are also time consuming and not of great use outside a research environment. In a clinical setting, goniometry (measurement of joint range) is at present the most commonly performed measurement of treatment efficacy, but this is probably not reliable other than at large joints. One of the few practical scales is the Modified Ashworth Scale (Bohannon and Smith, 1987), but even this scale is rarely accurate enough to be a useful monitor of a treatment goal. It is mainly a measurement of impairment and not a measurement of disability or handicap. It is better to use specific tests of impairment of relevant limb functioning, such as the Motoricity Index (Demeurisse *et al.*, 1980), a timed walking test (Bradstater *et al.*, 1983) or the nine-hole peg test (Mathiowetz *et al.*, 1985). More relevant to the individual would be the use of handicap and quality of life measures such as the Nottingham Health Profile (Hunt *et al.*, 1980) or the Newcastle Independence Assessment Form (Semlyen *et al.*, 1996). However, spasticity intervention is not likely to produce significant differences on such broad-based scales.

Non-pharmacological treatment of spasticity

In milder spasticity, the treatment goal will often be achieved by attention to relatively simple measures. It may, for example, be sufficient to reduce afferent sensory input due to inappropriate seating, tight catheter leg bags or poorly fitting orthoses, or by attention to painful skin conditions such as pressure sores. At this early stage, advice from a physiotherapist and/or orthotist regarding wheelchair and seating assessment and orthoses may be all that is required to achieve the desired outcome. There are a number of active physiotherapy techniques that are purported to be anti-spastic in nature, including the Bobath technique and the approach advocated by Carr and Shepherd (Edwards, 1996). There is little evidence that any particular technique is more advantageous than another in terms of anti-spastic efficacy, but both active and passive physiotherapy can clearly have a role in its management, particularly in terms of positioning, seating and mobility, and the appropriate use of splints, casts and orthoses. The reader is referred to a modern text on this subject for further detail (Edwards, 1996).

Pharmacological treatment

General points

Oral anti-spastic agents are generally more helpful in diffuse muscle spasticity rather than spasticity localized to one or just a few muscle groups. In the latter circumstances, a more focal approach to treatment such as phenol nerve blocks or botulinum toxin is often more appropriate. However, even in focal spasticity oral agents can sometimes be useful to give a 'background' muscle relaxation. In milder cases, oral agents can be sufficient in themselves to achieve the necessary treatment goal. However, in the majority of cases – and particularly those with moderate to severe spasticity – oral agents are often only part of the whole therapeutic approach. There are now three commonly used anti-spastic agents; baclofen, dantrolene and tizanidine. All of these agents have a clear anti-spastic effect, but all tend to share the same profile of side effects, particularly weakness, drowsiness and fatigue, and it is often these effects that limit their usefulness. They all tend to share a relatively narrow therapeutic window, with unacceptable side effects often appearing at roughly the same dosage level as the anti-spastic effects. In general, oral agents should be introduced at low doses and the dose increased slowly, with careful monitoring of optimal clinical effects and unhelpful side effects. The following section will illustrate that these drugs probably work at different pharmacological levels, and there is some limited evidence that using them in combination at low doses may produce the desired clinical outcome without the appearance of undesirable side effects.

A mention will also be made of the largely historical use of benzodiazepines and of some other agents that have shown some promise as anti-spastic agents but are not yet widely commercially available.

Finally, the use of intrathecal agents (particularly baclofen and phenol) that have a specialist place in the management of spasticity will be addressed.

Diazepam

Mechanism of action
It is likely that the anti-spastic effects of diazepam and other benzodiazepines are mediated through the $GABA_a$ receptor. Benzodiazepines are known to enhance the affinity of GABA binding to $GABA_a$ receptors. This has the effect of increasing the inhibitory post-synaptic effect of GABA, and it is thought that this is the main mechanism of action of the benzodiazepines (Schlosser, 1971).

Pharmacology

Diazepam is a well-established anti-spastic agent, and indeed was the first to be used in clinical practice, about 30 years ago (Wilson and McKechnie, 1966). It is a long-acting benzodiazepine, is well absorbed and obtains peak blood levels in 1–2 hours. It has active metabolites, N-desmethyl-diazepine and oxazepam, and quite a long half-life of around 20–50 hours. The active metabolite desmethyl-diazepine has a half-life up to 100 hours. Thus, there can be problems of withdrawal. It is also highly lipid-soluble and readily crosses the blood–brain barrier; it thus has a particularly wide range of central nervous system effects.

Clinical efficacy

Diazepam was introduced some time ago, and has not been subject to rigorous evaluation. However, there have been two high-quality, double-blind, cross-over studies that have demonstrated efficacy (Wilson and McKechnie, 1966; Verrier *et al.*, 1977), and there have also been a number of comparative studies against baclofen (Cartlidge *et al.*, 1974; Roussan *et al.*, 1987). In general, these studies have shown that both drugs are equally effective with regard to reduction of spasticity in multiple sclerosis and spinal cord injury, but day time sedation was significantly more common with diazepam. In addition, both clinicians and patients preferred baclofen in the majority of studies.

Dosage

Treatment is usually initiated at about 2 mg daily, slowly building up with 2 mg increments to a maximum dose of 40–60 mg per day in divided doses. However, the maximum dose is not often achieved, as the drug is significantly limited by side effects.

Side effects

The commoner adverse effects relate to central nervous system depression, and include drowsiness, fatigue and unsteadiness (Kendall, 1964; Cocchiarella *et al.*, 1967). The elderly are particularly sensitive to unpleasant side effects, as are those with a tendency to confusion (e.g. individuals with pre-senile dementia). The drug should also be used with care in those with an acquired brain injury because of potential adverse effects on concentration, attention and memory. There is a range of other less common side effects, including headache, visual disturbance, hypotension, gastrointestinal problems, skin rashes, vertigo and reduced libido. Regrettably, withdrawal symptoms are also quite common, and include anxiety, depression, nervousness, agitation, irritability, restlessness, tremor, sweating, nausea and diarrhoea. This unfortunate range of adverse effects usually follows abrupt cessation or rapid tapering of treatment, and the drug should therefore be withdrawn very slowly.

Conclusion

Although diazepam is an efficacious anti-spastic agent, it has no advantages over more modern alternatives and is significantly limited by central nervous system depressive side effects. It is no longer in widespread usage as an anti-spastic medication.

Other benzodiazepines

Other benzodiazepines have been subject to trials as anti-spastic agents. However, none have been subject to a range of rigorous double-blind studies, nor has there been any high-quality comparative study with more acceptable anti-spastic agents such as baclofen. Clonazepam (Cendrowski and Sobczyk, 1977) has been shown to be equally effective as diazepam but less well tolerated, due to a similar range of side effects such as sedation, fatigue and confusion. Clorazepate, ketazolam and tetrazepam have also been shown to be valid anti-spastic agents, but in general seem to share the same disadvantages as diazepam (Basmajan *et al.*, 1984; Lossius *et al.*, 1985; Milanov, 1992).

Baclofen

Mechanism of action
Baclofen is a structural analogue of GABA, which is known to be one of the main inhibitory transmitters in the central nervous system. Baclofen is known to bind to the bicuculline-insensitive $GABA_b$ receptors (Hwang and Wilcox, 1989). This has the effect of reducing the release of endogenous excitatory neurotransmitters such as glutamate and aspartate, but also inhibits gamma motor neurone activity and reduces intrafusal spindle muscle sensitivity, with the overall effect of inhibition of both monosynaptic and polysynaptic reflexes. Baclofen may also have some effect through its known analgesic and anti-nociceptive properties (Henry, 1980).

Pharmacology
Baclofen is well absorbed from the gastrointestinal tract, with a peak plasma level occurring 1–2 hours after administration. It has a relatively short half-life of approximately 3.5 hours, and thus should be taken in divided doses during a 24-hour period (Faigle and Keberle, 1972). Only small amounts cross the blood–brain barrier, and thus it tends to have less central nervous system depressive activity than diazepam. It is usually administered by mouth, although there are intrathecal formats available (see later).

Clinical efficacy
The drug has a long history, and it has been in clinical use as an anti-spastic agent for nearly as long as diazepam. However, as it was introduced into clinical practice some time ago it has not been subject to a rigorous clinical trial programme and most of the work has been in people with multiple sclerosis and spinal cord injury. There have been very few studies that have investigated the effect of baclofen in the treatment of spasticity of cerebral origin, and clinical practice would also suggest a more limited benefit in such people than for those with multiple sclerosis or spinal cord injury. There have been a few double-blind, cross-

over studies against placebo, which have shown that baclofen is effective in reducing spasticity, at least on the Ashworth Scale (Hudgson and Weightman, 1971; Duncan *et al.*, 1976; Levine *et al.*, 1977; Feldman *et al.*, 1978). Unfortunately, most studies have not looked in any detail at improvement in mobility or activities of daily living, and have largely used spasm frequency and/or the Ashworth Scale as the main outcome measure. A larger study of 106 patients conducted by Sachais *et al.* (1977) confirmed that baclofen was effective in relieving a variety of UMN symptoms such as flexor spasm, clonus, pain, resistance to passive movement, hyperactive stretch reflexes and stiffness.

Baclofen has been shown to be as effective as (or in some studies more effective than) diazepam but causes less sedation (Cartlidge *et al.*, 1974; Roussan *et al.*, 1987). There is no evidence of drug tolerance in any of the longer-term studies.

Dosage

It is usually recommended that the dosage begins with around 5 mg daily, increasing at approximately 4–5-day intervals by 5 mg increments to a normal dose of around 50–60 mg daily in divided doses. A maximum dose is around 100 mg daily but, in the author's experience, if there is no improvement at about 80 mg then improvement at higher levels is unlikely. As with all anti-spastic agents, the dose should be titrated in order to achieve an optimal clinical response with minimum side effects.

Side effects

The side effects are similar to those of the other anti-spastic agents, but are generally less severe than those with benzodiazepines. It is likely that a lower incidence of side effects is achieved by gradual introduction of the drug, and this is particularly important in the elderly. The commonest dose-limiting problems are drowsiness, sedation and fatigue, often combined with muscle weakness. A variety of other less common problems may occur, including gastrointestinal effects (such as dry mouth, nausea and constipation) and neurological effects (such as headache, dizziness, ataxia, insomnia, hallucinations, nightmares and dyskinesia) (Hattab, 1980). As with most such agents, care should be taken in elderly people or those with acquired brain injury who already have difficulty with concentration and memory. Sudden withdrawal should be avoided, as this may lead to seizures, hallucinations, confusional states and even psychotic reactions (Terrence and Fromm, 1981). A rare but important side effect is baclofen-induced asthmatic attacks (Dicpinigaitis *et al.*, 1993).

Overall side effects are common, but they can usually be kept under reasonable control by keeping the dosage as low as possible and introducing the medication slowly. However, there is still a clear overlap between the side effects and clinical effectiveness, which is difficult to manage.

Conclusion

Baclofen is a well-established and widely prescribed anti-spastic agent. It has the disadvantage of a significant range of side effects, and the dose is often limited by weakness and fatigue.

Dantrolene sodium

Mechanism of action
Dantrolene sodium, 1-(5-)p-nitrophenylfurfurylidene amino hydantoin sodium hydrate, is a hydantoin derivative and has a completely different mechanism of action to most other available anti-spastic agents. Dantrolene acts peripherally on muscle fibres, and the mechanism of action is probably through suppression of the release of calcium ions from the sarcoplasmic reticulum, which produces a disassociation of excitation/contraction coupling and thus diminishes the force of muscle contracture (Ellis and Carpenter, 1974). There may be an additional effect in alteration of muscle spindle sensitivity (Monster *et al.*, 1974).

Pharmacology
Dantrolene is available for oral administration, and is reasonably well absorbed in the small intestine before being mainly metabolized into 5-hydroxy dantrolene in the liver. The peak blood concentration occurs 3–6 hours after administration, and it has a half-life of approximately 15 hours (Herman *et al.*, 1972). It can cross the blood–brain barrier, as well as the placenta.

Clinical efficacy
Dantrolene has traditionally been used for spasticity of cerebral origin, such as that caused by stroke, brain injury or cerebral palsy. However, there is little hard evidence to support the assertion that it is a better anti-spastic agent in such conditions, and there is certainly conflicting evidence on whether people with stroke respond to dantrolene therapy (Ketel and Kolb, 1984; Katrak *et al.*, 1992). There have been a number of placebo-controlled studies that have confirmed dantrolene's superiority to placebo both in adults and children in a variety of conditions, including multiple sclerosis and cerebral palsy (Gelenberg and Poskanzer, 1973; Haslam *et al.*, 1974; Weiser *et al.*, 1978). There have been a few comparative studies, particularly with diazepam, which have shown that it is equally efficacious as an anti-spastic agent but has a significantly better side effect profile (Glass and Hannah, 1974; Schmidt *et al.*, 1976). In theory, a different site of action may indicate a potential synergistic effect with other more centrally acting agents. There is little confirmation of this theory, although in clinical practice dantrolene can often be introduced alongside baclofen, both at small doses, with apparently fewer side effects. However, there is little evidence to support this anecdotal experience.

Dosage
It is usual to start dantrolene at 25 mg per day, and this is slowly increased, at 25 mg increments, to the manufacturer's maximum recommended dose of 400 mg daily. It is usually taken in divided doses. However, it is unusual for

individuals to reach the maximum dose, and a reasonable clinical effect is usually apparent at 100–200 mg daily.

Side effects

Dantrolene has a range of central nervous system effects, including drowsiness, fatigue, anorexia and nausea. It occasionally produces a skin rash, and can also be associated with significant weakness and occasionally gastrointestinal disturbances (such as diarrhoea). It is usually muscle weakness rather than fatigue that is the main dose-limiting effect. Unfortunately dantrolene has been shown to cause transient abnormalities of liver function, with a risk of symptomatic hepatitis of approximately 0.5 per cent and occasional reports of fatal hepatitis in the order of 0.1 per cent (Utili et al., 1977; Wilkinson et al., 1979). The risk of hepatitis seems to be more prevalent in women over 35 years, and is possibly dose-related, being more common in those taking nearer the manufacturer's maximum dose of 400 mg. However, this does mean that liver function tests should be checked prior to the initiation of therapy and at periodic intervals during therapy. This is a minor but nevertheless important drawback to routine clinical usage.

Conclusion

Dantrolene is a well-established and effective anti-spastic agent, but its use is again limited by a range of side effects. Its mode of action at the muscle level is unique among anti-spastic agents. It has the slight clinical disadvantage of the need to monitor liver function tests.

Central alpha-2 adrenergic receptor agonists – clonidine and tizanidine

Mechanism of action

Both clonidine and tizanidine are imidazoline derivatives that affect central alpha-2 adrenergic receptors. The exact mechanism of action has yet to be clarified, and the effects on the central nervous system do seem to be varied. However, it is likely that the anti-spastic effects are mainly linked to the alpha-2 adrenergic agonist properties, although the effects on the imidazoline receptor may also play a role (Muramatsui and Kigoshi, 1992; Coward, 1994). Tizanidine acts predominantly pre-synaptically in the spinal cord, but it is possible that the depressant effect of tizanidine on the polysynaptic excitation of interneurones could be related to a post-synaptic reduction in the effectiveness of released excitatory transmitters. The compounds also possibly have an inhibitory action on alpha motor neurone excitability, and in vitro experiments have indicated that the release of excitatory amino acids from spinal interneurones may be inhibited (Curtis et al., 1983).

Pharmacology

Both compounds are well absorbed from the gastrointestinal tract. However, clonidine has quite a long half-life of about 23 hours, whereas the half-life of tizanidine is significantly shorter at 2–4 hours. Tizanidine is extensively metabolized in the liver, and only about 3 per cent of the administered dose is excreted unchanged in the urine.

Clinical efficacy

Tizanidine is now marketed throughout the world; it has been available in the European community for some years, but was only released in the United Kingdom in 1997. Tizanidine has thus been subject to a rigorous clinical trial programme. Regrettably there have been few clinical trials of clonidine, and most of these have been open-label studies or involved just small numbers of individuals (Sandford et al., 1988; Dall et al., 1996). However, it does seem clear that clonidine has definite anti-spastic effects. One study suggested that it may be useful in reducing spasticity in multiple sclerosis in individuals who have failed to respond to baclofen and diazepam (Khan and Olek, 1995). Transdermal patches of clonidine have been reported to have efficacy with few systemic side effects (Weingarden and Belen, 1992), but at the present time clonidine has not been specifically licensed as an anti-spastic agent.

The situation is dramatically different with tizanidine, and there have been a large number of randomized double-blind, placebo-controlled studies involving several hundred patients (Smith et al., 1994; UK Tizanidine Trial Group, 1994). The studies have confirmed a beneficial anti-spastic effect against placebo. There have also been a number of double-blind studies of tizanidine against baclofen (Hoogstraten et al., 1988) and against diazepam (Bes et al., 1988), which have generally shown a similar efficacy but often with a lesser range of side effects. In particular, muscle strength seems relatively more preserved than with either baclofen or diazepam.

Dosage

It is usual to start tizanidine at approximately 2 mg daily, and this can be increased at 4–7-day intervals in 2 mg increments. The maximum recommended dose is 36 mg daily in divided doses, but clinical experience indicates that most individuals are adequately controlled at around 24 mg daily.

Side effects

Although side effects are common, they are often of minimal impact. The commoner effects include dry mouth, drowsiness, tiredness, dizziness, postural hypotension and muscle weakness. However, it is important to emphasize that muscle weakness does seem to be significantly less on tizanidine therapy than with other anti-spastic agents (Wagstaff and Bryson, 1997), and this is an important clinical bonus. Unfortunately, it increases liver enzymes in a small number of individuals, although this is rarely of clinical importance. There have been a few cases of serious hepatic problems (de Graaf et al., 1996), but in very few people and generally only in those who have been additionally on other anti-spastic agents. However, measurement of liver function tests are recommended before initiation of tizanidine, after 1 month of treatment, and then at clinically determined intervals.

Conclusion

Clonidine may be a useful anti-spastic agent, but it has unfortunately not been subject to any rigorous trial programme. Tizanidine, however, is now actively marketed, and is clearly a useful and efficacious anti-spastic agent. It has a range of side effects, but these seem to be less troublesome than those of alternative agents; in particular, the drug seems to induce less muscle weakness. It has a slight disadvantage in the need to monitor liver function.

Other anti-spastic agents

There have been a number of other anti-spastic agents suggested in the literature. However, few have been subject to sufficiently extensive placebo-controlled studies, and most have simply appeared in the literature as anecdotal cases or open uncontrolled trials with small numbers of patients. Thus, none of the drugs yet have an established place in clinical practice. Agents that have shown some efficacy include: cyclobenzaprine (Ashby *et al.*, 1972); chlorpromazine (Cohan *et al.*, 1980) and a further phenothiazine derivative, dymethothiazine (Burke *et al.*, 1975); piracetam (Maritz *et al.*, 1978); and even the use of a topical anaesthetic spray (Sabbahi and Powers, 1981). A few agents are worthy of further consideration.

L-threonine

This is a precursor of glycine, which is an important post-synaptic inhibitory neurotransmitter in the spinal cord. There have been a few studies of the use of L-threonine in hereditary spastic paraparesis and multiple sclerosis, with modest success (Barbeau *et al.*, 1982).

GABA agonists

A number of GABA agonists have recently been introduced as anti-epileptic agents, which generally enhance inhibitory GABAergic neurotransmission. There have been a small number of studies indicating some benefit from these agents, but once again there have been very few high-quality controlled studies. Some of these agents appear to produce modest effects on spasticity (Jaeken *et al.*, 1991; Priebe *et al.*, 1997).

Orphenadrine

Orphenadrine blocks muscarinic acetylcholine receptors, and is occasionally used to treat Parkinsonism. A single double-blind, placebo-controlled trial reported a beneficial effect in individuals with spinal cord injuries (Casale *et al.*, 1995).

Cannabis

There has recently been significant media interest in the use of cannabis as an anti-spastic agent, particularly in multiple sclerosis. Delta-9-tetra-hydrocannabinol (THC) is a major ingredient, but this is only one of 66 active cannabinoid constituents of the *Cannabis Sativa* plant. There have been a number of anecdotal reports of a muscle relaxant effect after smoking marijuana (Dunn and Davis, 1974), but there have been few double-blind studies. In one double-blind, placebo-controlled, cross-over clinical trial of delta 9 THC in 30 patients with multiple sclerosis, there were significant improvements in subjective ratings of spasticity at a dosage of 7.5 mg (Ungerleider *et al.*, 1987).

Other studies have shown that posture and balance deteriorated following treatment (Greenberg *et al.*, 1994). At the present time there is little hard evidence of the efficacy of THC as an anti-spastic agent, but nevertheless further studies are clearly justified, given the wide-ranging anecdotal reports of benefit.

Intrathecal usage

Intrathecal baclofen

In recent years, baclofen has been available for administration by the intrathecal route using an implanted pump. Obviously this mechanism has theoretical advantages as the drug is delivered to the appropriate region, with a potential increase in efficacy and reduction in side effects. Very small doses can be given. A number of well-designed studies have now confirmed the efficacy of intrathecal baclofen in a number of different clinical situations, including intractable spasticity both in spinal cord injury and multiple sclerosis (Ochs *et al.*, 1989; Coffey *et al.*, 1993; Becker *et al.*, 1997). The drug is administered by means of an implanted subcutaneous pump. There are a variety of designs, but all include a drug reservoir and a delivery mechanism. The pump is connected via a catheter tunnelled under the skin, usually to the L3/4 intrathecal space. More modern devices are now externally programmable, allowing the dose to be titrated while the pump remains *in situ*. This method is usually reserved for those with severe functional disability or intractable pain and who have not responded to other modalities. Obviously the technique has risks, including infection, pump failure, catheter movement and the risk of over-dosage. The pump should only be put in place at recognized regional centres.

Intrathecal phenol

Phenol is a neurolytic agent that will impair nerve conduction when injected close to a nerve. It used to be one of the few available treatments for the management of severe intractable spasticity. In recent years it has rather fallen out of favour following the advent of safer techniques, including botulinum toxin and intrathecal baclofen. However, it is a technique that should be borne in mind for individuals with very severe spasticity and who may not be suitable for surgery. It should probably only be used in those with complete lack of motor and sensory function in the lower limbs, and preferably without bowel or bladder function. In such individuals phenol can be introduced intrathecally, and the effect is usually immediate and permanent (Kelly and Gautier-Smith, 1959).

Conclusion

This chapter has summarized the overall approach to the management of spasticity in multiple sclerosis. Pharmacological agents can be extremely useful but should nevertheless be used with caution, given the considerable range of side effects. Any treatment should only be initiated after careful discussion and planning of the treatment goals, and the patient should always be monitored in the long term in order to ensure that such goals are being met and are still necessary. Pharmacological management should rarely be used in isolation from an overall multidisciplinary assessment, and it is often used as part of a general treatment strategy that usually includes physiotherapy as well as more focal treatment such as botulinum toxin. However, with careful planning the management of spasticity can certainly be rewarding and of significant functional benefit to the person with multiple sclerosis.

References

Ashby, P., Burke, D., Rao, S. *et al.* (1972). Assessment of cyclobenzaprine in the treatment of spasticity. *J. Neurol. Neurosurg. Psychiatr.*, **35**, 599–605.

Bajd, T. and Bowmand, B. (1982). Testing and modelling of spasticity. *J. Biomed. Eng.*, **4**, 90–96.

Barbeau, A., Roy, M. and Chouza, C. (1982). Pilot study of threonine supplementation in human spasticity. *Can. J. Neurol. Sci.*, **9**, 141–5.

Basmajan, J. V., Shandarkass, K., Russell, D. *et al.* (1984). Ketazolam treatment for spasticity: double-blind study of a new drug. *Arch. Phys. Med. Rehabil.*, **65**, 698–701.

Becker, R., Alberti, O. and Bauer, B. L. (1997). Continuous intrathecal baclofen in severe spasticity after traumatic or hypoxic brain injury. *J. Neurol.*, **244**, 160–66.

Bes, A., Eyssette, M., Pierrot-Deseilligny, E. *et al.* (1988). A multicentre, double-blind trial of tizanidine: a new anti-spastic agent in spasticity associated with hemiplegia. *Curr. Opin. Med. Res.*, **10**, 709–18.

Bohannon, R. W. and Smith, M. B. (1987). Inter-rater reliability of a Modified Ashworth Scale in muscle spasticity. *Phys. Ther.*, **67**, 206–7.

Bradstater, M. E., de Bruin, H., Gowland, C. and Clarke, B. M. (1983). Hemiplegic gait: analysis of temporal variables. *Arch. Phys. Med. Rehabil.*, **64**, 583–7.

Brown, P. (1994). Pathophysiology of spasticity (editorial). *J. Neurol. Neurosurg. Psychiatr.*, **57**, 773–7.

Burke, D., Hammond, C., Skuse, N. *et al.* (1975). A pheno-thiazine derivative in the treatment of spasticity. *J. Neurol. Neurosurg. Psychiatr.*, **38**, 469–74.

Cartlidge, N. E. F., Hudgson, P. and Weightman, D. (1974). A comparison of baclofen and diazepam in the treatment of spasticity. *J. Neurol. Sci.*, **23**, 17–24.

Casale, R., Glynn, C. J. and Buonocore, M. (1995). Reduction of spastic hypertonia in patients with spinal cord injury. A double-blind comparison of IV orphrenadrine citrate and placebo. *Arch. Phys. Med. Rehabil.*, **76**, 660–65.

Cendrowski, W. and Sobczyk, W. (1977). Clonazepam, baclofen and placebo in the treatment of spasticity. *Eur. Neurol.*, **16**, 257–62.

Cocchiarella, A., Downey, J. A. and Darling, R. C. (1967). Evaluation of the effect of diazepam on spasticity. *Arch. Phys. Med. Rehabil.*, **49**, 393–6.

Coffey, R. J., Cahill, D., Steers, W. *et al.* (1993). Intrathecal baclofen for intractable spasticity of spinal origin: results of a long-term multicentre study. *J. Neurosurg.*, **78**, 226–32.

Cohan, S. L., Raines, A., Panagakos, J. *et al.* (1980). Phenytoin and chlorpromazine in the treatment of spasticity. *Arch. Neurol.*, **37**, 360–64.

Coward, D. M. (1994). Tizanidine: neuropharmacology and mechanism of action. *Neurology*, **44(Suppl. 9)**, S6–11.

Curtis, D. R., Leah, J. D. and Peet, M. J. (1983). Spinal interneurone depression by DS103-282. *Br. J. Pharmacol.*, **79**, 9–11.

Dall, J. T., Harmon, R. I. and Quinn, C. M. (1996). Use of clonidine for the treatment of spasticity arising from various forms of brain injury: a case series. *Brain Inj.*, **10**, 453–8.

de Graaf, E. M., Oosterveld, M., Tjabbes, T. *et al.* (1996). A case of tizanidine-induced hepatic injury. *J. Hepatol.*, **25**, 772–3.

Demeurisse, G., Demol, O. and Robaye, E. (1980). Motor evaluation in vascular hemiplegia. *Eur. Neurol.*, **19**, 382–9.

Dicpinigaitis, P. V., Nierman, D. M. and Miller, A. (1993). Baclofen-induced bronchoconstriction. *Ann. Pharmacother.*, **27(7–8)**, 883–4.

Duncan, G. W., Shahani, B. Y and Young, R. R. (1976). An evaluation of baclofen treatment for certain symptoms in patients with spinal cord lesions: a double-blind, cross-over study. *Neurology*, **26**, 441–6.

Dunn, M. and Davis, R. (1974). Perceived effects of marijuana on spinal cord injured males. *Paraplegia*, **12**, 175.

Edwards, S. (ed.) (1996). *Neurological Physiotherapy: Problem Solving Approach*. Churchill Livingstone.

Ellis, K. O. and Carpenter, J. F. (1974). Mechanisms of control of skeletal muscle contraction by dantrolene sodium. *Arch. Phys. Med. Rehabil.*, **55**, 362–9.

Faigle, J. W. and Keberle, H. (1971). The metabolism and pharmacokinetics of Lioresal. Spasticity: a topical survey. In: *An International Symposium, Vienna 1971* (W. Birkmayer, ed.), pp. 94–100. Huber.

Feldman, R. G., Kelly-Hayes, M., Conomy, J. P. and Foley, J. M. (1978). Baclofen for spasticity in multiple sclerosis: a double-blind, cross-over and three year study. *Neurology*, **28**, 1094–8.

Gelenberg, A. J. and Poskanzer, D. C. (1973). The effect of dantrolene sodium on spasticity in multiple sclerosis. *Neurology*, **23**, 1313–15.

Glass, A. and Hannah, A. (1974). A comparison of dantrolene sodium and diazepam in the treatment of spasticity. *Paraplegia*, **12**, 170–74.

Greenberg, H. S., Werness, A. S., Pugh, J. E. *et al.* (1994). Short-term effects of smoking marijuana on balance in patients with multiple sclerosis and normal volunteers. *Clin. Pharmacol. Ther.*, **55**, 324–8.

Haslam, R. H. A., Walcher, J. R., Lietman, P. S. *et al.* (1974). Dantrolene sodium in children with spasticity. *Arch. Phys. Med. Rehabil.*, **55**, 384–8.

Hattab, J. R. (1980). Review of European clinical trials with baclofen. In: *Spasticity: Disordered Motor Control* (R. G. Feldman, R. R. Young and W. P. Koella, eds), pp. 71–86. Year Book Medical Publishers.

Henry, J. L. (1980). Pharmacologic studies on baclofen in the spinal cord of the cat. In: *Spasticity: Disordered Motor Control* (R. G. Feldman, R. R. Young and W. P. Koella, eds), pp. 437–52. Year Book Medical Publishers.

Herman, R., Mayer, N. and Mecomber, S. A. (1972). Clinical pharmaco-physiology of dantrolene sodium. *Am. J. Phys. Med.*, **51**, 296–311.

Hoogstraten, M. C., van der Ploeg, R. J. O., van der Burg, W. *et al.* (1988). Tizanidine versus baclofen in the treatment of spasticity in multiple sclerosis patients. *Acta Neurol. Scand.*, **77**, 224–30.

Hudgson, P. and Weightman, D. (1971). Baclofen in the treatment of spasticity. *Br. Med. J.*, **4**, 15–17.

Hunt, S. M., McKenna, S. P. and McEwan, J. (1980). A quantitative approach to perceived health status: a validation study. *J. Epidem. Comm. Health*, **34**, 281–6.

Hwang, A. S. and Wilcox, G. L. (1989). Baclofen, gamma-aminobutyric acid-b receptors and substance P in the mouse spinal cord. *J. Pharmacol. Exp. Ther.*, **248**, 1026–33.

Jaeken, J., de Cock, P. and Casaer, P. (1991). Vigabatrin as a spasmolytic drug. *Lancet*, **338**, 8782–3.

Katrak, P. H., Cole, A. M. D., Poulos, C. J. and McCauley, J. C. K. (1992). Objective assessment of spasticity, strength and function with early exhibition of dantrolene sodium after cerebrovascular accident: a randomised, double-blind controlled study. *Arch. Phys. Med. Rehabil.*, **73**, 4–9.

Kelly, R. E. and Gautier-Smith, P. C. (1959). Intrathecal phenol in the treatment of reflex spasms in spasticity. *Lancet*, **ii**, 1102–5.

Kendall, H. P. (1964). The use of diazepam in hemiplegia. *Ann. Phys. Med.*, **7(6)**, 225–8.

Ketel, W. B. and Kolb, M. E. (1984). Long-term treatment with dantrolene sodium in stroke patients with spasticity limiting the return of function. *Curr. Med. Res. Opin.*, **9(3)**, 161–9.

Khan, O. and Olek, M. J. (1995). Clonidine in the treatment of spasticity in patients with multiple sclerosis. *J. Neurol.*, **242**, 712–15.

Levine, I. M., Jossmann, P. B. and de Angelis, V. (1977). Lioresal, a new muscle relaxant in the treatment of spasticity: a double-blind quantitative evaluation. *Dis. Nerv. Sys.*, **38**, 1011–15.

Lossius, R., Dietrichson, P. and Lunde, P. K. M. (1985). Effect of clorazepate in spasticity and rigidity: a quantitative study of reflexes and plasma concentrations. *Acta Neurol. Scand.*, **71**, 190–94.

Maritz, N. G., Muller, F. O. and Pompe van Meerdervoort, H. F. (1978). Piracetam in the management of spasticity in cerebral palsy. *S. Afr. Med. J.*, **53**, 889–91.

Mathiowetz, V., Weber, K., Kashman, N. and Weber, K. (1985). Adult norms for the nine-hole peg test of finger dexterity. *Occup. Ther. J. Res.*, **5**, 24–37.

Milanov, I. (1992). Mechanisms of tetrazepam action on spasticity. *Acta Neurol. Belgica.*, **92(1)**, 5–15.

Monster, A. W., Tamai, Y. and McHenry, J. (1974). Dantrolene sodium: its effects on extrafusal muscle fibres. *Arch. Phys. Med. Rehabil.*, **55**, 355–62.

Muramatsui, I. and Kigoshi, S. (1992). Tizanidine may discriminate between imidazoline-receptors and alpha-2-adrenoceptors. *Jpn. J. Pharmacol.*, **59**, 457–59.

Ochs, G., Struppler, A., Meyerson, B. A. *et al.* (1989). Intrathecal baclofen for long-term treatment of spasticity: a multicentre study. *J. Neurol. Neurosurg. Psychiatr.*, **52**, 133–9.

Priebe, M. M., Sherwood, A. M., Graves, D. E. *et al.* (1997). Effectiveness of gabapentin in controlling spasticity: a quantitative study. *Spinal Cord*, **35**, 171–5.

Roussan, M., Terrence, C. and Fromm, G. (1987). Baclofen versus diazepam for the treatment of spasticity and long-term follow-up of baclofen therapy. *Pharmatherapeutica*, **4(5)**, 278–84.

Sabbahi, M. A. and Powers, W. R. (1981). Topical anaesthesia: a possible treatment method for spasticity. *Arch. Phys. Med. Rehabil.*, **62**, 310–14.

Sachais, B. A., Logue, J. N. and Carey, M. S. (1977). Baclofen, a new anti-spastic drug: a controlled, multi-center trial in patients with multiple sclerosis. *Arch. Neurol.*, **34**, 422–8.

Sandford, P. R., Spengler, S. E. and Sawasky, K. B. (1988). Clonidine in the treatment of brainstem spasticity. *Am. J. Phys. Med. Rehabil.*, **71**, 301–3.

Schlosser, W. (1971). Action of diazepam on spinal cord. *Arch. Int. Pharmacodyn. Ther.*, **194**, 93–102.

Schmidt, R. T., Lee, R. H. and Spehlman, R. (1976). Comparison of dantrolene sodium and diazepam in the treatment of spasticity. *J. Neurol. Neurosurg. Psychiatr.*, **39**, 350–56.

Semlyen, J. K., Hurrell, E., Carter, S. and Barnes, M. P. (1996). The Newcastle Independence Assessment Form (Research): development of an alternative functional measure. *J. Neurol. Rehabil.*, **10(4)**, 251–7.

Shahani, B. T. and Cross, D. (1990). Neurophysiological testing in spasticity. In: *The Practical Management of Spasticity in Children and Adults* (M. B. Glenn and J. Whyte, eds), pp. 34–43. Lea & Febiger.

Smith, C., Birnbaum, G., Carter, J. T. *et al.* (1994). Tizanidine treatment for spasticity caused by multiple sclerosis: results of a double-blind, placebo-controlled trial. *Neurology*, **44(Suppl. 9)**, S34–43.

Terrence, D. V. and Fromm, G. H. (1981). Complications of baclofen withdrawal. *Arch. Neurol.*, **38**, 588–9.

UK Tizanidine Trial Group (1994). A double-blind, placebo-controlled trial of tizanidine in the treatment of spasticity caused by multiple sclerosis. *Neurology*, **44(Suppl. 9)**, S70–78.

Ungerleider, J. T., Andyrsiak, T., Fairbanks, L. *et al.* (1987). Delta-9-THC in the treatment of spasticity associated with multiple sclerosis. *Adv. Alcohol Subst. Abuse*, **7(1)**, 39–50.

Utili, R., Boitnott, J. K. and Zimmerman, H. J. (1977). Dantrolene-associated hepatic injury: incidence and character. *Gastroenterology*, **72**, 610–16.

Verrier, M., Ashby, P. and Macleod, S. (1977). Diazepam effect on reflex activity in patients with complete spinal lesions and in those with other causes of spasticity. *Arch. Phys. Med. Rehabil.*, **58**, 148–53.

Wagstaff, A. J. and Bryson, H. M. (1997). Tizanidine: a review of its pharmacology, clinical efficacy and tolerability in the management of spasticity associated with cerebral and spinal disorders. *Drugs*, **53(3)**, 435–52.

Weingarden, S. I. and Belen, J. G. (1992). Clonidine transdermal system for treatment of spasticity in spinal cord injury. *Arch. Phys. Med. Rehabil.*, **73**, 876–7.

Weiser, R., Terenty, T., Hudgson, P. *et al.* (1978). Dantrolene sodium in the treatment of spasticity in chronic spinal cord disease. *Practitioner*, **221**, 123–7.

Wilkinson, S. P., Portmann, B. and Williams, R. (1979). Hepatitis from dantrolene sodium. *Gut*, **20**, 33–6.

Wilson, L. A. and McKechnie, A. A. (1966). Oral diazepam in the treatment of spasticity in paraplegia: a double-blind trial and subsequent impressions. *Scot. Med. J.*, **11**, 46–51.

13

Management of spasticity – botulinum toxin

Introduction

Spasticity is a major feature of both primary and secondary progressive multiple sclerosis, and leads directly *per se* to disability. As noted in Chapter 12, it is often difficult to manage and frequently sub-optimally treated, yet it is one of the important considerations in the rehabilitation of the multiple sclerosis (MS) patient. Not only can its successful treatment lead to improved physical functioning in the individual, but just as importantly deterioration can be prevented and function preserved. A strategy for patients with chronic neurological disease is required, and this applies to spasticity. Therefore, its management should be part of the patient's and carer's rehabilitation goals, and the treatment objectives should be clearly known and communicated to all concerned.

Botulinum toxin is a relatively new option in anti-spasticity drug management. Its use is entirely for focal spasticity, i.e. in a functional unit, and this chapter will deal with the pharmacokinetics, indications and clinical uses for this novel and exciting drug, as well as giving practical information on its delivery and administration. Safety issues will also be addressed, and the place of botulinum toxin in the overall management of the spastic patient will be described.

MS patients often present with multiple problems due to increased tone, but there are specific difficulties requiring additional attention. This is where botulinum toxin is effective and, while it is not yet licensed for spasticity in acquired neurological disease, its common usage, its good safety record and the data from USA and UK studies make it a viable option for management in rehabilitation settings. A particular local problem can therefore be treated without recourse to increasing systemic therapy and the concurrent risk of more troublesome side effects.

Treatment of spasticity should be considered in MS patients only when it is causing harm. Neurological rehabilitation frequently uses its beneficial effects, particularly when limbs are becoming increasingly weak and patients can utilize their spasticity for support when their weakness would not otherwise allow it. It is thus very important to take a clear history and to observe patients during functional activities, e.g. walking, transferring, eating, etc. It is not enough to measure the range of joint movement in a limb, or the degree of tone. It is also important to have a clear idea of what patients wish to achieve from their treatment. They may be so severely disabled as to have no limb function, and treatment may be necessary to improve the ability of carers to provide their physical care. Issues such as getting arms through sleeves or legs through trousers and providing perineal hygiene are important, especially if carers have to 'fight' with spastic limbs to gain access, or recruit more help. The setting of rehabilitation goals in these patients should thus include carers' views and wishes. Table 13.1 shows the widespread effects of spasticity on patients with MS. In common with other features of the disease, the age, size and location of the plaques, disease severity and the rapidity of progression are important in its presentation. In some patients pain may be the dominant feature, and considerations for treatment will be addressed later in the chapter.

Table 13.1 The consequences of spasticity

Decreased mobility	
Contracture	
Pain	
Decreased personal function	
Increased carer burden	
Impaired life satisfaction in respect of:	• Poor mobility
	• Hygiene difficulties
	• Self-care problems
	• Cosmetic effect of limb deformities
	• Difficulties with sleep
	• Poor self-esteem
	• Effect on mood
	• Effect on sexuality and sexual functioning

History of botulinum toxin

Botulinum toxin is produced by the anaerobe *Clostridium botulinum*, and is responsible for the clinical features of botulism. These effects have been recognized since the end of the nineteenth century, when van Ermengem related botulism to the toxin produced by this anaerobic bacterium (van Ermengem, 1979). Botulism occurs through the ingestion of contaminated food or from wound infection. Its incidence in the Western world has fallen dramatically (Simpson, 1989a), as has its fatality, and this has been due to improvements in resuscitation. The neurotoxin is a powerful neuromuscular paralysing agent, and in botulism the clinical features include muscular weakness in the limbs, face, and extra-ocular and bulbar muscles. Smooth muscle is also affected, leading to constipation, ileus and urinary retention (Davis, 1993).

Burgen *et al.* (1949) described the theoretical foundation of the development of the toxin as a therapeutic tool, and its purification represents a dramatic paradox in modern medicine whereby a potential killer has been turned into a beneficial therapeutic agent. Different antigenically-distinct neurotoxins have been recognized, and human intoxication has been primarily due to types A, B, and E. Our knowledge now recognizes seven immunologically distinct types; A, B, C, D, E, F and G. Types C and D tend to affect other animals, particularly livestock, and Type F rarely affects humans. No outbreaks have been reported for Type G.

An advance in knowledge of botulinum toxin therapy came with the recognition in 1973 of its use in the treatment of strabismus in non-human primates (Scott *et al.*, 1973). The initial results were then applied to the treatment of humans in 1981, which showed this to be safe and efficient therapy for a large number of neurological and non-neurological diseases (Jankovic and Brin, 1991). Botulinum toxin Type A (BTX-A) received approval from the US Food and Drugs Administration in 1989 for the treatment of strabismus, blepharospasm and hemifacial spasm, and this was extended by the Committee for Safety of Medicines in Britain in 1991 for the same conditions. Its use in spasticity due to acquired disorders is still unlicensed, but its clinical uses and safety profile are now well established. The toxin is now licensed for the treatment of spastic lower leg problems in children with cerebral palsy over the age of 2 years and, after being granted a product licence in Ireland, Denmark and Portugal, the UK was included in September 1998. A wide number of applications have been suggested, and these are shown in Table 13.2. The safety, effectiveness, specificity and reversibility of botulinum toxin make it a powerful and versatile tool in a wide variety of upper motor neurone pathology.

Mechanism of action and pharmacology

Botulinum toxin acts at the neuromuscular junction by inhibiting the release of acetylcholine. The end effect is the same for all the seven serologically distinct toxins, and, although they are antigenically different, they possess similar molec-

Table 13.2 Clinical indications for botulinum toxin

Dystonias	**Involuntary movements**
Blepharospasm	Voice, head and limb tremor
Cervical dystonia	Palatal myoclonus
Laryngeal dystonia (spasmodic dystonia)	Hemifacial spasm
Occupational cramps	Tics
Other focal dystonias	

Other applications	
Achalasia	Back pain, muscle spasm and nerve root pain
Bruxism	Cosmesis (wrinkles, etc.)
Headaches (tension/muscular contraction)	Hyperhidrosis
Myokymia	Nystagmus
Pelvirectal spasms (anismus, vaginismus)	Ptosis (for corneal protection)
Spasticity (limb, bladder)	Rigidity
Stuttering	Other spastic disorders

ular weights and have a common sub-unit structure (Simpson, 1980, 1983). The complete amino acid sequences for the various serotypes are becoming known, and regions of sequence similarities among the serotypes and also between botulinum toxin and tetanus toxin suggest that they all employ similar methods of action (Binz et al., 1990; Campbell et al., 1993).

When botulinum neurotoxin is isolated from bacterial cultures it is frequently associated with proteins or nucleic acids, and type A associates non-covalently with haemagglutinin. As a result, when the toxin is administered orally these proteins enhance toxicity compared to the toxins without the proteins. It is thought that proteolytic enzymes in the gut protect the neurotoxin, but when administered parenterally these proteins do not protect the toxin and may interfere slightly (Simpson, 1989). However, they do enhance stability and retard diffusion, which benefits therapeutic control.

The toxins are synthesized as single chain polypeptides with a molecular mass of approximately 150 kda (DasGupta, 1994). Neurotoxicity occurs as a result of activation following modification in the tertiary structure of the protein. In the first step, the parent chain is cleaved to produce a heavy chain of approximately 100 kda and a light chain, to which it is attached by a disulphide bond. A single atom of zinc is associated with the light chain, and the molecule is cleaved to form the di-chain molecule with a disulphide bridge. The light chain acts as a zinc endopeptidase, with proteolytic activity concentrated at the N-terminal end, whereas the heavy chain provides cholinergic specificity and promotes light chain translocation across the endosomal membrane. The toxin enters the axon terminal in its cleaved form, and disulphide reduction occurs after internalization in the target cell.

For paralysis to occur, three steps are necessary (Figure 13.1).

1. *Internalization.* This occurs via an endocytotic/lysosomal vesicle pathway, and is mediated by receptors. The process is independent of the calcium concentration and, to a degree, of nerve stimulation (Nathan et al., 1985), but it is energy dependent (Simpson, 1989b). The process is accelerated in an acidic environment, and is temperature dependent. *In vitro* studies suggest that the specificity of the toxin attaches to various sites (Dolly, 1994) and the C-terminal half of the heavy chain determines the cholinergic specificity. It is also responsible for binding, while the light chain is the intracellular toxic component (Black and Dolly, 1986). The toxin is only active while the disulphide bond between the two chains is intact.

2. *Disulphide reduction and cleavage.* The mechanism of cleavage of the disulphide bond is at present unknown, and occurs after internalization. The N-terminal portion of the heavy chain is responsible for penetration and translocation of the light chain across the endosomal membrane, which eventually disrupts the secretory pathway for acetylcholine (Dolly et al., 1990). Botulinum toxin blocks acetylcholine release, but does not affect synthesis or storage (Dolly, 1994). As a result, nerve stimulation can be restored after the effect of toxin has finished, and this has important therapeutic connotations. Botulinum toxin is a zinc endopeptidase, whose proteolytic activity is located

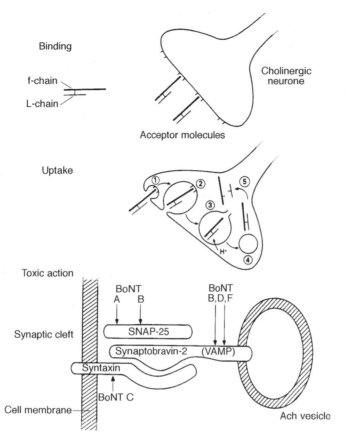

Figure 13.1 Diagram portraying the mechanisms of binding and uptake and the toxic actions of the botulinum neurotoxins within the cholonergic nerve terminal (from Hambleton, P. and Moore, A. P., Botulinum Neurotoxins: Origin, structure, molecular actions and antibodies, pp. 16–27. In Moore, A. P. (1995) *Butulinium Toxin Treatment*. Oxford: Blackwell Science.)

Binding. The heavy (H) chain is responsible for binding and uptake of the toxin, and the light (L) chain is the toxic portion.

Uptake is an active, energy-dependent process using endocytosis (1, 2) and escape of toxin into the cytoplasm (3, 4). It is not clear whether the two chains become dissociated *in vivo* before the L-chain produces its toxic effect (5).

Toxic action. Syntaxin is a protein that is embedded in the cell surface plasma membrane, and SNAP 25 (synaptosomal-associated protein of molecular weight 25 kDa) is a cytoplasmic protein that transiently associates with the membrane. Synaptobrevin-2 is embedded within the membrane of the synaptic vesicles. It is also known as VAMP (vesicle-associated membrane protein). Damage to these proteins by the botulinum neurotoxins blocks fusion of the vesicle with the cell membrane and release of acetylcholine (Ach) into the synaptic cleft. The sites of action of the toxins BoNT/A–F are indicated. BoNT/A and BoNT/B also inhibit resealing of the disrupted cell membrane.

in the N-terminal of the light chain. The binding of the zinc ion to the light chain is reversible and involves co-ordination with histidines, as occurs with other zinc endopeptidases such as tetanus toxin (Morante *et al.*, 1996). Acetylcholine release is inhibited when the endopeptidase cleaves one or more neuronal proteins of the vesicle transport pathway.

3. *Inhibition of neurotransmitter release.* Each of the toxin types has specific cellular substrates and a target site for inhibition of neurotransmitter function (Table 13.3). Translocation of an intact vesicle from the cytosol to the plasma membrane is dependent on specific proteins, and cleavage interferes with proper binding and fusion of a vesicle to the plasma membrane, which therefore impedes neurotransmitter release. Similarly, the steps for intracellular translocation have also become clearer (Barinaga, 1993). Attachment of the toxin to the inner membrane surface of the vesicle involves the formation of a complex, which includes cytoplasmic proteins, gamma SNAP, alpha SNAP, NSF, SNAP 25, vesicle proteins (VAMP/synaptobrevins) and proteins of the target membrane (syntaxin). Again, each toxin type has specificity for the location of these proteins. The intracellular substrate for both BTX-B and tetanus toxin is the vesicle protein, VAMP/synaptobrevin-2 (Schiavo *et al.*, 1992), and its light chain activity is specific for VAMP/synaptobrevin-2. Proteolysis thus inhibits the release of the neurotransmitter. BTX-D and BTX-F also cleave VAMP/synaptobrevin-2, but at a different site to BTX-B; BTX-A and BTX-E cleave another translocation protein, SNAP 25; and BTX-C acts by cleaving syntaxin (Blast *et al.*, 1993).

Table 13.3 Target proteins of botulinum toxin

Toxin type	Cellular substrate	Cleavage site	Target localization
BTX-A	SNAP 25	Gin 197–Arg 198	Presynaptic plasma membrane (PPM)
BTX-B	VAMP/synaptobrevin	Gin 76–Phe 77	Synaptic vesicle
BTX-C	Syntaxin 1A/1B	Lys 253–Ala 254 Lys 252–Ala 253	PPM + other regions
	SNAP 25		Neurone
BTX-D	VAMP/ Synaptobrevin	Lys 59–Leu 60 Ala 67–Asp 68	Synaptic vesicle
	Cellubrevin	Unknown	Vesicles of endocytosing /recycling system
BTX-E	SNAP 25	Arg 108–Ile 181	PPM
BTX-F	VAMP/ Synaptobrevin	Gin 58–Lys 59	Synaptic vesicle
	Cellubrevin	Unknown	Vesicles of endocytosing/recycling system
BTX-G	VAMP/synaptobrevin	Ala 81–Ala 82	Unknown

It is thought that in contrast to tetanus toxin, which reaches the central nervous system soon after its ingestion, botulinum toxin has only a weak presence. Some animal studies have shown that it is able to bind brain synaptosomes, but Weigand *et al.* (1976) injected iodine-labelled BTX-A into the gastrocnemius muscles of cats at doses of up to 91 per cent of the lethal feline dose. Accumulated radioactivity was noted in the spinal cord 3–4 days after the injection, suggesting some retrograde axonal transportation of the toxin from the injection site. However, it was not known whether the radioactivity was still bound to the toxin and, in subsequent testing, the cats did not demonstrate any spastic paralysis. Thus the evidence of spinal cord involvement is only circumstantial, although it would be expected to mimic that of tetanus toxin.

The clinical effect of the toxin is primarily due to its action at the neuromuscular junction, and this typically occurs up to about 3 days after administration of the toxin. The delay between the appearance of the toxin at the neuromuscular junction and the onset of paralysis is not understood, but may be due to a protracted effect of the protease on substrate metabolism or a proximal spread of the toxin, as suggested above. Long-term exposure to the toxin causes reversible denervation atrophy (Spencer and McNeer, 1987; Harris *et al.*, 1991; Borodic and Ferrante, 1992), and non-collateral sprouting can occur from the nodes of Ranvier of myelinated parent pre-terminal axons, unmyelinated terminal axons immediately proximal to the end plate, or ultraterminal axonal arborization over the end plate. Necrosis or inflammation is not seen and different activities are not only seen between different individuals, but between different muscles within the same person. Borodic (1992) showed that BTX-A diffuses up to 4.5 cm from the site of a single injection of 10 u per 0.1 ml injection into the longissimus dorsi muscle of rabbits. The denervation field is largely determined by the dose and the volume of the toxin and it was suggested that multiple point injections of smaller volumes along the muscle might better restrict the toxin's biologic effects to the boundaries of the target muscle. Shaari and Sanders (1993) tested the effects of dose, volume and injection site on paralysis in tibialis anterior muscles in rats, which were subjected to repetitive prolonged stimulation of the common peroneal nerve. The effect of the toxin was greatest when injected closest to the motor end plate band, and fell dramatically with distance. At a constant volume, a 10–25-fold increase in dose was needed to double the area of paralysis; at a constant dose, this same doubling could be achieved with a 100-fold increase in volume. A dose of 5 u in 25 ml produced an area of paralysis of 50 mm^2, the total cross-sectional area of the rat tibialis anterior muscle. Therefore in clinical practice divided doses are given in muscles, and it is recognized that increasing the dose will increase the area of paralysis but not necessarily the duration of weakness.

Commercial preparation of the toxin

Botulinum toxin cultures are established in a fermenter, grown, acidified, and harvested by centrifugation (Tonello *et al.*, 1996). The toxin is purified and monitored for its potency and protein content, and solubilization reduces any contamination. It is then added to a diluent containing human serum albumin and prepared in vials for freeze drying, sealing and storage. BTX-A is most commonly used, and is marketed throughout the world by Allergan Inc. as Botox®. It is prepared in the USA and Ireland, and shipped worldwide. Speywood Pharmaceuticals, a subsidiary of Beufour Ipsen, also produces BTX-A in the United Kingdom as Dysport®, and markets their product throughout Europe. The products have equal potency and efficacy and have been used with equivalent success in clinical trials.

A word of caution is necessary here. The unit of measurement for BTX-A is the mouse unit (mU), which is a unit of bioactivity or potency and not of weight (Harris *et al.*, 1991), and is determined according to published specifications of the amount of toxin required to kill 50 per cent of a group of 18–20-g Swiss–Webster mice (LD50) (Hatheway and Dang, 1994). A vial of Botox® contains 100 units, while a vial of Dysport® contains 500 units. One unit of Botox® is not equivalent to 1 unit of Dysport®, and studies have been undertaken to identify equivalent doses. There are significant differences of 3.5–10 times between the observed potencies of the various doses in differing clinical situations, and most workers agree an equivalence of 1 Botox® unit to 3–5 Dysport® units (Odergren *et al.*, 1998). It is important for clinicians to realize that the two preparations of BTX-A are therefore quite distinct and not generic. It is for this reason that many people suggest the use of one preparation only to avoid confusion, as the expectation of clinical effect can be quite different from one clinical situation to another. These differences in unit potency may be due in part to differences in the dilution vehicle and the scheme of potency testing. Dysport® is reconstituted in saline but tested in a gelatin–phosphate buffer, which has been shown to increase the BTX-A potency relative to saline, whereas Botox® is tested and administered in saline (Brin, 1997). The World Health Organization and National Institute of Biological Standards and Control have recently undertaken a study on the issue, and a new paralysis assay may result in the definition of an international unit system. Obviously this will be important to clinicians, and will resolve much of the potential confusion.

BTX-A is also produced in Japan, but this particular product has not been marketed in the USA or Europe. BTX-B has recently gone into commercial production for the treatment of spasmodic torticollis (Athena Neurosciences, USA). Recent clinical trials have used doses of between 2500 and 10 000 units, but again the units are of different potencies to those of BTX-A (Lew *et al.*, 1997). These compare to the usual doses of 150–250 units of Botox®. It is thus very important that the exact preparation is indicated whenever the dose of the toxin is written, in order to avoid confusion. Most people use the abbreviation BTX-A to describe the generic preparation.

Toxicity

Despite the fearful reputation of botulism and the toxin as the world's most powerful neurotoxin, the safety profile of the purified product has been quite remarkable. Scott and Suzuki (1988) determined the LD50 in monkeys to be approximately 39 units/kg body weight following intramuscular injection. Even intravenous injection showed a similar LD50 of 40 units/kg, and Scott also found that the lowest dose causing systemic toxicity was about 33 units/kg. The lethal dose of the toxin in humans is not known, but extrapolating data from two studies to a 70 kg human implies a LD50 of about 3000 units (Herrero *et al.*, 1967; Scott and Suzuki, 1988). Since the recommended maximum dose is 400 units at one sitting, there is a high safety margin. It is also suggested that further toxin should not be given within 3 months, which allows the product a further margin of safety. Morbidity is also low and cardiotoxicity is not a feature. ECG evidence of conduction defects was only seen in doses exceeding the lethal dose in animal studies, and accidental overdose requiring treatment is thus unlikely (Lamanna *et al.*, 1988). Anti-toxin is available to treat this, and the medical department at Allergan has a telephone information and advice line for this purpose. However, the anti-toxin is not risk-free, as it contains foreign immunoglobulins and produces anaphylaxis in up to 9 per cent of those receiving it (Tacket and Rogawski, 1989). Its effectiveness also diminishes within 1 day of the toxin overdose. Fortunately the toxin's safety record means that it really does not have to be used.

Non-response and antibody detection

Development of resistance to BTX-A is characterized by the absence of any beneficial effect and by the lack of muscular atrophy following the injection. Antibodies against toxin are presumed to be important and to be responsible for most cases of resistance. These have been shown in the small number of people who develop antibodies in response to treatment (Zuber *et al.*, 1993; Green *et al.*, 1994), and several types of assays are now available to detect their presence in serum. However, the most likely causes of non-response are insufficient dosage, incorrect assessment of the muscles at fault or poor needle localization/injection technique (Figure 13.2; Koko and Ward, 1997).

In vivo mouse neutralization assays are available to detect the presence of antibody in serum, and in its assay, BTX-A is titrated with human serum suspected of harbouring anti-BTX-A antibodies (Hatheway and Dang, 1994). After injection into mice, the binding of antibodies with the toxin prevents deaths from the toxin's effects. Immunosorbent assays have been used to detect anti-BTX antibody, including an enzyme-linked immunosorbent assay (ELISA) (Doellgast *et al.*, 1994; botulinum toxin type A antibody test, Athena Diagnostics Inc., USA), an enzyme-linked coagulation assay, a sphere-linked diagnostic assay (Siatkowski *et al.*, 1993), a Western blot assay and a combined fluoroscein and enzyme-linked assay (Doellgast *et al.*, 1997). However, correlation between positive results and clinical resistance has not been established and patients may well develop antibodies to parts of the toxin, which are functionally not important (Doellgast *et al.*, 1994).

Much of the work on antibodies and resistance has concerned patients with cervical dystonias, and between 3 per cent and 5 per cent of patients have been found

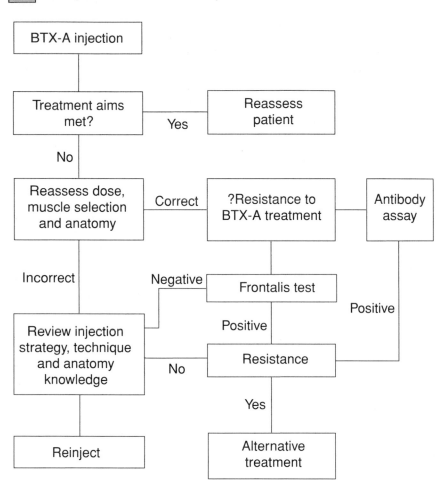

Figure 13.2 Response following botulinum toxin injection.

to have antibodies (Zuber *et al.*, 1993). However, it is the level of antibody titre that is important in human resistance, and this may be too low in many cases in animal studies. For instance, the mouse lethality assay reports much lower rates of antibody production, but probably underestimates the number of cases of immunoresistance. While a positive antibody result appears to correlate with a poor clinical response to treatment, a negative response is not necessarily predictive of a good clinical response (Greene *et al.*, 1993, 1994; Jankovic and Schwartz, 1995). In their study of 559 patients with cervical dystonia, Greene *et al.* did not test all non-responders, but showed that at least 24 developed antibodies (Greene *et al.*, 1993; Zuber *et al.*, 1993). They therefore suggested that the true prevalence of patients with antibodies may be more than 7 per cent. All seropositive patients were resistant to treatment, but some originally responsive patients who later developed resistance had no serological evidence of antibody production (Greene *et al.*, 1993). When comparing a second cohort of patients clinically resistant to treatment against non-resistant patients, the resistant patients had had a shorter interval between injections, more booster injections and a higher dose per 3-month interval, as well as a higher dose of non-booster injections. Of the eight patients who developed clinical resistance, three were seropositive and five were not. The inference therefore is that less frequent injections and a lower dose per 3-month interval results in less resistance, and this philosophy has been adopted in the treatment of spasticity. Jankovic and Wartz (1995) also reported resistance in dystonia patients, and some of these patients had only been treated once; 4.5 per cent showed an inadequate or lack of response, and a subset of patients were tested for seropositivity. These were probably at an earlier age of the onset of their dystonia and having a higher mean dose per visit. A higher total cumulative dose also correlated.

The frontalis test is a clinical test of toxin resistance, in which 15 units of BTX-A is injected into two sites on one side of the corrugator muscle (Hanna and Jankovic, 1998). If the muscle does not contract after 2 weeks and the patient cannot furrow that side of the forehead, the patient is not resistant; a lack of response suggests resistance. (This technique is also used widely in the USA and Europe for cosmesis of facial wrinkles.) Kessler and Benneke (1997) have also reported a neurophysiological challenge to patients suspected of resistance to treatment of their dystonia. Measuring muscle action potentials in extensor digitorum brevis muscle following common peroneal nerve stimulation has shown that seropositive non-responders remain unchanged for roughly 4 weeks after the injection, whereas in seronegative non-responders a marked decrease in amplitude was detected. This indicates that patients remained susceptible to the effects of BTX-A despite their clinical resistance, and suggests that the dose may have been suboptimal or the injection site inaccurate. This test may go on to be useful in conjunction with the antibody test in the diagnosis of truly resistant patients.

A number of studies have also shown that BTX-A resistance may be circumvented by injections with other serotypes. In particular, both BTX-B and BTX-F appear to give benefit, and studies have shown that the former appears to last for about a month (Jankovic and Schwartz, 1995) and that both seronegative and positive patients benefit (Greene and Fahn, 1996). A recent report on BTX-C shows it too has a similar duration of effect to BTX-A (Eleopra *et al.*, 1997).

In conclusion, therefore, the following are recommended in order to minimize the possibility of non-response and immunoresistance:

- the smallest possible effective dose should be used, and no more than 400 units per 3-month interval
- intervals between treatments should be as long as possible and not be less than 3 months
- booster injections should be avoided.

Figure 5 in the Spasticity Study Group's training syllabus demonstrates a useful method of investigating non-response in patients (Spasticity Study Group, 1997).

Contraindications and warnings

BTX-A is a safe drug, and there are no absolute contraindications. Patients with pre-existing dysfunction of the neuromuscular junction may be injected with caution; this includes those with myasthenia gravis (Emerson, 1994) or conditions affecting the anterior horn cell, such as motor neurone disease (Mezake *et al.*, 1996) and poliomyelitis. Similarly, patients with the Eaton–Lambert syndrome (Erbguth *et al.*, 1993) are of concern, and one patient had subclinical Eaton–Lambert syndrome unmasked by BTX-A injections for blepharospasm. Two patients with limb spasticity developed features of botulism (Bakheit *et al.*, 1997), and these were the first cases reported. While limb spasticity had been associated with injections around the neck (Brans *et al.*, 1995), it had not been associated with dysphagia. However, further data are required.

BTX-A is safe in both adults and children, but long-term studies are only just being published. Children do not appear to have adverse effects any more frequently than adults, and the commonest features are of greater widespread weakness than that expected from the injection. However, weakness and EMG changes in muscles distant to the site of the injection are not features (Koman *et al.*, 1993), and any detectable abnormalities of single fibre EMG have not had any clinical significance (Girlanda *et al.*, 1992). Transient weakness has been reported, such as urinary incontinence in twin boys lasting for 3 weeks, for lower limb spasticity (Boyd *et al.*, 1996). It is recommended that pregnant and lactating women are not injected due to lack of information on the potential effects. In one study of 16 pregnant women treated in the first trimester, there were two miscarriages and 14 normal deliveries. While there were no signs of toxin effects in the newborn, further evaluation is necessary (Moser *et al.*, 1997). An immune mechanism may underlie some cases of side effects (Glanzmann *et al.*, 1990); a brachial plexopathy was noted following a sternocleidomastoid muscle injection.

A transient flu-like syndrome lasting for a few days has been reported in a number of patients, but the cause for this is not known. Weakness appears to be the commonest effect, but lack of specificity of both assessment and injection is of far more significance than true side effects. For this reason, the American Academy of Neurology has recommended training for injectors of botulinum toxin and has released training guidelines (American Academy of Neurology, 1994). It has also indicated that this should be part of medical practice, and not delegated to other professions. Treatment should be part of an overall management of the spastic patient, and doctors should know the relevant anatomy and have some training in neurophysiology and electromyography.

Effectiveness of BTX-A in multiple sclerosis

Although BTX-A is not licensed for the treatment of spasticity in acquired disorders, there is little doubt that it is effective and has been fairly widely used in MS patients (Snow *et al.*, 1990; Borg-Stein *et al.*, 1993). Much of the work in adult spasticity has been performed in stroke and spinal cord injured patients, but the same principles apply, and MS is a good model for spasticity management for all disabling chronic neurological diseases. Several clinical scales have been utilized in MS patients, which include the validation of the original Ashworth Scale (Ashworth, 1964). Two uncontrolled studies have been undertaken in MS patients, reporting the effect of BTX-A in reducing lower limb spasticity (Borg-Stein *et al.*, 1993; Benecke, 1994), but the randomized cross-over study by Snow and colleagues has stood the test of time as one of the few double-blind placebo-controlled trials of BTX-A for spasticity in MS (Snow *et al.*, 1990). The patient cohort was made up of 10 non-ambulatory patients with thigh adductor spasticity that interfered with their posture in a wheelchair, their perineal hygiene and ease of urethral catheterization. Four hundred units of BTX-A or placebo were injected into both thigh adductor muscle groups, and patients were followed up for 6 weeks and then reinjected at 12 weeks with the alternate BTX-A or placebo. There was a significant benefit of BTX-A over the placebo in reducing the spasticity score and hygiene score. In addition, no adverse effects were noted in the BTX-treated patients.

Studies of BTX-A treatment in other conditions also support its use for the treatment of spasticity in MS patients (Shakta *et al.*, 1996). Bohlega *et al.* (1995) took 11 patients with spastic hereditary paraplegia in an open-label study and injected lower limb muscles, and 10 of them improved on at least one measure of tone, range of joint movement, gait or global change. Upper and lower limb studies in spasticity following stroke showed an improvement on the modified Ashworth Scale of at least one grade, a reduction in muscle spasm frequency and a beneficial change in the level of pain. However, changes in activities of daily living scores, such as the Functional Independence Measurement (FIM), were not significant, although this is perhaps not surprising because they are global scales and BTX-A is a focal treatment (Barnes, 1997).

Cost-effectiveness

The priority now is to show that BTX-A is a cost-effective addition to anti-spastic treatment. Although the toxin is expensive it is known to be an effective treatment, and one method of demonstrating its place in management is through the establishment of a spasticity service. The main cost relates to the price of the toxin, whereas other specialized treatments (such as nerve blockade with phenol and intrathecal baclofen) have considerable manpower costs as well. While phenol may be very cheap, nerve blockade may take quite a while to perform; therefore the doctor's time must be added to the cost of the procedure. In contrast, BTX-A administration literally takes only a few minutes. Training costs must also be added for all these techniques, and these are considerable for intrathecal baclofen. As stated above, doctors should be trained in these procedures, but there should be general training for all practitioners involved in spasticity management.

A number of pharmaco-economic studies concentrating on acquired brain injury due to stroke and trauma have commenced, but as far as the author is aware there are no specific studies concerning multiple sclerosis. A German study

(Wallesch *et al.*, 1997) looked at the cost of three treatment strategies following stroke; physiotherapy only, BTX-A plus physiotherapy, and oral baclofen plus physiotherapy. Decisions and costs regarding medical intervention were based on a Delphi panel survey of 13 neurologists, and the panel estimated that the average extent of improvement with BTX-A with physiotherapy, as measured by the Ashworth Scale, was three times greater than for baclofen plus physiotherapy, and 10 times greater than for physiotherapy alone. The total direct medical costs did not differ markedly, but it was felt that the overall cost was about DM 3000 (~£1000) per additional unit improvement on the Ashworth Scale. While it is difficult to make direct comparisons to real-life clinical situations for other conditions, and while the Ashworth Scale has major flaws, the overall consequence of this study is interesting in terms of defining a role for BTX-A in spasticity management. Other cost-effectiveness studies have compared the cost of care, the level of personal functioning and the placement of patients, but have lacked definitive health gain outcomes; this complicates the message given to health care payers. One of the real issues in this equation is the amount of toxin used, and further information on dosage is given below.

Treatment rationale in MS

Botulinum toxin is effective in the treatment of spasticity in MS, as in other conditions. As noted above, its success depends on accurate patient assessment and in defining the underlying problems as the goals for treatment. The spasticity found in MS patients presents considerable difficulties as, unlike in brain injury, spinal cord injury or cerebral palsy, the patient has a progressive disorder that can change rapidly. BTX-A tends to be used for severe disease when patients have moved into a progressive phase and problems relate to mobility, posture, continence and pain, and Table 13.4 lists some of the indications for treatment.

Aim of treatment

The aim of treating MS patients with BTX-A is to produce selective muscle weakness with the smallest possible dose and thereby reduce the harmful effects of spasticity in order to achieve the rehabilitation objectives. The toxin is given by accurate intramuscular injection, with or without the use of electromyography, to produce a flaccid paralysis. It is one of a range of available treatments, and can be used in combination with other medication (Koko and Ward, 1997). It is an adjunct to physical treatment, and the scheme is given in Figure 13.3.

Patient assessment

Certain decisions are required during treatment (Table 13.5). The scope of the problem must be defined and the difficulty experienced by the patient in carrying out a particular task must, if possible, be quantified. The degree of the problem and the way in which it is interfering with life must also be clarified. Patients must

Table 13.4 Indications for botulinum toxin treatment in spasticity

To achieve rehabilitation objectives	
Improve function – Personal	Mobility – quality and speed, wheelchair propulsion
	Transfers
	Seating/positioning/comfortable fitting of casts
	Dexterity and reaching
	Sexuality and sexual functioning
	Self-care and hygiene
	Promote continence
	Other activities of daily living
– Carer	Positioning
	Care and hygiene
	Dressing
	Decrease care time to allow quality time
Pain relief	
Improve sleep	
Contracture prevention	
Cosmesis	Improve body image
	Fitting of clothes

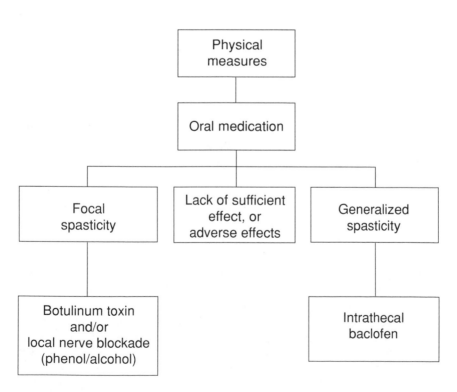

Figure 13.3 Management strategy.

Table 13.5 Treatment decisions

Patient characteristics	Size of patient (weight and muscle bulk)
	Degree of spasticity (based on Ashworth or Tardieu Score)
	Overall health status
Scope of the problem	What is the problem? (focal, regional or generalized spasticity)
	Severity of the spasticity – induced disability
Therapeutic objectives	Within context of rehabilitation programme
Cost–benefit and risk–benefit analysis of treatment	

be in reasonable health to benefit from the treatment, for while this may reduce energy costs for mobility, it is important that patients will be able to use the benefits to their advantage. The aims of treatment depend on both the rehabilitation aims for that particular patient and on the underlying condition. Clearly they will be different for someone trying to maintain ambulation as compared to a patient with little or no independent function. Experience needs to be gained regarding when to treat patients with BTX-A, and what combination of agents to use.

Assessment is based on identifying the muscle or group of muscles that is causing the immediate problem. Four scenarios come to mind in multiple sclerosis patients:

• the spastic upper arm and shoulder
• flexed wrist and clawed hand
• flexor and thigh adductor spasticity
• talipes equinovarus deformity.

Gaining skill in assessing and treating patients with these four clinical pictures will account for the great majority of problems encountered. Doctors must have a good knowledge of muscle anatomy and function and, of course, of surface anatomy. They must know the origin, insertion and action of muscles, and the location of relevant injection sites. In chronic spasticity, changes occur in myocyte structure and function and muscle contracture occurs due to enhanced velocity-independent plastic resistance, which leads to changes in muscle type (Hufschmidt and Mauritz, 1985; Dattola *et al.*, 1993). Slow oxidative conversion of longstanding spastic muscle from fast glycolytic allows easier recruitment, and may not only sustain but also enhance the spastic state (Dattola *et al.*, 1993). This eventually leads to tendon, soft tissue and joint capsule contracture, with subsequent deformity. It is sometimes very difficult to distinguish severe Ashworth Grade 4 stiffness from contracture in deformed limbs, and it may be necessary to use sedation to assess the patient. Intravenous benzodiazepines perform this task very well, are quick and easy to give, and have the advantage of being themselves good anti-spastic agents. A general anaesthetic may be used, but this is potentially problematic and gives a very artificial situation. Nerve blockade is also possible, but time-consuming and painful. BTX-A is not helpful in the treatment of contractures, and muscles may switch off during this period; it is only useful for spasticity, which explains the need to distinguish contracture from severe Ashworth Grade 4 spasticity.

Treatment success depends on the expected outcomes, which will be specific to individual patients. In other words, treatment is part of the rehabilitation process and comes within the goals that have been agreed between the team, patient and carer. It is thus vital that everyone has a clear idea of the expected outcome and aims of the injection. It is necessary to state this over and over again in order to arrive at realistic and achievable goals and important to employ the most relevant outcome measures before injection in order to gain a baseline against which to compare the effect of treatment. Treatment may or may not affect function, and both body and personal functions are useful measures of outcome. For reasons given above, patients may have little or no function and treatment may be aimed at reducing carer burden; in these cases, the most appropriate measurement may be of carer function. As in all rehabilitation lateral thinking is required, and measures of the impact of a procedure along the lines of impairments, disability and handicap or, in ICIDH-2 terms, of impairments, activity and participation (WHO, 1997). The following are some of the measures used in MS patients.

Impairment	Measurement of disability
Modified Ashworth Scale	Walking speed, e.g. 10 m walking time
Joint range of movement	Functional abilities, e.g. nine-hole peg test
Gait patterns and deviations	Rivermead Behavioural Mobility Test
Pain	Activities of daily living, e.g.. Barthel, FIM
Mood	Carer burden

Many measures can be employed, and Wade's book *Measurement in Neurological Rehabilitation* (Wade, 1996) is useful. The most important outcome measure is, however, goal attainment and with experience, rehabilitationists get better at predicting valid, valuable and achievable goals with sufficient ambition to benefit the patient and carer. Therefore, if spasticity is interfering with function to a point where climbing stairs has become impossible, what better outcome measure is there than restoring this function?

Hesse *et al.* (1997) showed that uptake of the toxin is increased in active muscles and that exercise and functional electrical stimulation can enhance the toxin's paralytic effect. It is therefore wise to stimulate the muscle as much as possible around the time of the injection and for a period thereafter.

Injection technique

Doctors who wish to inject BTX-A must be especially trained, as gaining the necessary skills requires time and commitment. The accurate placing of the injection is straightforward, but careful thought is required to achieve good results. BTX-A has a great propensity to seek neuromuscular junctions, but placing the toxin as near as practical to them may achieve better results, and a sound knowledge of anatomy is necessary. This is particularly important for regions where the target muscles require selective weakness and adjacent muscles should be spared.

Should EMG guidance be used to inject muscles? This is certainly unnecessary for large, superficial, easily visible muscles, but it is advisable for smaller and deep muscles, particularly forearm and lower leg muscles, hip flexors (psoas major) and small inaccessible muscles around the jaw. The aim is to record muscle action potentials and their interference patterns on voluntary activation. This can sometimes be difficult to interpret in view of mass synergies in spasticity, and either active contraction of the muscle or passive movements will indicate the correct placement. EMG guidance is particularly useful in flexor digitorum profundus and extensor digitorum communis muscles, which are organized into muscular fascicles supplying each digit. Correct placement of the needle can therefore allow neuromuscular blockade for each fascicle and hence accurate denervation.

The procedure is carried out using a hollow Teflon®-coated EMG needle with a sideport for syringe attachment. Motor point stimulation can also be carried out to activate small intramuscular fascicles. This is time consuming but it does place the toxin as closely as possible to the binding area, the motor end plate; however, increased effectiveness has not been shown in human studies. Animal studies support a relationship between dose-related diffusion and the muscle response (Borodic *et al.*, 1994), and a study in humans is now required. At present, the avid binding of toxin to presynaptic nerve terminals does not necessarily make motor stimulation vital for clinical practice. Motor stimulation has been used primarily for nerve blockade, where the immediate expected response can authenticate the accuracy of the procedure. It is possible that accurate localization through EMG guidance can reduce the dose of toxin, which is obviously important for patients with progressive disorders such as multiple sclerosis and for those requiring repeated injections. In this way, costs will be contained and the chance of antibody-mediated non-responsiveness decreased. Motor point injection with phenol takes longer, and the increased procedure time taken should be included in cost comparisons.

The four clinical scenarios described earlier require treatment of specific groups of muscles, and these are described below. The commonly injected muscles and dosages are detailed in Table 13.6.

The spastic upper arm and shoulder

This typically results in adduction and internal rotation of the upper arm, with flexion of the elbow and pronation of the forearm. With increasing spasticity, contractures occur at the shoulder and elbow and difficulties arise in maintaining axillary hygiene. The clinical findings are due to spasm in all groups, but particularly the subscapularis muscle, pectoralis group and, to a lesser extent, the latissimus dorsi muscle and teres minor muscle. Injection of these muscles is indicated, followed by physical therapy. Pronator teres and pronator quadratus muscles are responsible for the pronation deformity.

The flexed wrist and clawed hand

In the flexed wrist and clawed hand, the flexor muscles exert a greater influence than the extensors. This results in flexion deformities of the wrist and small joints of the hand, as well as pronation of the forearm. The flexor carpi radialis and ulnaris muscles are responsible for flexion of the wrist, and the lumbrical muscles for flexion of the fingers at the metacarpophalangeal joints. The flexor digitorum superficialis muscle flexes the fingers at the proximal interphalangeal joints, and the flexor digitorum profundus muscle is responsible for flexion of the terminal phalanges. It is important to differentiate between these muscles in order to localize the injection accurately. Thumb flexion deformity should be dealt with, as hand function is not possible with an adducted flexed thumb in the palm. This is caused by the flexor pollicis longus and brevis, the opponens pollicis and the adductor pollicis muscles.

Hip flexor and thigh adductor spasticity

Scissoring of the legs is a common feature in non-ambulant severely disabled people with MS. They are usually obligate wheelchair users, and their legs are not sufficiently stretched to overcome flexor muscle shortening. With time, they assume a typical 'wheelchair user' shape, and difficulties arise with perineal hygiene, dressing and undressing, and with transfers. These problems have significant care implications. Patients may also complain of considerable pain. Injection of adductor muscles is useful in patients with true adductor spasm, but in a significant proportion of people this is not the answer and adductor muscle injection is not very effective. In such patients, hip flexor spasticity and shortening are responsible for the problem. The action of the psoas major muscle is to flex the hip and internally rotate and adduct the thigh, mimicking adductor spasticity and also results in patients being unable to stand erect; it is most important to deal with this muscle prior to the adductor group. Because the psoas major muscle is segmentally innervated, injection is required at each individual level, and 50 units is placed at L2, L3 and L4 to a total of 150 units per muscle. The psoas major arises from the lateral aspect of the vertebral bodies from T12–L5, but the muscle is thin at T12 and L1 and lies posterior to the kidney. It is thus wise to avoid injecting here, but the muscle is thick and well rounded at L2–5 before forming its tendon as it enters the pelvis and joining that of iliacus muscle to form the ilio-psoas tendon, which inserts into the lesser trochanter. The lumbo-sacral plexus is closely applied at the L5 level, and it is advisable to steer clear of this area as well. A considerable effect is achieved by injecting at L2, 3 and 4, which deals with hip flexor spasticity more than adequately. The most sensitive measures are hip flexion deformity angle changes (demonstrated by the Thomas test), and the stride length and walking speed (tested by a 10 m walking time) in ambulant patients and by a modified Ashworth Scale in non-ambulant patients. Less commonly, rectus femoris muscle shortening results in loss of hip extension (demonstrated by the Staheli test), since it crosses both hip and knee joints.

Table 13.6 Commonly injected muscles

Clinical pattern	Muscles involved	Origin	Insertion	Action	No. of injection sites	Dose (units Botox)
Upper limb						
Spastic shoulder	Pectoralis major	Clavicle and third to eighth anterior ribs	Greater tubercle of humerus	Adducts and medially rotates arm	4	100
	Latissimus dorsi	Tips of lower six thoracic spines and iliac crest	Intertubular groove of humerus	Adducts, retracts, medially rotates arms	4	100
	Subscapularis	Anterior aspect scapula	Lesser tubercle of humerus	Medially rotates arm	1	50
Flexed arm	Biceps brachii	Short: coracoid process; Long: s/glenoid tubercle of scapula	Bicipital aponeurosis	Supination and elbow flexion	4	100–150
	Brachialis	Anterior distal humerus	Ulnar coronoid process	Flexes elbow in pronation	2	50–75
	Brachioradialis	Supracondylar ridge of humerus	Lateral surface distal radius	Flexes elbow	2	50
Pronated forearm	Pronator teres	MHE and ulnar coronoid process	Middle radius	Pronates forearm	1	40
	Pronator quadratus	Distal ulna	Distal radius	Pronates forearm	1	25
Flexed wrist	Flexor carpi radialis	MHE	Base second metacarpal	Flexes wrist and elbow	1	40
	Flexor carpi ulnaris	MHE and olecranon	Pisiform bone in wrist	Flexes and adducts hand	1	40
Clenched fist	Flexor digit profundus	Proximal two-thirds of ulna	Terminal phalanges	Flexes all finger joints	1	40
	Flexor digit superficialis	MHE, coronoid, upper half of radius	Middle phalanges	Flexes PIP and MCP joints	1	40
	Flexor pollicis longus	Upper two-thirds of radius	Terminal phalanx of thumb	Flexes all joints of thumb	1	25

Lower limb

	Muscle	Origin	Insertion	Action		Dose
Flexed hip	Psoas major	T12–L5 vertebral bodies	Lesser trochanter	Flexes hip, medial rotation of leg	3	150 (50 U at L2, L3 and L4)
	Iliacus	Floor of ilium	Lesser trochanter	Flexes hip, medial rotation of leg	2	100
Adducted thigh	Rectus femoris	Anterior inferior iliac spine	Tibial tubercle	Flexes hip and extends knee	4	100
	Adductor magnus	Ischial tuberosity	Posterior two-thirds of leg	Adducts and laterally rotates thigh	4	150–200 into adductor group
	Adductor longus	Pubic body and symphysis	Linea alba, femur	Adducts thigh	4	
Flexed knee	Medial hamstrings	Ischial tuberosity	Pes anserinus	Flexes knee	4	150
	Biceps femoris	Ischial tuberosity and linea aspera, femur	Pes anserinus	Flexes knee	4	150
Equino varus foot	Medial and lateral heads of gastrocnemius	Medial and lateral femoral condyles	Calcaneum	Plantar flexes foot	4	150
	Soleus	Posterior tibia and fibula	Calcaneum	Plantar flexes foot	2	150
	Tibialis posterior	Interosseous membrane and posterior tibia and fibula	Base of fifth metatarsal	Inverts foot in plantar flexion	2	75
Extended toes	Flexor hallucis longus	Posterior fibula	First terminal phalanx	Flexes great toe	1	50
	Flexor digitalis longus	Posterior tibia	Terminal phalanges	Flexes toes	1	50
	Tibialis anterior	Upper half of tibia	Medial cuneiform bone	Dorsiflexes foot	2	75
	Extensor hallucis longus	Middle half of fibula	Base of terminal phalanx	Extends great toe	1	50
	Extensor digitalis longus	Upper three-quarters of fibula	Second to fifth phalanges	Extends toes	1	50

MHE, medial humeral epicondyle; PIP, proximal interphalangeal; MCP, metacarpophalangeal.

Talipes equino-varus foot

A common feature of a spastic lower limb is an inverted plantar-flexed foot, and it is important to demonstrate that this is due to spasticity rather than to an imbalance between the plantar flexor/inverter and dorsiflexor/everter muscles, because BTX-A will not be effective if the deformity is simply due to weakness. Where spasticity is the major feature, injection of the tibialis posterior and posterior calf muscles is useful for the purpose of achieving a straight foot to allow weight bearing or fitting of an orthosis. This facilitates standing transfers and allows the patient to stand on a flat foot, which is essential for safe walking. The best outcome measures are the range of active and passive dorsi- and plantar-flexion at the ankle, and walking speed in ambulant patients. It is often necessary to inject all the muscles, but differentiation between the contributions from gastrocnemius and soleus muscles and Achilles tendon contracture is easy, and expertise comes with practice. An effective alternative is to carry out a posterior tibial nerve blockade with 6 per cent phenol in aqueous solution, but this is time consuming and may give rise to a troublesome dysaesthesia in the sole of the foot.

Post-injection care

Since the treatment of spasticity is essentially physical, one of the aims of BTX-A is to enhance the effect of physical therapy by utilizing the maximal effect of the toxin (or any nerve blockade) to allow promotion of further physical improvement. In order to maximize its effect, a treatment strategy is necessary. Intensive physiotherapy in the form of stretching and strengthening is thus required for at least 4 weeks immediately following the procedure. As a result, it has been noted anecdotally that the effect of a single dose of BTX-A can be prolonged beyond its action duration, and repeat injections, which are necessary for MS patients, can be reduced to a minimum. Limbs should be stretched to a functional position, but should not be traumatized because this will provide a nociceptive stimulus to increase spasticity in non-injected muscles. Therapy should be given every day for a period of at least 4 weeks, but the benefit, duration and optimal regimen requires scientific evaluation. Similarly, there is anecdotal information that, to be effective, stretching should be carried out for several hours every day. Clearly this cannot be done on a one-to-one basis, and splinting and casting are therefore very useful; skills in this technique need to be improved. Casting expertise has traditionally been in locomotor rehabilitation, but this treatment in neurological rehabilitation depends on different principles in order to prevent further spasticity. Effective casting can provide a stretch for several hours, and night resting casts are thus of particular value because they achieve this purpose without interfering with daily activities.

Follow-up is important to identify whether or not the treatment objectives have been met and to plan further treatment. As stated above, it is important to identify those muscles requiring injection at the start of treatment episode and to re-inject 3–4 months later if necessary. At each follow-up the relevant outcome measures should be recorded, and it is worth having a separate page in the clinical notes for this purpose, noting the date of the injection, the muscles injected and the outcome measures used. Multiple sclerosis patients, like others with chronic spasticity, may require repeated injections, and it is important to have clear documentation of previous treatment. A trend may thus be observed to aid further management.

Conclusion

This chapter has described the place of botulinum toxin treatment in the management of spasticity in patients with multiple sclerosis. Physicians and surgeons wishing to learn this technique should contact the representatives of manufacturers of the toxin to participate in the relevant training courses. In Great Britain and Ireland, the British Society of Rehabilitation Medicine has a database of doctors involved in BTX-A treatment of spasticity, and 1-day training courses are held in Stoke on Trent several times per year. These are open both to trainees and to doctors wishing to undertake continuing medical education in this subject. In the USA and Canada, both the American Academy of Neurology and the American Academy of Physical Medicine and Rehabilitation have databases of forthcoming seminars, including those on spasticity management and botulinum toxin treatment. Those interested may contact the relevant Academy directly, or use their web pages for further information (http://www.ana.org and http://ww.aapmr.org). The use of BTX-A is variable in Europe, but is growing rapidly. The author is not aware of formal national training programmes, but has given lectures and run seminars in Sweden, Finland, Holland, the Czech Republic and Russia.

BTX-A has certainly increased interest in the management of spasticity, not only in terms of the injection technique, but also in other aspects of care and rehabilitation.

References

American Academy of Neurology (Therapeutics and Technology Assessment Subcommittee) (1994). Training guidelines for the use of botulinum toxin for the treatment of neurologic disorders. *Neurology*, **44**, 2401–3.

Ashworth, B. (1964). Preliminary trial of carisoprodal in multiple sclerosis. *Practitioner*, **192**, 540.

Bakheit, M., Ward, C. D. and McLellan, D. L. (1997). Generalised botulism-like syndrome after intramuscular injections of botulinum toxin type A: a report of two cases (letter). *J. Neurol. Neurosurg. Psychiatr.*, **62**, 198.

Barinaga, M. (1993). Secrets of secretion revealed. *Science*, **260**, 487–9.

Barnes, M. P. (1997). Experience of botulinum toxin in the management of spasticity. *Eur. J. Neurol.*, **4(Suppl. 2)**, S33–S36.

Benecke, R. (1994). Botulinum toxin for spasms and spasticity in the lower extremities. In: *Therapy with Botulinum Toxin* (J. Jankovic and M. Hallett, eds), pp. 557–65. Marcel Dekker.

Bhakta, B. B., Cozens, J. A., Bamford, J. M. and Chamberlain, M. A. (1996). Use of botulinum toxin in stroke patients with severe upper limb spasticity. *J. Neurol. Neurosurg. Psychiatr.*, **61(1)**, 30–35.

Binz, T., Kurazono, H., Wille, M. *et al.* (1990). The complete sequence of botulinum neurotoxin type A and comparison with other clostridial neurotoxins. *J. Biol. Chem.*, **265**, 9153–8.

Black, J. D. and Dolly, J. O. (1986). Interaction of 125-labelled botulinum toxins with nerve terminals. I. Ultrastructural autoradiographic localisation and quantitation of distinct membrane receptors for types A and B on motor nerves. *J. Cell Biol.*, **103**, 521–34.

Blast, J., Chapman, E. R., Yamasaki, S. *et al.* (1993). Botulinum toxin C1 blocks neurotransmitter release by means of cleaving IIPC 1/syntaxin. *EMBO J.*, **12**, 4821–8.

Bohlega, S., Chaud, P. and Jacob, P. C. (1995). Botulinum toxin A in the treatment of lower limb spasticity in hereditary spastic paraplegia (abstract). *Movement Disorders*, **10**, 399.

Borg-Stein, J., Pine, Z. M., Miller, J. R. and Brin, M. F. (1993). Botulinum toxin for the treatment of spasticity in multiple sclerosis: new observations. *Am. J. Phys. Med. Rehabil.*, **72**, 364–8.

Borodic, G. E. and Ferrante, R. (1992). Effects of repeated botulinum toxin injections on orbicularis oculi muscle. *J. Clin. Neuro-ophthalmol.*, **12**, 121–7.

Borodic, G. E., Ferrante, R., Pearce, L. B. and Smith, K. (1994). Histologic assessment of dose related diffusion and muscle fibre response after therapeutic botulinum A toxin injections. *Movement Disorders*, **9**, 31–9.

Boyd, R. N., Britton, T. C., Robinson, R. O. and Borzyskowski, M. (1996). Transient urinary incontinence after botulinum A toxin (letter). *Lancet*, **348**, 481–2.

Brans, J. W., de Boer, I. P., Aramideh, M. *et al.* (1995). Botulinum toxin in cervical dystonia: low dosage with electromyographic guidance. *J. Neurol.*, **242(8)**, 529–34.

Brin, M. F. (1997). Botulinum toxin: chemistry, pharmacology, toxicity and immunology. *Muscle Nerve*, **Suppl. 6**, S146–S168.

Burgen, A. F. V., Dickens, F. and Zatman, L. J. (1949). The action of botulinum toxin on the neuromuscular junction. *J. Physiol.*, **109**, 10–24.

Campbell, K., Collins, M. D. and East, A. K. (1993). Nucleotide sequence of the gene coding for *Clostridium botulinum* (*Clostridium argentinense*) type G; nucleotoxin genealogical comparison with other clostridial neurotoxins. *Biochim. Biophys. Acta*, **1216**, 487–91.

DasGupta, B. R. (1994). Structures of botulinum neurotoxin, its functional domains and perspectives on the crystalline type A toxin. In: *Therapy with Botulinum Toxin* (J. Jankovic and M. Hallett, eds), pp. 15–39. Marcel Dekker.

Dattola, R., Girland, P., Vita, G. *et al.* (1993). Muscle rearrangement in patients with hemiparesis after stroke: an electrophysiological and morphological study. *Eur. J. Neurol.*, **33**, 109–14.

Davis, D. (1993). Botulinum toxin: from poison to medicine. *W. J. Med.*, **158**,

25–9.

Doellgast, G. J., Beard, G. A., Bottoms, J. D. *et al.* (1994). Enzyme-linked immunosorbent assay and enzyme-linked coagulation assay for detection of *Clostridium botulinum* neurotoxin A, neurotoxin B and neurotoxin E and solution phase complexes with dual label antibodies. *J. Clin. Microbiol.*, **32**, 105–11.

Doellgast, G. J., Brown, J. E., Koufman, J. A. and Hatheway, C. L. (1997). Sensitive assay for measurement of antibodies to *Clostridium botulinum* neurotoxins A, B and E: use of hapten labelled antibody elution to isolate specific complexes. *J. Clin. Microbiol.*, **35**, 570–83.

Dolly, J. O. (1994). General properties and cellular mechanisms of neurotoxins. In: *Therapy with Botulinum Toxin* (J. Jankovic and M. Hallett, eds), pp. 168–83. Marcel Dekker.

Dolly, J. O., Ashton, A. C., McInnes, C. *et al.* (1990). Clues to the multi-phasic action of botulinum neurotoxins on release of transmitters. *J. Physiol.*, **84**, 237–46.

Eleopra, R., Tugnoli, V., Rossetto, O. *et al.* (1997). Botulinum neurotoxin serotype C: a novel, effective botulinum toxin therapy in humans. *Neurosci. Lett.*, **224**, 91–4.

Emerson, J. (1994). Botulinum toxin for spasmodic torticollis in a patient with myasthenia gravis. *Movement Disorders*, **9**, 367.

Erbguth, F., Claus, D., Engelhardt, A. and Dressler, D. (1993). Systemic effect of local botulinum toxin injections unmasks subclinical Lambert–Eaton myasthenic syndrome. *J. Neurol. Neurosurg. Psychiatr.*, **56**, 1235–6.

Girlanda, P., Vita, G. and Nicolosi, C. (1992). Botulinum toxin therapy: distant effects on neuromuscular transmission and autonomic nervous system. *J. Neurol. Neurosurg. Psychiatr.*, **55**, 844–5.

Glanzmann, R. L., Gelb, D. J., Drury, I. *et al.* (1990). Brachial plexopathy after botulinum toxin injections. *Neurology*, **40**, 1143.

Greene, P. and Fahn, S. (1993). Development of antibodies to botulinum toxin type A in patients treated with injections of botulinum toxin type A. In: *Botulinum and Tetanus Neurotoxins: Neurotransmission and Biomedical Aspects* (B. R. DasGupta, ed.), pp. 651–4. Plenum Press.

Greene, P. E. and Fahn, S. (1996). Response to botulinum toxin type F in seronegative botulinum toxin type A resistant patients. *Movement Disorders*, **11**, 181–4.

Greene, P., Fahn, S. and Diamond, B. (1994). Development of resistance to botulinum toxin type A in patients with torticollis. *Movement Disorders*, **9**, 213–17.

Hanna, P. and Jankovic, J. (1998). Mouse bioassay versus Western blot assay for botulinum toxin antibodies: correlation with clinical response. *Neurology*, **50(6)**, 1624–9.

Harris, C. P., Alderson, K., Nebeker, J. *et al.* (1991). Histologic features of human orbicularis oculi treated with botulinum A toxin. *Arch. Ophthalmol.*, **109**, 393–5.

Hatheway, C. G. and Dang, C. (1994). Immunogenicity of the neurotoxins of

Clostridium botulinum. In: *Therapy with Botulinum Toxin* (J. Jankovic and M. Hallett, eds), pp. 93–108. Marcel Dekker.

Herrero, B. A., Ecklund, A. E., Street, C. S. *et al.* (1967). Experimental botulism in monkeys, a clinical pathological study. *Exp. Mol. Pathol.*, **6**, 84–95.

Hesse, S. and Mauritz, K.-H. (1997). Management of spasticity. *Curr. Opin. Neurol.*, **10(6)**, 498–501.

Hufschmidt, A. and Mauritz, K.-H. (1985). Chronic transformation of muscle in spasticity: a peripheral contribution to increased muscle tone. *J. Neurol. Neurosurg. Psychiatr.*, **48**, 676–87.

Jankovic, J. and Brin, M. (1991). Therapeutic uses of botulium toxin. *N. Engl. J. Med.*, **324**, 1186–94.

Jankovic, J. and Schwartz, K. (1995). Reponse and immunoresistance to botulinum toxin injections. *Neurology*, **45**, 1743–5.

Kessler, K. R. and Benecke, R. (1997). The EDB test – a clinical test for detection of antibodies to botulinum toxin type A. *Movement Disorders*, **12**, 95–9.

Koko, C. and Ward, A. B. (1997). Management of spasticity. *Br. J. Hosp. Med.*, **58(8)**, 400–405.

Koman, L. A., Mooney, J. F. III, Smith, B. P. *et al.* (1993). Management of cerebral palsy with botulinum A toxin: preliminary investigation. *J. Paediatr. Orthopaed.*, **13**, 489–95.

Lamanna, C., El Hage, A. N. and Vick, J. A. (1988). Cardiac effects of botulinum toxin. *Arch. Int. Pharmacodyn. Ther.*, **293**, 69–83.

Lew, M. F., Adornato, B. T., Duane, D. D. *et al.* (1997). Botulinum toxin type B (BotB): a double-blind placebo-controlled safety and efficacy study in cervical dystonia. *Neurology*, **49(3)**, 701–7.

Mezaki, T., Kaji, R., Kohara, N. and Kimura, J. (1996). Development of generalised weakness in a patient with amyotrophic lateral sclerosis after focal botulinum toxin injection. *Neurology*, **46**, 845–6.

Morante, S., Furenlid, L., Schiavo, G. *et al.* (1996). X-ray absorption spectroscopy study of zinc coordination in tetanus neurotoxin, astacin, alkaline protease and thermolysin. *Eur. J. Biochem.*, **235**, 606–12.

Moser, E., Ligon, K. M., Singer, C. and Sethi, K. D. (1997). Botulinum toxin (Botox) therapy during pregnancy (abstract). *Neurology*, **48**, 399.

Nathan, P., Dimitrijevic, M. R. and Sherwood, A. M. (1985). Reflex path length and clonus frequency (letter). *J. Neurol. Neurosurg. Psychiatr.*, **48**, 7–25.

Odergren, T., Hjaltason, H., Kaakkola, S. *et al.* (1998). A double-blind placebo-controlled study to investigate the dose equivalence of Dysport and Botox in the treatment of cervical dystonia. *J. Neurol. Neurosurg. Psychiatr.*, **64(1)**, 6–12.

Schiavo, G., Benfenati, F., Poulain, B. *et al.* (1992). Tetanus and botulinum B neurotoxins block neurotransmitter release by proteolytic cleavage of synaptobrevin. *Nature*, **359**, 832–5.

Scott, A. B. and Suzuki, D. (1988). Systemic toxicity of botulinum toxin by intramuscular injection in the monkey. *Movement Disorders*, **3**, 333–5.

Scott, A. B., Rosenbaum, A. and Collins, C. C. (1973). Pharmacologic weakening of extraocular muscles. *Inv. Ophthalmol. Vis. Sci.*, **12**, 924–7.

Shaari, C. M. and Sanders, I. (1993). Quantifying how location and dose of botulinum toxin injections affect muscle paralysis. *Muscle Nerve*, **16**, 964–9.

Siatkowski, R. M., Tyutyunikov, A., Biglan, A. W. *et al.* (1993). Serum antibody production to botulinum A toxin. *Ophthalmology*, **100**, 1861–6.

Simpson, L. L. (1980). Kinetic studies on the interaction between botulinum toxin A and the cholinergic neuromuscular junction. *J. Pharmacol. Exp. Ther.*, **212**, 16–21.

Simpson, L. L. (1983). Botulinum neurotoxin type E: studies on mechanism of action and on structure activity relationships. *J. Pharmacol. Exp. Ther.*, **224**, 135–40.

Simpson, L. L. (ed.) (1989a). *Botulinum Toxin and Neurotoxin*. Academic Press.

Simpson, L. L. (1989b) Peripheral action of the botulinum toxins. In *Botulinum Toxin and Tetanus Toxin* (L. L. Simpson, ed.), pp. 153–78. Academic Press.

Snow, B. J., Tsui, J. K., Bhatt, M. H. *et al.* (1990). Treatment of spasticity with botulinum toxin: a double-blind study. *Ann. Neurol.*, **28**, 512–15.

Spasticity Study Group (1997). Spasticity: aetiology, evaluation, management and the role of botulinum toxin type A. *Muscle Nerve*, **Suppl. 6**, S158.

Spencer, R. F. and McNeer, K. W. (1987). Botulinum toxin paralysis of adult monkey extraocular muscle. Structural alterations in orbital, singly innervated muscle fibres. *Arch. Ophthalmol.*, **105**, 1703–11.

Tacket, C. O. and Rogawski, M. A. (1989). In: *Botulinum Neurotoxin and Tetanus Toxin* (L. L. Simpson, ed.), pp. 351–78. Academic Press.

Tonello, F., Morante, S., Rossetto, O. *et al.* (1996). Tetanus and botulism neurotoxins: a novel group of zinc endopeptidases. *Adv. Exp. Med. Biol.*, **389**, 251–60.

van Ermengem, E. (1979). Classics in infectious diseases. A new anaerobic bacillus and its relationship to botulism. *Rev. Inf. Dis.*, **1**, 701–19.

Wade, D. T. (1996). *Measurement in Neurological Rehabilitation*. Oxford University Press.

Wallesch, C. W., Maes, E., Lecomte, P. and Bartels, C. (1997). Cost-effectiveness of botulinum toxin type A injection in patients with spasticity following stroke: a German perspective. *Eur. J. Neurol.*, **4(Suppl 2)**, S53–S57.

WHO (1997). *Impairments of Impairments, Disabilities and Handicaps (ICIDH-2)*. World Health Organization.

Wiegand, H., Erdmann, G. and Wellhoener, H. H. (1976). 125-I-labelled botulinum toxin A neurotoxin; pharmacokinetics in cats after intramuscular injection. *Naunyn Schmiedebergs Arch. Pharmacol.*, **292**, 161–5.

Zuber, M., Sebald, M., Bathien, N. *et al.* (1993). Botulinum antibodies in dystonic patients treated with type A botulinum toxin: frequency and significance. *Neurology*, **43**, 1715–18.

14

Symptomatic management: ataxia, tremor and fatigue

Introduction

Ataxia, tremor and fatigue are some of the most difficult symptoms to manage effectively in the care of people with multiple sclerosis (MS). The pathological basis of these problems is not well understood. Ataxia, tremor and fatigue may be due directly to demyelination and associated damage, such as later axonal loss and atrophy, i.e. they may be primary deficits. Fatigue may also arise from other impairments such as spasticity and weakness, i.e. as a secondary deficit not directly due to demyelination but consequent upon it.

Ataxia and tremor

Classification of ataxia and tremor

In 1902, Dejerine defined tremor as 'an involuntary, rhythmical and symmetrical movement about an axis of equilibrium' (Dejerine, 1902). This clearly differentiates tremor from ataxia, which occurs during voluntary movement and consists of irregular, asymmetrical and non-rhythmic oscillations.

From the second century AD, Galen classified two types of tremor; one occurring at rest and one during movement. These correspond to the two types distinguished by Charcot (1887), rest and intention tremor. In 1928, Thomas described a tremor occurring when the subject maintained a position against the force of gravity, such as holding up the arms (Thomas and Long-Landry, 1928). Adapting an early classification (Molina-Negro and Hardy, 1975) these forms of tremor may be summarized as:

1. Tremor
   a. Resting – occurring in the absence of voluntary activity in the resting limb.
   b. Attitudinal – occurring when the subject maintains a static position or posture against the force of gravity. Attitudinal tremor has wide amplitude

and progressively increases in amplitude with attempts to maintain posture (Sabra and Hallett, 1981).

2. Movement tremor – occurring during movement, intermittent and increasing in amplitude as the movement nears completion. It ceases when the movement is finished, and does not occur during automatic movements such as arm swing when walking.

3. Physiological tremor – a fine, rapid, 8–9 Hz movement confined to the extremities.

The two forms of tremor commonly experienced by people with MS are attitudinal (or postural) tremor, occurring during attempts to maintain posture against gravity, and movement (or intention) tremor, with voluntary movements. Actions affected by movement tremor show delayed initiation, increased action duration and a 3–5 Hz terminal tremor (Francis *et al.*, 1986). Forty to fifty per cent of chronic patients have movement tremor (Muller, 1949; Kurtzke, 1970). Upper limb weakness complicates the assessment of attitudinal and movement tremor.

A review of movement disorders in MS showed that tremor was the most common, but that paroxysmal dystonias, ballism/chorea and palatal myoclonus might also result from demyelination. However, parkinsonism, dystonia and other types of myoclonus were felt to be coincidental (Tranchant *et al.*, 1995). This chapter concerns ataxia and tremor only, and oscillopsia and other eye movement disorders, sometimes referred to as ocular ataxia, are not included.

Basis of ataxia and tremor

Several different techniques have been used to explore the anatomical basis of ataxia and tremor in MS. Surface electromyography of limbs showing tremor demonstrates that an alternating or synchronous activation of antagonist muscles may be responsible (Nakamura *et al.*, 1993). The site of damage during this activation is uncertain. The cerebellum and its outflow tracts have been implicated by MR scanning (Nakamura *et al.*, 1993) and the basal ganglia by post-mortem studies (Riechert *et al.*, 1975).

Proton magnetic resonance spectroscopy in MS patients with severe cerebellar ataxia was compared to that of age-matched MS patients with similar disease duration but without cerebellar disease, and with healthy controls (Davie *et al.*, 1995). These studies showed that in severely ataxic MS patients N-acetylaspartate, a neuronal marker, is significantly decreased in cerebellar white matter. There is a significantly greater lesion volume in the posterior fossa, and marked cerebellar atrophy. These results suggest that axonal loss, as well as demyelination, is important in ataxia.

Surgical interventions indicate the importance of the pathway from the dentate nucleus of the cerebellum to the thalamic nucleus ventrolateralis via the superior cerebellar peduncle and the red nucleus (Cooper, 1967; Arsalo *et al.*, 1973; Zager, 1987; Goldman and Kelly, 1992; Whittle and Haddow, 1995). Secondary functional changes in the thalamic nucleus ventrointermedius (Vim) may also play a role (Andrew *et al.*, 1974; Narabayashi, 1994).

Management of ataxia and tremor

There are several different approaches, which may be used singly or in combination. Broadly, these are pharmacological, invasive (surgery and electrostimulation) or physical (orthoses and therapy).

Pharmacological treatments

Various drugs have been proposed but few tested in well-designed trials in people with MS. No trials in MS patients of agents such as primidone were identified by literature review.

Isoniazid

Literature search revealed five papers, published between 1982 and 1987, which described 39 patients treated with isoniazid for MS tremor. The results are summarized in Table 14.1.

All participants suffered from tremor, but the type of tremor varied between studies and, occasionally, within studies. There were 21 evaluable patients with attitudinal tremor, whereas one pilot study of five patients (Francis *et al.*, 1986) looked at movement tremor. The largest single study reported on four patients with attitudinal tremor and nine with movement tremor; in addition all patients were described as having moderate to severe cerebellar symptoms (Duquette *et al.*, 1985). Close reading of some trials suggests patients had both attitudinal and movement tremor, although the titles refer to one tremor type only (Hallett *et al.*, 1985; Bozek *et al.*, 1987).

Sabra *et al.* (1982) reported on four cases who were considered by their unblinded physician to have shown a change in functional ability. This group proceeded to a double-blind cross-over trial of seven patients with severe postural cerebellar tremor. As well as patient ratings and videoed examination, tremor was quantitatively assessed using electronic measurement of upper limb position and forearm acceleration (Hallett *et al.*, 1985). The four patients who improved by at least two outcome measures all had 'moderate or severe postural tremors that interfered with their ability to move their arms away from their bodies'. Symptomatic improvement occurred in only one patient, who became able to hold a glass. The authors concluded that isoniazid might inhibit attitudinal (postural) tremor, reducing injury to upper limbs and easing nursing, but that it rarely benefited movement tremor and thus upper limb function.

Duquette *et al.* (1985) carried out a larger open-label study, with blinded reporting of serial video recordings of a standard examination. This study recruited two types of tremor; movement and attitudinal. Furthermore, all participants had moderate to severe cerebellar damage and nine had paraparesis. The Expanded Disability Status Scale (EDSS) of the patients was not given, but they clearly had severe disease because 10 lived in 'chronic care institutions' and two were felt unable to give informed consent.

As well as videoed examinations, two other outcome measures were employed; clinical assessment and patient opinion. Results for an individual were frequently

Table 14.1 Studies on isoniazid in the treatment of tremor in multiple sclerosis

	Open-label	Open-label, blinded assessor	Open-label, quantitative measure	Double-blind cross-over	
	Sabra et al. (1982) Attitudinal	Duquette et al. (1985) Attitudinal 4/13 Movement 9/13	Francis et al. (1986) Movement	Hallett et al. (1985) Attitudinal	Bozek et al. (1987) Attitudinal
Males : females	1:3	10:3	1:4	3:3	4:6
Age range (mean) (years)	30–41 (35.25)	24–47 (40)	25–51 (35.2)	34–51 (42.3)	28–49 (36.5)
Disease duration (years)	6–18 (11.5)	4–21 (13)	3–15 (9.6)		
Other signs:					
Cerebellar	4/4	13/13	4/5		
Paraparesis	4/4	9/13	4/5		
UL weakness	3/4	11/13			
Isoniazid, dose escalation	800–1200 mg, unspecified	1000 mg, from 400 mg over 2 weeks	1200 mg, from 300 mg over 6 weeks	1200 mg, from 300 mg over 4 weeks	600–1600 mg; 12 or 20 mg/kg per day
Pyridoxine	100 mg	200 mg	100 mg	100 mg	100 mg
Outcome measures and improvement	Subjective assessment by unblinded observer – 4/4	(i) patient rating – 3/10; (ii) unblinded examination – 7/12; (iii) videoed examination, blinded assessor – 8/12	(i) patient rating – 5/5; (ii) unblinded examination – 5/5; (iii) polarized light goniometry – 4/5	(i) patient rating – 4/6; (ii) videoed examination, blinded assessor – 4/6; (iii) quantitative tremor recording – 5/5	(i) patient rating – 6/8; (ii) blinded examination – 6/8; (iii) tremograms – 3/8
Withdrawals and side effects	One withdrawal – obtunded with abnormal LFTs	One withdrawal with UTI. Drowsy 8/12, dysphagia 6/12, MS temporarily worse 3/12	Anorexia and nausea 3/5	None	One withdrawal – rash, fever, obtunded and one withdrawal for lack of efficacy
Acetylators fast : slow	Unstated	2:10	2:3	Unstated	4:6

not consistent across the three outcome measures, beneficial effects being most common on objective assessment (8/12). Six patients were felt to improve on clinical and/or video assessment, although they reported no benefit. Only one patient improved on all three measures, a patient with attitudinal tremor who reported side effects of fatigue and discontinued the drug at trial close. None of the assessors were impressed with the level of improvement, which was slight and rarely produced change in daily function.

A second double-blind cross-over study was performed by Bozek *et al.* (1987) in 10 patients, attitudinal tremor being assessed by clinical evaluation and the movement component by tremograms (Bozek *et al.*, 1987). Tremor was measured by an accelerometer attached to a hand grip while patients tracked an oscillating target on a screen.

The attitudinal tremor showed minimal objective improvement on video recordings reported blind. The tremograms showed improvement for isoniazid compared to pre-treatment values in three patients, but only one showed a significant effect. It is interesting that the tremograms of a further four patients had an improvement on isoniazid compared to placebo, which arose from a worsening of tremor on placebo. The authors believed these patients could identify the active agent, implying that tremograms are not as objective a measure as might be supposed.

Francis *et al.* (1986) conducted a pilot study showing benefit from isoniazid in 'severe cerebellar dysfunction' and 'action tremor'. Objective assessment was by limb movement when a seated subject reached to touch a static target, with a polarized light source detecting two photosensitive transducers on the upper limb. The authors felt this equipment might be useful in evaluating intention tremor objectively.

With regard to the mechanism of isoniazid, it is known to inhibit gamma-aminobutyric acid (GABA) aminotransferase, an enzyme involved in the degradation of GABA (Enna and Maggi, 1979). Patients with MS and cerebellar degeneration have low gamma-aminobutyric acid levels in cerebrospinal fluid (Achar *et al.*, 1976; Kuroda *et al.*, 1983), and it has been shown that there is a four-fold increase in free and unconjugated GABA levels in humans taking isoniazid 900 mg daily (Manyam and Tremblay, 1984). In the cerebellar Purkinje cells, GABA may be an important inhibitory neurotransmitter (Defeadis, 1975).

Glutethimide

Aisen *et al.* (1991) conducted a pilot study of glutethimide in eight patients, six with MS and two with traumatic brain injury. All the patients (four of whom were male) had disabling tremor; their average age was 41.3 years (range 34–50) and their disease duration 14 years (5–24).

Doses of glutethimide were gradually increased to a range of 750–1250 mg daily. There were two broad measures of efficacy; functional and quantitative tremor severity. Functional assessment involved a series of clinical tests conducted by a blinded occupational therapist, such as a timed keyboard test, handwriting, tracing an Archimedes spiral, eating soup, etc. The quantitative tests involved a pursuit-tracking task on a computer screen, where the subject could move a tracking image using a manipulator attached to a wrist splint. The aim was to superimpose the tracking image onto a randomly moving target image.

Of the MS patients, five showed functional improvement 7–14 days after achieving a stable dose of glutethimide, and one was unchanged. Of the five MS patients able to attempt the tracking task, four improved and one deteriorated. Three patients elected to continue medication at trial close; three discontinued due to sedation, although they had benefit on functional and/or quantitative testing.

Ondansetron

A reduction in tremor was noted during an open-label study of ondansetron for vertigo, and this led to a double-blind placebo-controlled cross-over study of a single dose of 8 mg ondansetron intravenously, or placebo, a week apart (Rice *et al.*, 1997). Principal outcome measures were blinded assessment of Archimedes spiral copying done at baseline and 1 hour after infusion. Patients who were capable also did a nine-hole peg test.

Sixteen of the 20 subjects had MS, three cerebellar degeneration and one lithium intoxication. All had movement tremor. Thirteen patients on ondansetron were felt to have improved spiral copying by a blinded panel, compared to one patient on placebo ($P = 0.00024$). Twelve patients able to do a nine-hole peg test were faster on ondansetron (79 s compared to 87 s for placebo; $P = 0.08$). Twelve patients preferred ondansetron, and none placebo ($P = 0.00098$).

Carbamazepine

A single-blind controlled trial of carbamazepine 600 mg daily suggested improvement in attitudinal and movement tremor as assessed by tremograms and clinical evaluation (Sechi *et al.*, 1989). Seven MS patients, mean disease duration 11 years (range 5–16) and mean EDSS 5.3 (range 3–7) were included in the series of 10 patients. While there were no significant abnormalities of blood count or electrocardiogram in any patient, four MS patients experienced asthenia.

Four MS patients elected to continue treatment. During 2–10 months follow-up, beneficial effects on writing and eating were sustained. Trials of dose reduction led to a deterioration in tremor.

Propranolol

One small single-blind cross-over trial of propranolol on cerebellar tremor in MS and primary cerebellar degeneration yielded negative results (Koller, 1984).

Cannabinoids and tetrahydrocannabinol

A pilot study was undertaken in MS and ataxia using the major active ingredient of marijuana, tetrahydrocannabinol. Eight patients (four male) who all had disabling tremor and ataxia took part in a single-blind placebo-controlled trial (Clifford, 1983).

The mean age of the patients was 32.7 years (range 21–49), and the mean EDSS was 6.88 (range 5–9). Half had used marijuana previously, and two were regular users.

After a 5 mg test dose, patients received 5 mg increments until they showed therapeutic response or experienced side effects. Assessment was three-fold; first, video recordings were made of clinical assessment, including neurological examination for cerebellar function, use of a spoon, handwriting and spiral drawing done at baseline, 2 and 4 hours after each dose; next, mental state was assessed by requiring the subject to recall three objects and repeat a number sequence; and finally, there was a subjective assessment of psychological effects, such as sedation or being 'high'. To examine placebo responses, patients received a single-blind placebo dose. The minimum time between doses was 6 hours.

Patients received 5–15 mg of the drug. All experienced a subjective high with the largest dose used, two becoming dysphoric. Five reported a subjective benefit, but there was no objective change. Two had both subjective and objective benefits, one with 5 mg and one with 15 mg. No benefit was seen with placebo, on which one patient reported being 'high', but rechallenge with the active drug produced an objective response. The patient showing response to 5 mg had a decrease in hand tremor confirmed by recording movement artefact from EEG leads.

Some further objective evidence of a possible effect of cannabis on ataxia is provided by a case report. A 30-year-old male with a 2-year history of MS reported a benefit from regular marijuana use sufficient to significantly influence ambulation and hence EDSS (Meinck *et al.*, 1989). He was tested before and after a single marijuana cigarette used after a 10-day period of no drug use. Neither patient nor observer was blinded in clinical assessment, EMG recordings of flexor reflex to a painful electrical shock to the foot, and recording of finger movement when the patient pointed at a target.

All three outcome measures appeared to improve. Before treatment, the movement tremor was a 3 Hz coarse tremor with amplitude of 1–3 cm, persisting throughout a 10 cm reach. After treatment, this tremor was virtually abolished with no significant effect on movement velocity. These results may have been influenced by placebo effect, but the positive results of the flexor reflex test are supported by animal experiments in dogs (Gilbert, 1981) and rats (Yaksh, 1981) that showed attenuation of polysynaptic reflexes with exposure to tetrahydro-cannabinol derivatives.

Invasive treatments

Stereotactic thalamotomy
Stereotactic thalamotomy has been widely used to treat tremor in people with MS. Since 1960, 15 papers describing 280 patients have been published. The proportion of patients having short-term improvement (up to 8 weeks after surgery) was 73–100 per cent, and long-term benefit (at least 1 year post-surgery) was seen in 50–94 per cent (Haddow *et al.*, 1997).

However, there are several difficulties in interpreting these apparently beneficial results. Evaluation of tremor was highly variable, and several methods were potentially subject to observer bias as they involved questioning the patient, doctor or carer. In some studies the assessing doctor was the surgeon, while in others there was clinical examination by a neurologist. The same doctor did not always rate patients before and after surgery. Tremor and disability scales were frequently designed by the trialists. Their intra- and inter-observer variability is unknown.

The operative procedure was similarly variable, with different methods of target localization and lesion formation. The target was usually the ventro-lateral nuclear complex in general (Cooper, 1960; Samra *et al.*, 1970; Arsalo *et al.*, 1973; van Manen, 1974; Kandel and Hondcarian, 1985; Goldman and Kelly, 1992; Whittle and Haddow, 1995), or a specific area such as the nucleus Vim (Andrew *et al.*, 1974) or ventro-oralis (Andrew *et al.*, 1974; Wester and Haughlie-Hanssen, 1990). Some studies did not describe the operative procedure used (Krayenbuhl and Yasargil, 1962; Hauptvogel *et al.*, 1975; Speelman and van Manen, 1984; Kandel and Hondcarian, 1985; Hitchcock *et al.*, 1987), or used more than one operative procedure in the same series (Shahzadi *et al.*, 1995).

The duration of follow-up was variable and, when stated, long-term outcomes in terms of disability and general function were often poor, either because of disease progression or sequelae of surgery (Arsalo *et al.*, 1973; van Manen, 1974; Hauptvogel *et al.*, 1975; Speelman and van Manen, 1984; Hitchcock *et al.*, 1987; Wester and Haughlie-Hanssen, 1990; Goldman and Kelly, 1992; Whittle and Haddow, 1995). Complications were common, although usually transient. A summary of those commonly recorded in the literature is detailed in Table 14.2.

Table 14.2 Common complications recorded in the literature after stereotactic thalamotomy for MS tremor (*n* = 221)

Complication	Frequency	
	Transient	Permanent
Cognitive	15	2
Speech difficulties	20	18
Motor	27	18
Ataxia or gait	3	3
Subdural or intracerebral haematoma	3	

After Haddow *et al.* (1997) and Shahzadi *et al.* (1995).

A particular difficulty for the neurologist when contemplating the possibility of surgery for a given patient is the lack of data on patient selection in the published literature. This makes it very difficult to know if particular subgroups are more likely to show benefit. Series sometimes include no data on selection criteria (van Manen, 1974; Hauptvogel *et al.*, 1975; Hitchcock *et al.*, 1987; Goldman and Kelly, 1992; Shahzadi *et al.*, 1995) or provide no details beyond the fact that the patient was disabled with tremor and/or advanced MS (Cooper, 1960; Krayenbuhl and Yasargil, 1962; Kandel and Hondcarian, 1985; Wester and Haughlie-Hanssen, 1990). There may be no information provided on age range (Samra *et al.*, 1970;

Andrew *et al.*, 1974; van Manen, 1974; Hitchcock *et al.*, 1987; Wester and Haughlie-Hanssen, 1990), gender (Riechert and Richter, 1972; Andrew *et al.*, 1974; van Manen, 1974; Hitchcock *et al.*, 1987; Wester and Haughlie-Hanssen, 1990) or clinical examination (Andrew *et al.*, 1974; Kandel and Hondcarian, 1985; Hitchcock *et al.*, 1987; Wester and Haughlie-Hanssen, 1990; Shahzadi *et al.*, 1995).

Thalamic stimulation

This technique may have theoretical advantages over thalamotomy, causing less neural damage (Caparros-Lefebvre *et al.*, 1994) and side effects that are reversible by discontinuing stimulation (Niclot *et al.*, 1993). Despite these considerations, there is relatively less published work on stimulators.

Brice and McLellan (1980) described three patients with MS who showed reduction in severe intention tremor on stimulation of the contralateral midbrain and basal ganglia by bipolar electrodes. Later, development of more sophisticated electrodes with four contact points allowed stimulation to be tailored to the individual patient. A series of four patients, one with MS, had electrode placement checked by intraoperative stimulation while conscious. The MS patient showed benefit to tremor of head and limbs maintained for 17 months (Nguyen and Degos, 1993).

This technique of quadripolar leads with intraoperative assessment was used in a larger series of 13 patients (Geny *et al.*, 1996). The mean age of the patients was 37 years (range 25–56), and the gender ratio showed female predominance (eight females). Mean disease duration was 9 years (range 2–21). All were severely disabled with MS (mean EDSS 6.8; range 4.5–9). Twelve of the patients had severe attitudinal tremor of upper limbs, head and trunk. One patient had moderate movement tremor.

The electrode was placed in the Vim nucleus at a locus where tremor was suppressed with active stimulation at the lowest electrical intensity. Outcome measures were clinical examination by a neurologist, including EDSS and video recordings, rating of the amplitude of upper limb tremor and a functional scale derived from Speelman and van Manen (1984).

Patients showed improvement in tremor amplitude (9/13) and functional ability (12/13). Degree of change in function depended on baseline EDSS and associated cerebellar dysfunction. Four patients (EDSS 5–7) became able to eat and drink independently. Of the eight more severely disabled patients, seven could manipulate an object such as a remote control and two could eat and drink alone. Three patients showed an increase in EDSS of 1 point by 3 months post-surgery, which may have been due to disease progression. Side effects were mild, asthenia in one patient and transient weakness in another.

Physical treatments

Orthoses

Tremor and ataxia may be treated by using mechanical loads to reduce amplitude of oscillation. In occupational therapy practice, weighted wristbands are used.

However, constant loads may enhance tremor, as opposed to viscous loads, which suppress it (Aisen *et al.*, 1993).

Energy dissipating orthoses, which generate resistive viscous loads by means of computer-controlled magnetic particle brakes, have been used in research situations. Patients with cerebellar action tremor due to MS or traumatic brain injury may show benefit (Aisen *et al.*, 1993). The principle of damping tremor while permitting slower purposeful movements has been used in simpler mechanical forms in the design of feeding aids for ataxic patients (Broadhurst and Stammers, 1990).

Physiotherapy and occupational therapy

Physiotherapy and occupational therapy, provided on a daily inpatient basis to MS patients with ataxia of upper limbs and/or trunk, may improve activities of daily living and patient and assessor visual analogue scales (Jones *et al.*, 1996). Therapy was aimed towards improving dynamic posture and encouraging appropriate adaptation of the environment. Assessment was independent of treatment, with the second measure being performed just 1 day after treatment ended.

Fatigue

The term fatigue has a range of meanings to both clinicians and lay people. To clinicians, fatigue may be a symptom of exhaustion out of keeping with effort expended, or a much narrower physiological definition comprising 'inability of a muscle or group of muscles to sustain the required or expected force' (Bigland-Ritchie *et al.*, 1978).

Research and clinical experience have shown that the term fatigue covers an even broader range of problems for patients than for their doctors. Chronic fatigue syndrome offers a condition in which fatigue is prominent and well studied. For patients, fatigue proved to have many dimensions; subjective feelings of fatigue, psychological wellbeing, functional impairment, the level of physical activity, sleep problems, social functioning, neuropsychological functioning, and self-efficacy (Vercoulen *et al.*, 1994).

It is hardly surprising that such a broadly defined symptom is common to a variety of clinical states and diagnoses. Fatigue occurs in depression (American Psychiatric Association, 1987), rheumatoid arthritis (Katon *et al.*, 1991), systemic lupus erythematosus (Krupp *et al.*, 1989a) and renal failure (Cardenas and Kutner, 1982), among other conditions. Finally, fatigue is common in healthy adults (Krupp *et al.*, 1988).

Considerations of loose clinical definition and multiple aetiology mean that epidemiological and therapeutic data may be difficult to interpret. Prevalence studies may be based on disparate definitions of fatigue, and scales designed to measure the severity of fatigue vary in the dimensions they study. Therapeutic trials frequently do not rigorously define fatigue as used as an eligibility criterion.

Fatigue in MS

Acknowledging the limitations of available data, fatigue is a common symptom in MS. Krupp *et al.* (1988) interviewed 32 consecutive MS clinic patients and 33 healthy controls recruited from the patients' friends or family, or hospital workers not acquainted with the study. Controls were comparable for residential area, education, age and gender. Defining fatigue as 'a sense of physical tiredness and lack of energy, distinct from sadness or weakness', 87.5 per cent (28/32) of MS patients reported being bothered by fatigue compared to 51 per cent (17/33) of controls (Krupp *et al.*, 1988).

Freal *et al.* (1984) sent questionnaires to 656 patients with MS, and found that 78 per cent of respondents reported fatigue. Among patients surveyed in a Canadian MS research clinic, 40 per cent reported fatigue as their most serious symptom (Murray, 1985). A survey in an Italian hospital clinic screened 507 consecutive patients with clinically definite MS attending during 1 calendar year. Patients were designated fatigued if they agreed with at least two statements from three abstracted from the Fatigue Severity Scale; (a) I am easily fatigued, (b) exercise brings on my fatigue, and (c) fatigue interferes with my work, family or social life. Fifty-three per cent (269/507) fell into the fatigue group (Colosimo *et al.*, 1995).

In a population-based study in Norway of an incident cohort of all patients with disease onset over a 10-year period, 38.7 per cent of respondents (48/124) reported fatigue. Fatigue was defined as 'preventing sustained physical function' (Midgard *et al.*, 1996).

Definition of MS fatigue

MS fatigue may be described as 'a sense of physical tiredness and lack of energy, greater than expected for the degree of effort required for a usual task' (Freal *et al.*, 1984). Fatigue may be subdivided into general and focal fatigue (Latash *et al.*, 1996). General fatigue persists throughout the day, and is improved only by extended periods of rest or sleep. Focal fatigue occurs with activity, and is relieved by brief rest; examples include visual blurring with prolonged reading or leg weakness after a short walk. Most of the epidemiological and treatment studies seem to relate to general fatigue.

Distinction from fatigue of healthy adults

Comparison of MS patients and healthy controls provides information on the similarities and differences in fatigue in these two groups (Krupp *et al.*, 1988). In both groups, fatigue was worsened by exercise, depression and towards the end of the day. Both groups found fatigue caused a loss of motivation and patience, and led to a need to rest. Fatigue was improved by sex, rest, sleep and positive experiences.

However, there were significant differences between MS fatigue and that of normal healthy adults. The paper states that 89 per cent of MS patients reported fatigue preventing sustained physical functioning, and 67 per cent reported fatigue interfering with responsibilities, whereas no healthy controls agreed with these statements ($P < 0.001$). Other characteristics significantly more common in MS fatigue were easy onset (MS 82 per cent, controls 22 per cent, $P < 0.001$), interference with physical functioning (79 per cent, 28 per cent, $P < 0.01$), and causing frequent problems (63 per cent, 17 per cent, $P < 0.01$).

A major difference between MS fatigue and that of healthy controls concerned temperature sensitivity, with exacerbation of fatigue by heat in the MS group (MS 92 per cent, controls 17 per cent, $P < 0.001$; Krupp et al., 1988). MS fatigue was worsened by heat in 69–92 per cent of patients in three different studies (Krupp et al., 1988; Fisk et al., 1994a; Bergamaschi et al., 1997). A possible mechanism is the slowing of conduction with heat in demyelinated axons (Matthews et al., 1979).

Physiological basis of fatigue in MS

The basis of fatigue may be central or peripheral. In central fatigue, central drive to muscle activity is not sustained (Macefield et al., 1993), whereas in peripheral fatigue there is a loss of force-generating capacity within the muscle itself (Merton, 1954). There is evidence that fatigue in MS has both central and peripheral components.

It has been shown that patients with MS have normal baseline strength but exhibit a significantly greater decline in strength during a sustained force (Sheean et al., 1997). Analysis of response to magnetic stimulation suggested that this inability to sustain force was central in origin. This reduction in central drive may be related to impaired motor drive, whether due to abnormalities of pyramidal tract, motor cortex, or the facilitatory afferent pathways that contribute up to 30 per cent of central motor drive during a maximal voluntary isometric contraction (Gandevia et al., 1990; Macefield et al., 1993). Comparisons of sustained muscle contractions in people with MS and age- and gender-matched volunteers gave further evidence of fatiguability (Latash et al., 1996). This appeared to be due to central neurogenic mechanisms, as electrical stimulation induced considerable increments in muscle contraction.

Central effects may include the perception of fatigue as well as reduced motor drive. Treatment with amantadine may improve attention, with benefits to alertness and subjective feelings of fatigue (Cohen and Fisher, 1989). Conversely, a study of memory task reaction times in MS patients showed prolongation when subjects were fatigued. This slowing of performance may lead to a perception of fatigue (Sandroni et al., 1992). A fatigue-inducing task was given to people with MS and healthy controls, and physiological muscular fatigue was similar in the two groups; however, perceived fatigue levels were higher in MS patients (Kersten and McLellan, 1996).

In relation to this evidence of the importance of central drive and perception of fatigue, it is interesting to examine positron emission tomography (PET) studies in fatigued and non-fatigued MS patients compared to healthy controls. Evidence from PET studies on cerebral glucose metabolism suggests fatigue in MS is associated with frontal cortex and basal ganglia dysfunction (Roelcke et al., 1997).

There may also be peripheral abnormalities of metabolism or excitation–contraction coupling. Fatiguability in terms of reduced oxidative capacity (Kent-Braun *et al.*, 1994a), impaired metabolic response to exercise (Sharma *et al.*, 1995) and impaired peripheral muscle activation (Kent-Braun *et al.*, 1994b) have been demonstrated in MS patients.

The metabolic changes in muscle fibres may be due to disuse or to altered patterns of use such as spasticity, and not specific to MS. Similar abnormalities were found in spastic paraplegia due to spinal cord injury and other neurological conditions (Lenman *et al.*, 1989; Miller *et al.*, 1990). Similar changes were also observed in healthy subjects after deconditioning (Duchateau and Hainaut, 1991).

Measurement of fatigue

One of the purposes of measurement is to allow the clinician to assess treatment efficacy by measuring the target variable before and after treatment. Before discussing management, it is worthwhile reviewing the measurement of fatigue. Apart from simple measures such as visual analogue scales, fatigue may be measured by a variety of self-report questionnaires. In some, fatigue is one dimension in a wide battery of subscales examining health status or quality of life, e.g. SF36 (Ware and Sherbourne, 1992) or Profile of Mood States (McNair *et al.*, 1992). There are also specific fatigue scales such as the Fatigue Impact Scale, Fatigue Assessment Instrument and Fatigue Severity Scale.

Fatigue Impact Scale

This is a 40-item questionnaire covering the effects of fatigue on cognitive function (10 items), physical function (10 items) and psychosocial function (20 items). These 40 items, detailed in Table 14.3, were chosen from existing questionnaires and interviews with people with MS. For each item the respondent rates the extent to which fatigue has caused problems within the last month, with 0 indicating no problems and 4 extreme problems. Score range is therefore 0–160 (Fisk *et al.*, 1994b).

Table 14.3 Fatigue impact scale

The fatigue impact scale asks subjects to rate how much of a problem fatigue has caused them during the past month, including the day of testing, in reference to the statements listed below. The subject is asked to circle the appropriate response for each: 0 = no problem; 1 = small problem; 2 = moderate problem; 3 = big problem; 4 = extreme problem. The item number in parentheses following each statement indicates the order in which it is presented in the fatigue impact scale.

Cognitive dimension
Because of my fatigue:
• I feel less alert (1)
• I have difficulty paying attention for a long period (5)

- I feel that I cannot think clearly (6)
- I find that I am more forgetful (11)
- I find it difficult to make decisions (18)
- I am less motivated to do anything that requires thinking (21)
- I am less able to finish tasks that require thinking (26)
- I find it difficult to organize my thoughts when I am doing things at home or at work (30)
- I feel slowed down in my thinking (34)
- I find it hard to concentrate (35)

Physical dimension

Because of my fatigue:
- I am more clumsy and unco-ordinated (10)
- I have to be careful about pacing my physical activities (13)
- I am less motivated to do anything that requires physical effort (14)
- I have trouble maintaining physical effort for long periods (17)
- My muscles feel much weaker than they should (23)
- My physical discomfort is increased (24)
- I am less able to complete tasks that require physical effort (31)
- I worry about how I look to other people (32)
- I have to limit my physical activities (37)
- I require more frequent or longer periods of rest (38)

Social dimension

Because of my fatigue:
- I feel that I am more isolated from social contact (2)
- I have to reduce my workload or responsibilities (3)
- I am more moody (4)
- I work less effectively (this applies to work inside or outside the home) (7)
- I have to rely more on others to help me or do things for me (8)
- I have difficulty planning activities ahead of time (9)
- I am more irritable and more easily angered (12)
- I am less motivated to engage in social activities (15)
- My ability to travel outside my home is limited (16)
- I have few social contacts outside of my own home (19)
- Normal day-to-day events are stressful for me (20)
- I avoid situations that are stressful for me (22)
- I have difficulty dealing with anything new (25)
- I feel unable to meet the demands that people place on me (27)
- I am less able to provide financial support for myself and my family (28)
- I engage in less sexual activity (29)
- I am less able to deal with emotional issues (33)
- I have difficulty participating fully in family activities (36)
- I am not able to provide as much emotional support to my family as I should (39)
- Minor difficulties seem like major difficulties (40)

From Fisk *et al.* (1994b).

Fatigue Assessment Instrument

This is a 29-item scale that attempts to assess quantitative and qualitative components of fatigue in general medical conditions (Schwartz *et al.*, 1993). Items were drawn from clinical experience and open-ended interviews of patients.

The questionnaire begins by defining fatigue in order to promote consistency across responders (see Table 14.4). The respondent is asked to answer each statement with a seven-point Likert scale (1 = completely disagree, 7 = completely agree) for a time scale of the previous 2 weeks.

Table 14.4 The fatigue assessment instrument

INSTRUCTIONS: Below are a series of statements regarding your fatigue. By fatigue, we mean a sense of tiredness, lack of energy or total body give-out. Please read each statement and choose a number from 1–7, where 1 indicates that you completely disagree with the statement and 7 indicates that you completely agree. Please answer these questions as they apply to the past TWO WEEKS.

1. I feel drowsy when I am fatigued
2. When I am fatigued, I lose my patience
3. My motivation is lower when I am fatigued
4. When I am fatigued, I have difficulty concentrating
5. Exercise brings on my fatigue
6. Heat brings on my fatigue
7. Long periods of inactivity bring on my fatigue
8. Stress brings on my fatigue
9. Depression brings on my fatigue
10. Work brings on fatigue
11. My fatigue is worse in the afternoon
12. My fatigue is worse in the morning
13. Performance of routine daily activities increases my fatigue
14. Resting lessens my fatigue
15. Sleeping lessens my fatigue
16. Cool temperatures lessen my fatigue
17. Positive experiences lessen my fatigue
18. I am easily fatigued
19. Fatigue interferes with my physical functioning
20. Fatigue causes frequent problems for me
21. My fatigue prevents sustained physical functioning
22. Fatigue interferes with carrying out certain duties and responsibilities
23. Fatigue predated other symptoms of my condition
24. Fatigue is my most disabling symptom
25. Fatigue is among my three most disabling symptoms
26. Fatigue interferes with my work, family or social life
27. Fatigue makes other symptoms worse
28. Fatigue that I now experience is different in quality or severity to the fatigue I experienced before I developed this condition
29. I experienced prolonged fatigue after exercise

From Schwartz *et al.* (1993).

Factor analysis shows four dimensions. The first is the fatigue severity subscale (11 items), which shares eight items with the nine-item Fatigue Severity Scale (see below). The second concerns whether the fatigue is situation-specific (e.g. heat, stress), the third fatigue consequences (e.g. poor concentration), and the fourth response to rest and sleep. Group means and standard deviations are shown in Table 14.5 for each subscale in MS patients and normal controls.

Table 14.5 Group means (and standard deviations) on four subscales of Fatigue Assessment Instrument for people with MS and normal controls

	Normal controls	MS
Number of subjects	37	40
Severity subscale	2.53 (1.18)	5.48 (1.22)
Situation specific	4.12 (1.45)	5.0 (1.09)
Consequences	5.01 (1.47)	5.27 (1.5)
Response to rest and sleep	5.5 (1.11)	5.6 (1.59)

From Schwartz *et al.* (1993).

Fatigue Severity Scale

This is a nine-item scale that describes the impact of fatigue on physical function (items 2, 4 and 6) and psychosocial aspects (items 1, 7 and 9) with three general statements (items 3, 5 and 8) (see Table 14.6). Respondents answer on a seven-point scale (1 = strong disagreement, 7 = strong agreement). The score is a mean score of all nine responses, range 1–7. Reliability and internal consistency are good in MS and other conditions (Krupp *et al.*, 1989a).

Table 14.6 Fatigue severity scale (FSS)*

1. My motivation is lower when I am fatigued
2. Exercise brings on my fatigue
3. I am easily fatigued
4. Fatigue interferes with my physical functioning
5. Fatigue causes frequent problems for me
6. My fatigue prevents sustained physical functioning
7. Fatigue interferes with carrying out certain duties and responsibilities
8. Fatigue is among my three most disabling symptoms
9. Fatigue interferes with my work, family, or social life

*Patients are instructed to choose a number from 1–7 that indicates their degree of agreement with each statement, where 1 indicates strongly disagree and 7 indicates strongly agree.
From Krupp *et al.* (1989b).

There is no cut-off value and only limited published comparison work with normal healthy controls. Thus the clinical significance of particular scores in patients with MS are difficult to evaluate. Bergamaschi *et al.* (1997) assessed the Fatigue Severity Scale (FSS) in MS outpatients with EDSS less than 6 and a stable clinical state in the previous 6 months (i.e. no relapses, no steroids or immunosuppressives, no progression of EDSS). Mean score was 4.12, range 1–7 (Bergamaschi *et al.*, 1997).

In the original paper describing the FSS, Krupp *et al.* (1989a) found similar values of mean FSS 4.8 in patients with chronic progressive MS, EDSS 3–6.5. Scores of 4 or higher were found in 91 per cent of MS patients but in only 5 per cent of healthy controls (Krupp *et al.*, 1989a).

MS-Specific Fatigue Scale

This is derived from the Fatigue Assessment Instrument, and consists of six items relatively specific to MS fatigue (Krupp *et al.*, 1995). Subjects rate each statement on a seven-point Likert scale from 'disagree' to 'agree'. The mean of the six items is the final score. A 2-week period preceding questionnaire completion is specified.

Use of scales in clinical trials

These scales vary in their definitions of fatigue and the dimensions of fatigue studied. This may explain why research studies using more than one outcome scale may yield both positive and negative results.

One randomized study of exercise showed a significant reduction in fatigue as measured by the Profile of Mood States, but not on the Fatigue Severity Scale (Petajan *et al.*, 1996). The authors found the Fatigue Severity Scale insensitive to change, commenting that their patients agreed with statements such as 'fatigue interferes with my physical functioning' irrespective of their actual level of fatigue around the time of assessment. A double-blind placebo-controlled drug trial exploring treatment effects of amantadine found a benefit on the MS Specific Fatigue Scale and not on the Fatigue Severity Scale (Krupp *et al.*, 1995).

Distinction from fatigue of chronic illness and disability

It has been postulated that the problem of fatigue in MS is related to the work load of performing self care and mobility tasks with physical disability. Under this hypothesis, fatigue is not a particular symptom complex in MS but a by-product of chronic disease.

Studies comparing fatigue in people with MS or systemic lupus erythematosus (SLE) and healthy adults show that fatigue has greater impact on lifestyle in both chronic conditions compared to controls. On the original 28-item scale from which the FSS is drawn there were five items that showed significant differences in responses between MS and SLE. Fatigue did not appear to be a uniform, non-specific consequence of chronic illness. However, none of these five items were retained for the final nine-item FSS, and mean FSS scores were similar for MS (4.8) and SLE (4.7) (Krupp *et al.*, 1989a).

Studies exploring the relation (if any) between disability and fatigue in MS are of limited assistance. Results are contradictory between studies, possibly because different methodologies and statistical approaches are used. Krupp *et al.* (1988) measured fatigue on a 10-cm visual analogue scale (VAS) from 'none' to 'severe', and compared the result against EDSS by Pearson correlation coefficients (Krupp *et al.*, 1988). The result was not statistically significant at a 0.05 level.

Fisk and colleagues found no relation between a specific scale, the Fatigue Impact Scale and either disease classification or neurological impairment in 85 MS patients (Fisk *et al.*, 1994a). Another study assessed fatigue severity using a subscale from a generic multidimensional tool, the Subjective Fatigue Subscale of the Checklist of Individual Strength (Vercoulen *et al.*, 1994). No significant differences by MS type or EDSS score were determined in 50 MS patients (Vercoulen *et al.*, 1996). However, although two MS types were represented (progressive 19, relapsing–remitting 31) with a wide EDSS range, 75 per cent of the total sample fell between EDSS 2–3.5. This may have hidden any relation to EDSS.

Colosimo *et al.* (1995) divided 507 consecutive MS outpatients into fatigued and non-fatigued groups on the basis of two positive responses to three questions from the FSS. Logistic regression analysis showed that higher EDSS scores (odds ratio (OR) 1.55, 95 per cent confidence interval (CI) 1.38–1.75) and progressive disease (OR 2.9, 95 per cent CI 1.67–5.05) were associated with fatigue (Colosimo *et al.*, 1995).

A second large outpatient study was performed by Bergamaschi *et al.* (1997), who restricted their study population to those with definite MS of 1 year's duration, a stable clinical course in the previous 6 months (no relapses, steroids, other immunosuppressive drugs, or progression) and an EDSS less than 6. These criteria aimed to exclude patients whose disease activity or medication might alter their responses, and to restrict assessment to independently ambulant patients in case aid or wheelchair use affected the experience of fatigue. Of 255 consecutive patients, 100 fulfilled the criteria (80 relapsing–remitting, 20 chronic progressive, of whom four were primary progressive). A multiple regression analysis of FSS score showed a single significant co-factor of EDSS ($P < 0.0001$). Mean FSS was significantly higher in the patients with an EDSS of at least 3.5 compared to those with a score of less than 3.5, 5.42 vs 3.71 respectively ($P < 0.0001$). Mean FSS was higher in progressive compared to relapsing–remitting patients, 5.43 vs 3.78 ($P < 0.0001$) (Bergamaschi *et al.*, 1997).

Multifactorial causation of fatigue

It must not be assumed that a person with MS who complains of fatigue is experiencing MS-related fatigue. The term fatigue has a multitude of meanings to patients, and furthermore MS-specific fatigue may co-exist with related symptoms such as sleepiness. A careful history is particularly important for therapeutic success. The clinician must clarify the complaint in order to develop a successful approach to management.

MS fatigue should be differentiated from drowsiness, which is often related to high-dose or rapidly escalating anti-spasticity drugs, anticonvulsants or analgesics. It differs from sedation, which is usually a side effect of anxiolytics or some of the older antidepressants, or a sequel to hypnotics. Tiredness may be due to higher energy expenditure, such as occurs in ambulant patients with a spastic paraparesis (Olgiati *et al.*, 1988). Tiredness also follows sleep disturbance, due to nocturia, nocturnal spasms, pain or anxiety.

Patients sometimes describe other MS impairments as tiredness. Muscle weakness ('My leg is always tired') or temperature sensitivity ('I feel like a wet rag and am just wiped out') may elicit a positive response to questions on tiredness and fatigue.

Fatigue may also reflect many psychological factors. The most clinically important is depression, where careful questioning may show fatigue as part of a syndrome of anhedonia, apathy and a sense of defeat. Fatigue may be used as a reason for passivity in patients who suffer anxiety, low self-esteem or frank illness behaviour. Fatigue may be more severe for patients with a low sense of control over their MS symptoms (Vercoulen et al., 1996).

Approach to management

Fatigue and medication
Drowsiness and sedation are usually related to medication, and should be treated by adjusting drugs, dose or timing. Many drugs commonly used in the treatment of MS symptoms may predispose to sedation or drowsiness, including baclofen, dantrolene, tizanidine, diazepam, oxybutynin, tolterodine, carbamazepine, sodium valproate and amitriptyline. General principles are to increase doses slowly and titrate against overall clinical state. On the other hand, fatigue may be erroneously attributed to medication, a suspicion best validated by a trial of withdrawal of therapy in an informed patient. Some of the disease modifying agents also cause fatigue and asthenia, such as interferon beta-1a and -1b (IFNB Multiple Sclerosis Study Group, 1993; Jacobs *et al.*, 1996) and mitoxantrone (Edan *et al.*, 1997).

Fatigue and sleep
Sleep disturbance may be improved by treating the underlying cause. Nocturia may be helped by intermittent self-catheterization, especially before bed. Nocturnal spasms may require a bedtime dose of an anti-spasticity agent such as baclofen 20–30 mg orally. Paroxysmal symptoms that interrupt sleep, such as trigeminal neuralgia or tonic spasms are better treated with carbamazepine. Pain that disturbs sleep can be treated with analgesics or, if neuropathic, with tricyclic antidepressants or anticonvulsants. Early morning wakening or poor sleep due to depression may be treated with tricyclic antidepressants at bedtime, when any side effect of sedation may be beneficial.

Fatigue and disability
As people with MS develop disabilities, fatigue may worsen because of two interlinked processes. Disabled people become deconditioned, and yet may need more energy to achieve an activity than non-disabled people.

Deconditioning results from inactivity, particularly common in MS because mobility is often affected and temperature sensitivity of demyelinated nerves may cause exercise to transiently worsen symptoms. As disability progresses, the feasibility of physical exercise or leisure sports diminishes, and normal activities such as walking, climbing stairs, housework or gardening are curtailed.

Comparison using an accelerometer of activity levels of MS patients, median EDSS 3 (range 1.5–6), and sedentary controls confirmed lower activity levels in MS ($P = 0.01$). Eighty-two per cent (14/17) of this MS sample had an EDSS of less than 4.5, i.e. were fully ambulant (Ng and Kent-Braun, 1997).

Studies of metabolic cost of exercise in MS patients with minimal disability (EDSS 0–2) showed reduced exertional capacity compared to age- and gender-matched controls. This impairment of ability appeared to be due to poor training (Tantucci et al., 1996). Such subjects with little physical disability may particularly benefit from exercise programmes.

Reduced activity levels in people with MS who have few impairments may reflect personal, family or societal expectations. Many clinicians have experience of patients and their families who curtail activity after the diagnosis of MS because of beliefs about rest and activity in illness. It is not known whether patient education programmes may improve this problem.

As people develop impairments such as spasticity, they expend disproportionate energy to perform activities. This was demonstrated by high energy expenditure in ambulant paraparetics (Olgiati et al., 1988). In addition, it should not be underestimated how mentally and physically tiring it may be to use newly learned skills to perform activities of daily living. For example, a non-disabled person may rise, bathe and dress following automatic routines. The disabled person may need to recall techniques learned from therapists and nurses, plan each step, struggle with newly learned skills, monitor performance, and fear the consequences of any error. Carers sometimes inadvertently increase the burden of this type of fatigue by trivializing it. It may help to draw comparisons with the fatigue following the first day in a new job before routines become familiar and less taxing.

The dual basis of fatigue relating to disability necessitates a dual approach to management.

Deconditioning

Deconditioning should be minimized. Patients may be taught home exercise regimens by physiotherapists, and some MS patient groups sponsor exercise classes. Temperature-sensitive patients may swim, or sometimes they are able to continue exercising once they understand the phenomenon.

Randomized controlled trials of exercise have shown benefits to people with MS. Petajan et al. (1996) randomized 54 subjects with an EDSS of 6 or less to aerobic training with combined arm and leg cycle ergometer or a control group who continued doing no regular physical activity. After 15 weeks of thrice-weekly sessions of 30 minutes at 60 per cent of VO_2 max, the exercise group showed significant increases in maximal aerobic capacity, upper and lower limb strength, and physical dimensions of Sickness Impact Profile (SIP). The EDSS did not change for either group over the 15 weeks of the study, nor did the baseline EDSS correlate with changes in maximum aerobic capacity; participants with EDSS greater than 5 showed equal improvement to those with EDSS less than or equal to 3.5.

This randomized trial showed that people with MS experienced significant decreases in skin fold thickness, triglyceride and VLDL following exercise. They may be expected to have similar benefits with regard to cardiovascular health and obesity as are recognized in non-disabled people taking regular exercise (American College of Sports Medicine, 1983, 1993; Powell *et al.*, 1987).

Serial measures of muscle structure, fatigue, work and power indicated some benefits in MS patients following an exercise programme (Gehlsen *et al.*, 1984; Svensson *et al.*, 1994).

Activity modification and lifestyle change

Patients may benefit from advice from the occupational therapist on planning their activities and their environment to conserve energy and simplify work. A diary detailing activities and fatigue, and a home assessment, may be helpful.

A range of time management skills, principally pacing but also planned relaxation periods, may be beneficial. Many of these techniques increase the patient's environmental mastery, defined as 'the ability to manipulate, control or change the environment to suit personal psychological needs'. Environmental mastery appears the best predictor of both global fatigue and fatigue-related distress for people with MS (Schwartz *et al.*, 1996). The beneficial effects of multidisciplinary outpatient therapy on MS fatigue may be related to improved skills for self-management and enhanced environmental mastery (Fabio *et al.*, 1998).

Pharmacological treatments for fatigue

It is worth reviewing a few of the more influential treatment trials to show some of the difficulties in assessing response to medication. Outcome measures, whether VAS or measurement scales, give disparate results. Placebo effects appear significant.

Amantadine

Evidence from case reports (Schapira, 1974) and a 32 patient cross-over study (Murray, 1985) suggested a benefit from amantadine. This was tested in a randomized, double-blind, placebo-controlled cross-over trial of 165 patients with a range of MS types and levels of disability (Canadian MS Research Group, 1987).

The patients were screened as having at least a 3-month history of chronic persistent daily fatigue of moderate to severe severity. A 2-week placebo period was used to collect baseline data on fatigue severity (with a VAS) and rate ability to perform 13 activities of daily living (ADL). Following this placebo period, 71/165 (43 per cent) were ineligible because VAS scores over the 2 weeks were less than 50 per cent, attributed by the trialists to problems with the VAS or placebo response. Twenty-one of these ineligible patients were randomized in error and completed the study.

Patients had two 3-week periods of either amantadine or placebo, separated by a 2-week washout period. Fatigue scores, patient and physician ratings, ADL scores and patient preferences were all in favour of amantadine 100 mg orally bd. Adverse experiences were matched between the two groups, apart from insomnia, which was more common in the treated group.

A similar double-blind, randomized cross-over study was conducted in 22 MS patients, and included neuropsychological measures assessing the effect of fatigue on memory, attention, visual–motor performance, etc. Participants gave a history of daily fatigue for at least 3 months, had an EDSS less than 6.5 and were not depressed or taking confounding medication such as betablockers (Cohen and Fisher, 1989).

Amantadine 100 mg orally bd was associated with improvements in daily diary fatigue ratings. There was no effect detected on any of the psychological measures except for the Stroop Interference Test, a measure of attention and freedom from distractibility (Stroop, 1935).

Pemoline

Pemoline is another central nervous system stimulant, and was reported to show amelioration of fatigue in an open-label pilot study of 10 MS patients (Krupp *et al.*, 1989b). A double-blind, placebo-controlled cross-over study of pemoline, in doses of up to 75 mg daily, was conducted on 41 patients with at least 3 months' history of severe fatigue, defined as abnormal tiredness out of proportion to effort and significantly interfering with basic daily functions. Outcome was assessed using a daily VAS comparing fatigue to that at entry (Weinshenker *et al.*, 1992).

Mean VAS showed a modest improvement with pemoline of 6.7 ±18.5 mm on a 50-mm scale by the fourth week compared to baseline. 21/41 (51.2 per cent) patients preferred pemoline compared to 19/41 (46.3 per cent) placebo, which did not reach statistical significance.

Side effects were experienced by more than 25 per cent of pemoline-treated patients. Pemoline was significantly more likely to be associated with irritability, insomnia, dizziness, anorexia, nausea and headache. Overall, the authors anticipated 'some long-term benefit in 7/41 (17 per cent) patients for whom it is prescribed'.

Relative efficacy of amantadine and pemoline

A randomized, double-blind, placebo-controlled study with parallel group design compared pemoline and amantadine (Krupp *et al.*, 1995). Ninety-three patients completed the study. All participants had an EDSS of 6 or less and a baseline Fatigue Severity Score (FSS) of at least 4 persisting over a 2-week run-in phase. To avoid possible confounding factors, patients who had used drugs such as azathioprine, cyclophosphomide or benzodiazepines in the previous 2 months were excluded, as were those with depressive symptoms.

Patients were randomized to amantadine, pemoline or placebo groups, receiving amantadine 100 mg bd and placebo pemoline, placebo amantadine and placebo pemoline, or placebo amantadine and pemoline. Pemoline was increased from 18.75 mg daily in week 1 by 18.75 mg per week until week 3, when the maximum dose of 56.25 mg was reached. All groups were treated for 6 weeks.

Change in FSS was a primary outcome measure. During the 2-week pre-treatment phase, FSS significantly declined in all three groups; this was attributed to trial participation. FSS declined more markedly during the treatment course, attributed to placebo effects.

The other two primary outcome measures of MS Fatigue Scale and patient's self-report showed an improvement in fatigue with amantadine. After treatment, 79 per cent (15/19) of the amantadine group, 32 per cent (7/22) of the pemoline group and 52 per cent (13/25) of the placebo group recalled feeling better on medication. The pemoline group showed no significant differences compared with placebo on any fatigue measure. However, when interpreting the negative results for pemoline from this study it must be noted that the dose used was somewhat lower than Weinshenker's study (56.25 mg *cf.* 75 mg) (Weinshenker *et al.*, 1992).

Aminopyridines

Many of the trials of aminopyridines do not report effect on fatigue, using EDSS (van Diemen *et al.*, 1992; Panitch and Bever, 1993) or visual and motor signs as endpoints (Davis *et al.*, 1990).

However, Polman and colleagues compared the effect of 4-aminopyridine and 3-4 diaminopyridine on a range of neurological functions and symptoms, including fatigue (Polman *et al.*, 1994a). On a VAS, 4-aminopyridine was more effective than 3-4 diaminopyridine in reducing fatigue. Systemic side effects of 3-4 diaminopyridine were more pronounced.

This group reported long-term efficacy and safety of 4-aminopyridine. Twenty-three patients taking daily oral doses of up to 0.5 mg of 4-aminopyridine per kg body weight were followed for 6–32 months. Patients reported improvements in fatigue (57 per cent, 13/23) and ambulation (57 per cent, 13/23). In 406 patient months of follow-up, there were three major side effects; seizures in two patients and hepatitis in one (Polman *et al.*, 1994b).

Sheean *et al.* (1998) studied the effects of 3-4 diaminopyridine on both fatigue (as measured by Fatigue Severity Scale) and motor performance. Baseline tests showed abnormal motor function and central fatigue. After a 3-week course of 25–60 mg daily 3-4 diaminopyridine, 75 per cent (6/8) patients reported less fatigue and showed slightly less fatigue on more objective testing.

Possible basis of pharmacological effect

The mechamism of action of all these agents is not established. Amantadine and pemoline both act as central stimulants. Amantadine has been shown to significantly increase levels of the pituitary hormone beta-endorphin, perhaps through the central release of catecholamines (Rosenberg and Appenzeller, 1988).

In normal individuals, beta endorphin shows a circadian rhythm, highest in the morning and lowest in the evening (Dent *et al.*, 1981). With amantadine, evening levels are elevated and are higher than morning levels (Rosenberg and Appenzeller, 1988). While stress and exercise cause beta endorphin release (Appenzeller *et al.*, 1980; Carr *et al.*, 1981), the evening rise is unlikely to be due to decreased fatigue promoting activity because levels rose in all subjects, whether or not they reported less fatigue. Increases were greater in patients who reported a decrease in fatigue.

The positive effects of aminopyridines may be due to their ability to prolong action potential duration and partially reverse conduction block (Sherratt *et al.*, 1980).

References

Achar, V. S., Welch, K. M., Chabi, E. *et al. (*1976). Cerebrospinal fluid gamma-aminobutyric acid in neurologic disease. *Neurology*, **26**, 777–80.

Aisen, M. L., Holzer, M., Rosen, M. *et al.* (1991). Glutethimide treatment of disabling action tremor in patients with multiple sclerosis and traumatic brain injury. *Arch. Neurol.*, **48**, 513–15.

Aisen, M. L., Arnold, A., Baiges, I. *et al.* (1993). The effect of mechanical damping loads on disabling action tremor. *Neurology*, **43**, 1346–50.

American College of Sports Medicine (1983). Position statement on proper and improper weight loss programs. *Med. Sci. Sports Exer.*, **15**, 1–13.

American College of Sports Medicine (1993). Physical activity, physical fitness and hypertension. *Med. Sci. Sports Exer.*, **25**, 1–10.

American Psychiatric Association (1987). *Diagnostic and Statistical Manual of Mental Disorders*. American Psychiatric Association.

Andrew, J., Rice Edwards, J. M. and Rudolf, N. (1974). The placement of stereotaxic lesions for involuntary movements other than in Parkinson's disease. *Acta Neurochir. Suppl. (Wien)*, **21**, 49–55.

Appenzeller, O., Standefer, J., Appenzeller, J. *et al.* (1980). Neurology of endurance training: V. Endorphins. *Neurology*, **30**, 418.

Arsalo, A., Hanninen, A. and Laitinen, L. (1973). Functional neurosurgery in the treatment of multiple sclerosis. *Ann. Clin. Res.*, **5**, 74–9.

Bergamaschi, R., Romani, A., Versino, M. *et al.* (1997). Clinical aspects of fatigue in multiple sclerosis. *Funct. Neurol.*, **12**, 247–51.

Bigland-Ritchie, B., Jones, D. A., Hosking, G. P. and Edwards, R. H. T. (1978). Central and peripheral fatigue in sustained maximum voluntary contractions of human quadriceps muscle. *Clin. Sci. Mol. Med.*, **54**, 609–14.

Bozek, C. B., Kastrukoff, L. F., Wright, J. M. *et al.* (1987). A controlled trial of isoniazid therapy for action tremor in multiple sclerosis. *J. Neurol.*, **234**, 36–9.

Brice, J. and McLellan, L. (1980). Suppression of intention tremor by contingent deep-brain stimulation. *Lancet*, **1(8180)**, 1221–2.

Broadhurst, M. J. and Stammers, C. W. (1990). Mechanical feeding aids for patients with ataxia: design considerations. *J. Biomed. Eng.*, **12**, 209–14.

Canadian MS Research Group (1987). A randomized controlled trial of amantadine in fatigue associated with multiple sclerosis. *Can. J. Neurol. Sci.*, **14**, 273–8.

Caparros-Lefebvre, D., Ruchoux, M. M., Blond, S. *et al.* (1994). Long-term thalamic stimulation in Parkinson's disease: postmortem anatomical study. *Neurology*, **44**, 1856–60.

Cardenas, D. D. and Kutner, N. G. (1982). The problem of fatigue in dialysis patients. *Nephron*, **30**, 336–40.

Carr, D. B., Bullen, B. A., Skrinar, G. S. *et al.* (1981). Physical conditioning facilitates the exercise-induced secretion of beta-endorphin and beta-lipotropin in women. *N. Engl. J. Med.*, **305**, 560–63.

Charcot, J. M. (1887). *Lecons sur les Maladies du Systeme Nerveux.* V. Adrien Delahaye.

Clifford, D. B. (1983). Tetrahydrocannabinol for tremor in multiple sclerosis. *Ann. Neurol.*, **13**, 669–71.

Cohen, R. A. and Fisher, M. (1989). Amantadine treatment of fatigue associated with multiple sclerosis. *Arch. Neurol.*, **46**, 676–80.

Colosimo, C., Millefiorini, E., Grasso, E. *et al.* (1995). Fatigue in multiple sclerosis is associated with specific clinical features. *Acta Neurol. Scand.*, **92**, 353–5.

Cooper, I. S. (1960). Neurosurgical alleviation of intention tremor of multiple sclerosis and cerebellar disease. *N. Engl. J. Med.*, **263**, 441–4.

Cooper, I. S. (1967). Relief of intention tremor due to multiple sclerosis by thalamic surgery. *J. Am. Med. Assoc.*, **199**, 689–94.

Davie, C. A., Barker, G. J., Webb, S. *et al.* (1995). Persistent functional deficit in multiple sclerosis and autosomal dominant cerebellar ataxia is associated with axon loss. *Brain*, **118**, 1583–92.

Davis, F. A., Stefoski, D. and Rush, J. (1990). Orally administered 4-aminopyridine improves clinical signs in multiple sclerosis. *Ann. Neurol.*, **27**, 186–92.

Defeadis, F. V. (1975). Amino acids as central neurotransmitters. *Ann. Rev. Pharmacol. Toxicol.*, **15**, 105–30.

Dejerine, J. (1902). *Semiologie du Systeme Nerveux.* Masson.

Dent, R. M. M., Guilleminault, C., Albert, L. H. *et al.* (1981). Diurnal rhythm of plasma immunoreactive beta-endorphin and its relationship to sleep stages and plasma rhythms of cortisol and prolactin. *J. Clin. Endocrinol. Metab.*, **52**, 942–6.

Duchateau, J. and Hainaut, K. (1991). Effects of immobilization on electromyogram power spectrum changes during fatigue. *Eur. J. Appl. Physiol.*, **63**, 458–62.

Duquette, P., Pleines, J. and de Souich, P. (1985). Isoniazid for tremor in multiple sclerosis: a controlled trial. *Neurology*, **35**, 1772–5.

Edan, G., Miller, D., Clanet, M. *et al.* (1997). Therapeutic effect of mitoxantrone combined with methylprednisolone in multiple sclerosis: a randomised multicentre study of active disease using MRI and clinical criteria. *J. Neurol. Neurosurg. Psychiatr.*, **62**, 112–18.

Enna, S. J. and Maggi, A. (1979). Biochemical pharmacology of GABAergic agonists. *Life Sci.*, **24**, 1727–38.

Fabio, R. P., Soderberg, J., Choi, T. *et al.* (1998). Extended outpatient rehabilitation: its influence on symptom frequency, fatigue, and functional status for persons with progressive multiple sclerosis. *Arch. Phys. Med. Rehabil.*, **79**, 141–6.

Fisk, J. D., Pontefract, A., Ritvo, P. G. *et al.* (1994a). The impact of fatigue in patients with multiple sclerosis. *Can. J. Neurol. Sci.*, **21**, 9–14.

Fisk, J. D., Ritvo, P. G., Ross, L. *et al.* (1994b). Measuring the functional impact of fatigue: initial validation of the fatigue impact scale. *Clin. Inf. Dis.*, **18**, S79–S83.

Francis, D. A., Grundy, D. and Heron, J. R. (1986). The response to isoniazid of action tremor in multiple sclerosis and its assessment using polarised light goniometry. *J. Neurol. Neurosurg. Psychiatr.*, **49**. 87–9.

Freal, J. E., Kraft, G. H. and Coryell, J. K. (1984). Symptomatic fatigue in multiple sclerosis. *Arch. Phys. Med. Rehabil.*, **65**, 135–8.

Gandevia, S. C., Macefield, G., Burke, D. and McKenzie, D. K. (1990). Voluntary activation of human motor axons in the absence of muscle afferent feedback. The control of the deafferented hand. *Brain*, **113**, 1563–81.

Gehlsen, G. M., Grigsby, S. A. and Winant, D. M. (1984). Effects of an aquatic fitness program on the muscular strength and endurance of patients with multiple sclerosis. *Phys. Ther.*, **64**, 653–7.

Geny, C., Nguyen, J. P., Pollin, B. *et al.* (1996). Improvement of severe postural cerebellar tremor in multiple sclerosis by chronic thalamic stimulation. *Movement Disorders*, **11**, 489–94.

Gilbert, P. E. (1981). A comparison of THC, nantradol, nabilone, and morphine in the chronic spinal dog. *J. Clin. Pharmacol.*, **21**, 311–19.

Goldman, M. S. and Kelly, P. J. (1992). Symptomatic and functional outcome of stereotactic ventralis lateralis thalamotomy for intention tremor. *J. Neurosurg.*, **77**, 223–9.

Haddow, L. J., Mumford, C. and Whittle, I. R. (1997). Sterotactic treatment of tremor due to multiple sclerosis. *Neurosurg. Q.*, **7**, 23–34.

Hallett, M., Lindsey, J. W., Adelstein, B. D. and Riley, P. O. (1985). Controlled trial of isoniazid therapy for severe postural cerebellar tremor in multiple sclerosis. *Neurology*, **35**, 1374–7.

Hauptvogel, H., Poser, S., Orthner, H. and Roeder, F. (1975). Indikationen zur stereotaktischen Operation bei Patienten mit Multipler Sklerose. *J. Neurology*, **210**, 239–51.

Hitchcock, E., Flint, G. A. and Gutowski, N. J. (1987). Thalamotomy for movement disorders: a critical appraisal. *Acta Neurochir. Suppl.*, **39**, 61–5.

IFNB Multiple Sclerosis Study Group (1993). Interferon beta-1b is effective in relapsing-remitting multiple sclerosis. I. Clinical results of a multicenter, randomized, double-blind, placebo-controlled trial. *Neurology*, **43**, 655–61.

Jacobs, L. D., Cookfair, D. L., Rudick, R. A. *et al.* (1996). Intramuscular interferon beta-1a for disease progression in relapsing multiple sclerosis. *Ann. Neurol.*, **39**, 285–94.

Jones, L., Lewis, Y., Harrison, J. and Wiles, C. M. (1996). The effectiveness of occupational theapy and physiotherapy in multiple sclerosis patients with ataxia of the upper limb and trunk. *Clin. Rehabil.*, **10**, 277–82.

Kandel, E. I. and Hondcarian, O. A. (1985). Surgical treatment of the hyperkinetic form of multiple sclerosis. *Acta Neurol. Napoli*, **7**, 345–7.

Katon, W. J., Buchwald, D. S., Simon, G. E. *et al.* (1991). Psychiatric illness in patients with chronic fatigue and those with rheumatoid arthritis. *J. Gen. Intern. Med.*, **6**, 277–85.

Kent-Braun, J. A., Sharma, K. R., Miller, R. G. and Weiner, M. W. (1994a). Post-exercise phosphocreatinine resynthesis is slowed in multiple sclerosis. *Muscle Nerve*, **17**, 835–41.

Kent-Braun, J. A., Sharma, K. R., Weiner, M. W. and Miller, R. G. (1994b). Effects of exercise on muscle activation and metabolism in multiple sclerosis. *Muscle Nerve*, **17**, 1162–9.

Kersten, P. and McLellan, D. L. (1996). Evidence for a central mechanism in the process of fatigue in people with multiple sclerosis. *Clin. Rehabil.*, **10**, 233–9.

Koller, W. C. (1984). Pharmacologic trials in the treatment of cerebellar tremor. *Arch. Neurol.*, **41**, 280–81.

Krayenbuhl, H. and Yasargil, M. G. (1962). Relief of intention tremor due to multiple sclerosis by stereotaxic thalamotomy. *Confinia Neurol.*, **22**, 368–74.

Krupp, L. B., Alvarez, L. A., LaRocca, N. G. and Scheinberg, L. C. (1988). Fatigue in multiple sclerosis. *Arch. Neurol.*, **45**, 435–7.

Krupp, L. B., LaRocca, N. G., Muir-Nash, J. and Steinberg, A. D. (1989a). The fatigue severity scale: application to patients with multiple sclerosis and systemic lupus erythematosus. *Arch. Neurol.*, **46**, 1121–3.

Krupp, L. B., Coyle, P. K., Cross, A. H. *et al.* (1989b). Amelioration of fatigue with pemoline in patients with multiple sclerosis. *Ann. Neurol.*, **26**, 155–6.

Krupp, L. B., Coyle, P. K., Doscher, N. P. *et al.* (1995). Fatigue therapy in multiple sclerosis. *Neurology*, **45**, 1956–61.

Kuroda, H., Yamamoto, M., Otsuki, S. and Ogawa, N. (1983). Isoniazid effects on choreiform movement and on GABA, HVA and 5-HIAA in CSF. *Acta Neurol. Scand.*, **67**, 124–7.

Kurtzke, J. F. (1970). Clinical features of multiple sclerosis. In: *Handbook of Clinical Neurology. Vol. 9: Multiple Sclerosis and other Demyelinating Diseases* (P. J. Vinken and G. W. Bruyn, eds), North-Holland, Amsterdam, pp. 161–216.

Latash, M., Kalugina, E., Nicholas, J. *et al.* (1996). Myogenic and central neurogenic factors in fatigue in multiple sclerosis. *Multiple Sclerosis*, **1**, 236–41.

Lenman, A. J. R., Tulley, F., Vrbova, G. *et al.* (1989). Muscle fatigue in some neurological disorders. *Muscle Nerve*, **12**, 938–42.

Macefield, V. G., Gandevia, S. C., Bigland-Ritchie, B. *et al.* (1993). The firing rates of human motorneurones voluntarily activated in the absence of muscle afferent feedback. *J. Physiol. (Lond.)*, **471**, 429–43.

Manyam, B. V. and Tremblay, R. D. (1984). Free and conjugated GABA in human cerebrospinal fluid: effect of degenerative neurologic diseases and isoniazid. *Brain Res.*, **307**, 217–23.

McNair, D. M., Lorr, M. and Droppleman, L. F. (1992). *Profile of Mood States (POMS)*. Educational and Industrial Testing Service.

Matthews, W. B., Read, D. J. and Pountney, E. (1979). Effect of raising body temperature on visual and somatosensory evoked potentials in patients with multiple sclerosis. *JNNP*, **42**(3), 250–5.

Meinck, H. M., Schonle, P. W. and Conrad, B. (1989). Effect of cannabinoids on spasticity and ataxia in multiple sclerosis. *J. Neurol.*, **236**, 120–22.

Merton, P. A. (1954). Voluntary strength and fatigue. *J. Physiol. (Lond.)*, **123**, 553–64.

Midgard, R., Riise, T. and Nyland, H. (1996). Impairment, disability and handicap in multiple sclerosis. *J. Neurol.*, **243**, 337–44.

Miller, R. G., Green, A. T., Moussavi, R. S. *et al.* (1990). Excessive muscle fatigue in patients with spastic paraparesis. *Neurology*, **40**, 1271–4.

Molina-Negro, P. and Hardy, J. (1975). Semiology of tremors. *J. Can. Sci. Neurol.*, **2**, 23–9.

Muller, R. (1949). Studies on disseminated sclerosis with special reference to symptomatology, course and prognosis. *Acta Med. Scand.*, **133**, 1–214.

Murray, T. J. (1985). Amantadine therapy for fatigue in multiple sclerosis. *Can. J. Neurol. Sci.*, **12**, 251–4.

Nakamura, R., Kamakura, K., Tadano, Y. *et al.* (1993). MR imaging findings of tremors associated with lesions in cerebellar outflow tracts; report of two cases. *Movement Disorders*, **8**, 209–12.

Narabayashi, H. (1994). Analysis of intention tremor. *Clin. Neurol. Neurosurg.*, **94(Suppl.)**, 130–32.

Ng, A. V. and Kent-Braun, J. A. (1997). Quantitation of lower physical activity in persons with multiple sclerosis. *Med. Sci. Sports Exer.*, **29**, 517–23.

Nguyen, J. P. and Degos, J. D. (1993). Thalamic stimulation and proximal tremor. *Arch. Neurol.*, **50**, 498–500.

Niclot, P., Pollin, B., Nguyen, J. P. *et al.* (1993). Traitement du tremblement par chirurgie stereotaxique. *Rev. Neurol. (Paris)*, **149**, 755–63.

Olgiati, R., Burgunder, J. M. and Mumenthaler, M. (1988). Increased energy cost of walking in multiple sclerosis: effect of spasticity, ataxia and weakness. *Arch. Phys. Med. Rehabil.*, **69**, 846–9.

Panitch, H. S. and Bever, C. T. Jr (1993). Clinical trials of interferons in multiple sclerosis. What have we learned? *J. Neuroimmunol.*, **46**, 155–64.

Petajan, J. H., Gappamaier, E., White, A. T. *et al.* (1996). Impact of aerobic training on fitness and quality of life in multiple sclerosis. *Ann. Neurol.*, **39**, 432–41.

Polman, C. H., Bertelsmann, F. W., De Waal, R. *et al.* (1994a). 4-Aminopyridine is superior to 3, 4-diaminopyridine in the treatment of patients with multiple sclerosis. *Arch. Neurol.*, **51**, 1136–9.

Polman, C. H., Bertelsmann, F. W., van Loenen, A. C. and Koetsier, J. C. (1994b). 4-aminopyridine in the treatment of patients with multiple sclerosis. Long-term efficacy and safety. *Arch. Neurol.*, **51**, 292–6.

Powell, K. E., Thompson, P. D., Caspersen, D. J. and Kendrick, J. S. (1987). Physical activity and the incidence of coronary heart disease. *Ann. Rev. Publ. Health*, **8**, 253–87.

Rice, G. P. A., Lesaux, J., Vandervoort, P. *et al.* (1997). Ondansetron, a 5-HT3 antagonist, improves cerebellar tremor. *J. Neurol. Neurosurg. Psychiatr.*, **62**, 282–4.

Riechert, T. and Richter, D. (1972). Stereotaktische operationen zur behandlung des tremors der multiplen sklerose. *Schwiz. Arch. Neurol. Psychiatr.*, **111**, 411–16.

Riechert, T., Hassler, R., Mundinger, F. *et al.* (1975). Pathologic–anatomical findings and cerebral localization in stereotactic treatment of extrapyramidal motor disturbances in multiple sclerosis. *Confinia Neurol.*, **37**, 24–40.

Roelcke, U., Kappos, L., Lechner-Scott, J. *et al.* (1997). Reduced glucose metabolism in the frontal cortex and basal ganglia of multiple sclerosis patients with fatigue: an 18F-fluorodeoxyglucose positron emission tomography study. *Neurology*, **48**, 1566–71.

Rosenberg, G. A. and Appenzeller, O. (1988). Amantadine, fatigue and multiple sclerosis. *Arch. Neurol.*, **45**, 1104–6.

Sabra, A. and Hallett, M. (1981). Action tremor with alternating muscle activity in antagonist muscles. *Neurology*, **31**, 103.

Sabra, A. F., Hallett, M., Sudarsky, L. and Mullally, W. (1982). Treatment of action tremor in multiple sclerosis. *Neurology*, **32**, 912–13.

Samra, K., Waltz, J. M., Riklan, M. *et al.* (1970). Relief of intention tremor by thalamic surgery. *J. Neurol. Neurosurg. Psychiatr.*, **33**, 7–15.

Sandroni, P., Walker, C. and Starr, A. (1992). 'Fatigue' in patients with multiple sclerosis: motor pathway conduction and event-related potentials. *Arch. Neurol.*, **49**, 517–24.

Schapira, M. (1974). Treating multiple sclerosis with amantadine hydrochloride. *J. R. Coll. Gen. Pract.*, **24**, 411–12.

Schwartz, J. E., Jandorf, L. and Krupp, L. B. (1993). The measurement of fatigue: a new instrument. *J. Psychosom. Res.*, **37**, 753–62.

Schwartz, C. E., Coulthard-Morris, L. and Zeng, Q. (1996). Psychosocial correlates of fatigue in multiple sclerosis. *Arch. Phys. Med. Rehabil.*, **77**, 165–70.

Sechi, G. P., Zuddas, M., Piredda, M. *et al.* (1989). Treatment of cerebellar tremors with carbamazepine: a controlled trial with long-term follow-up. *Neurology*, **39**, 1113–15.

Shahzadi, S., Tasker, R. R. and Lozano, A. (1995). Thalamotomy for essential and cerebellar tremor. *Stereotac. Funct. Neurosurg.*, **65**, 11–17.

Sharma, K. R., Kent-Braun, J., Mynhier, M. A. *et al.* (1995). Evidence of an abnormal intramuscular component of fatigue in multiple sclerosis. *Muscle Nerve*, **18**, 1403–11.

Sheean, G. L., Murray, N. M. F., Rothwell, J. C. *et al.* (1997). An electrophysiological study of the mechanism of fatigue in multiple sclerosis. *Brain*, **120**, 299–315.

Sheean, G. L., Murray, N. M. F., Rothwell, J. C. *et al.* (1998). An open-labelled clinical and electrophysiological study of 3, 4-diaminopyridine in treatment of fatigue in multiple sclerosis. *Brain*, **121**, 967–75.

Sherratt, R. M., Bostock, H. and Sears, T. A. (1980). Effects of 4-aminopyridine on normal and demyelinated mammalian nerve fibres. *Nature (Lond.)*, **283**, 570–72.

Speelman, J. D. and van Manen, J. (1984). Stereotactic thalamotomy for the relief of intention tremor of multiple sclerosis. *J. Neurol. Neurosurg. Psychiatr.*, **47**, 596–9.

Stroop, J. R. (1935). Studies of interference in serial verbal reactions. *J. Exp. Psychol.*, **18**, 643–62.

Svensson, B., Gerdle, B. and Elert, J. (1994). Endurance training in patients with multiple sclerosis. *Phys. Ther.*, **74**, 1017–26.

Tantucci, C., Massucci, M., Piperno, R. *et al.* (1996). Energy cost of exercise in multiple sclerosis patients with low degree of disability. *Multiple Sclerosis*, **2**, 161–7.

Thomas, A. and Long-Landry, M. (1928). Deux cas de tremblement d'attitude du membre superieur. *Rev. Neurol.*, **1**, 585–7.

Tranchant, C., Bhatia, K. P. and Marsden, C. D. (1995). Movement disorders in multiple sclerosis. *Movement Disorders*, **10**, 418–23.

van Diemen, H. A., Polman, C. H., van Dongen, T. M. *et al.* (1992). The effect of 4-aminopyridine on clinical signs in multiple sclerosis: a randomized, placebo-controlled, double-blind, cross-over study. *Ann. Neurol.*, **32**, 123–30.

van Manen, J. (1974). Stereotaxic operations in cases of hereditary and intention tremor. *Acta Neurochir. Suppl.*, **21**, 49–55.

Vercoulen, J. H., Hommes, O. R., Swanink, C. M. *et al.* (1996). The measurement of fatigue in patients with multiple sclerosis. A multidimensional comparison with patients with chronic fatigue syndrome and healthy subjects. *Arch. Neurol.*, **53**(7), 642–9.

Ware, J. E. and Sherbourne, C. D. (1992). The MOS 36-item short-form health survey (SF-36): 1. Conceptual framework and item selection. *Med. Care*, **30**, 473–83.

Weinshenker, B. G., Penman, M., Bass, B. *et al.* (1992). A double-blind random-ized, cross-over trial of pemoline in fatigue associated with multiple sclero-sis. *Neurology*, **42**, 1468–71.

Wester, K. and Haughlie-Hanssen, E. (1990). Stereotactic thalamotomy – experi-ences from the levodopa era. *J. Neurol. Neurosurg. Psychiatr.*, **53**, 427–30.

Whittle, I. R. and Haddow, L. J. (1995). CT guided thalamotomy for movement disorders in multiple sclerosis: problems and paradoxes. *Acta Neurochir. Suppl.*, **64**, 13–16.

Yaksh, T. L. (1981). The antinociceptive effects of intrathecally administered lev-onantradol and desacetyllevonantradol in the rat. *J. Clin. Pharmacol.*, **21**, 334–40.

Zager, E. L. (1987). Neurosurgical management of spasticity, rigidity and tremor. *Neurol. Clin.*, **5**, 631–647.

15

The cause and management of bladder, sexual and bowel symptoms

Introduction

An intact neural pathway from higher brain centres to the distal segments of the spinal cord is required for normal bladder, bowel and sexual function. In multiple sclerosis, inflammation affecting the spinal cord is probably the main cause of pelvic organ dysfunction.

The predominant symptoms of bladder dysfunction are frequency and urgency, sometimes associated with urge incontinence. Both incomplete bladder emptying and bladder over-activity may give rise to these symptoms, and it is therefore essential to bladder management to establish the post-void residual urinary volume and elicit symptoms of bladder over-activity. A combination of bladder drainage by clean intermittent self-catheterization and pharmacological suppression of the over-active bladder with anticholinergic medication can be highly effective for the management of the MS bladder.

The introduction of non-invasive therapies for erectile failure has altered the climate of opinion in discussing sexual matters. Both men and women suffering from MS are likely to welcome the opportunity to discuss their sexual problem and seek treatment. Unfortunately, although there is an increasing range of therapies available for erectile failure, there is still little that can be done to help women with sexual dysfunction; however, it is likely that drugs may become available to treat women in future. After all, the innervation and composition of erectile tissue is similar in both sexes.

The prevalence of bowel dysfunction is higher in patients with MS than in the general population, and there are a number of possible pathophysiological mechanisms for the constipation and faecal incontinence that occurs. However, there are as yet few specific, effective treatments.

In recent years much has been learnt about the neural control of bladder, bowel and sexual function, although our knowledge is far from complete. It is quite clear that bladder and sexual function at least depend on an intact innervation between cerebral controlling centres and the conus of the cord. It is from the sacral level of the spinal cord that first order afferents enter and lower motor neurones innervating the pelvic structures arise. In multiple sclerosis there are many sites within the central nervous system where demyelination and subsequent axonal loss can occur in the neural pathways. The clinical evidence is that bladder problems and male sexual dysfunction are particularly likely in patients with spinal cord pathology that also impairs mobility, so some correlation between a patient's lower limb disability, bladder and sexual dysfunction can be demonstrated. The cause of bowel dysfunction is less clear.

Bladder dysfunction

Neural control of the bladder

Evidence from mammalian animal experiments shows that bladder function is controlled by centres in the brain stem. In the cat there are regions in the dorsal tegmentum of the pons that, when stimulated under experimental conditions, either cause the bladder to empty in a co-ordinated fashion or cause contraction of the pelvic floor (de Groat, 1990; Griffiths *et al.*, 1990). Some remarkable studies using PET scanning in human volunteers show that very similar controlling centres exist in humans (Blok *et al.*, 1997). These regions, sometimes referred to as the pontine micturition centres, have been likened to a central 'flip flop' switch (de Groat, 1990). The bladder is either in the storage phase or in the emptying phase, and activity of higher centres (the frontal region in particular) switches activity between the two states. For the pontine micturition centres to exert their regulatory effect, intact connections between these sites and the sacral part of the spinal cord are necessary. Interruption of spinal tracts will result in both impaired bladder storage and disruption of normal emptying mechanisms. The reorganization of the neuronal control of bladder function following spinal cord disease (de Groat *et al.*, 1990) has important therapeutic implications, and is discussed in the section describing the use of intravesical capsaicin to deafferent the bladder.

Symptoms

Bladder dysfunction is very common in patients with multiple sclerosis. In health, the bladder has two primary functions, urinary storage and voiding, and both may become dysfunctional.

The study by Miller *et al.* (1965) demonstrated that 75 per cent of patients with MS had bladder symptoms at some time, and in 50 per cent these were persistent and troublesome. The commonest urinary symptom in MS patients is urgency. Many urodynamic studies have shown that this is due to underlying detrusor hyper-reflexia (Betts *et al.*, 1993; Chancellor and Blaivas, 1995). In this condition, instead of the bladder acting as a compliant reservoir storing urine until a reasonable capacity has been achieved, the detrusor muscle becomes overactive and contracts spontaneously, often at a low volume (Figure 15.1). The subject senses imminent micturition at the onset of the contraction. If the detrusor con-

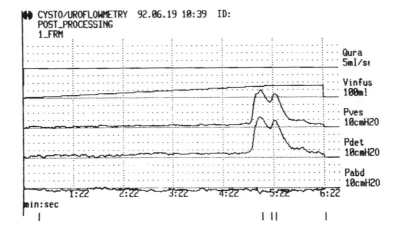

Figure 15.1 Cystometry showing detrusor hyper-reflexia. The detrusor pressure remains less than 10 cm water until the bladder has been filled to just over 150 ml, when a spontaneous rise in intravesical pressure is recorded. There is no rise in intra-abdominal pressure at this time – the pressure rise is due to a contraction of the detrusor muscle. The patient will sense impending micturition and urgency at the onset of this contraction and, if unable to 'hold on', will experience urge incontinence. (Pabdo, intra-abdominal pressure measured with a rectal catheter; Pves, measured intravesical pressure; Pdet, Pves–Pabdo; Vinfus, infusion volume, 50 ml/min.)

traction is mild, the patient may be able to suppress it and reach the toilet in time. If, however, the detrusor contraction is sudden and in addition the patient has a paraparesis, urge incontinence is likely. Urinary frequency is due to the reduced bladder capacity. A combination of urgency and frequency means that many patients are reluctant to be far away from a toilet.

Symptoms of urgency, frequency and urge incontinence in a patient with a mild or moderate paraparesis due to MS can reasonably be assumed to be due to detrusor hyper-reflexia. It has been argued that cystometry is not necessary in such a patient (Betts *et al.*, 1993), since some form of anticholinergic medication can be given to treat the complaint and the dosage adjusted according to the patient's response rather than the cystometric findings.

In addition to symptoms of detrusor hyper-reflexia, there may also be symptoms indicating that the neurological process of voiding has been affected. These are often less significant, and may only be elicited by direct questioning. However, since impaired emptying contributes in such a major way to the overall bladder dysfunction, it is important to assess the extent of this problem. Patients may volunteer information or admit on direct questioning to hesitancy of micturition, and the more disabled may find themselves unable to initiate micturition voluntarily, only emptying their bladders when an involuntary hyper-reflexic contraction occurs. Patients may also report an interrupted urinary flow pattern and complain of incomplete emptying. Evidence of the latter is often not the persistent sensation of incomplete emptying, but rather that the patient notices that having passed urine once, they need to do so again within 5–10 minutes. These symptoms of abnormal voiding are due to the presence of detrusor sphincter dyssynergia, together with poor neural drive on detrusor efferents during voiding. Detrusor sphincter activity is co-ordinated in the pontine micturition centre, and this must have intact connections with the sacral cord for there to be relaxation of the striated muscle of the urethral sphincter at the onset of micturition and, some seconds later, contraction of the detrusor smooth muscle. If the connections between the sacral cord and the pons are interrupted, the sphincter tends to contract simultaneously with the detrusor contraction.

Management

When a patient with MS complains of urinary urgency and urge incontinence, a prescription of an anticholinergic drug to lessen the effect of the parasympathetics on the detrusor muscle might seem reasonable. However, the effect of such medication is inevitably continuous, and although it will lessen detrusor hyperreflexia it may also reduce the already compromised efficiency of bladder emptying (Figure 15.2). A persistent residual urine volume acts as a stimulus to repeated hyper-reflexic contractions, so anticholinergic medication alone is unlikely to be effective if the patient also has incomplete bladder emptying. For this reason, the single most important investigation is to measure the post-micturition residual volume (Figure 15.3; Kornhuber and Schultz, 1990; Fowler, 1996). This can be done either using a small ultrasound device or by in–out catheterization. If the post-micturition residual volume is raised (more than 100 ml is usually agreed to be a significant figure), efforts must be made to improve bladder emptying before anticholinergic therapy is started. If a patient reports

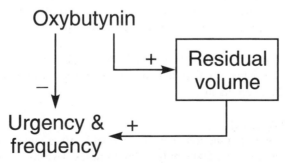

Figure 15.2 Although oxybutynin is effective in lessening detrusor hyperreflexia, it may also impair bladder emptying. The resulting increase in post-micturition residual volume may then lead to worsening symptoms of urgency and frequency.

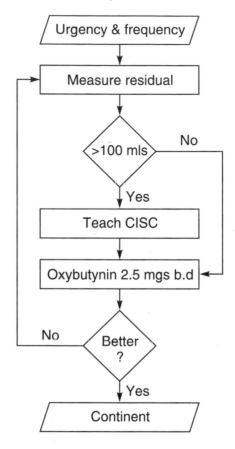

Figure 15.3 Algorithm for management of neurogenic incontinence.

initial benefit with an anticholinergic, which is then lost, it is advisable to repeat the measurement of the post-micturition residual urine volume because this may have increased as a result of the anticholinergic therapy and be exerting a significant effect.

The management algorithm outlined in Figure 15.3 is recommended as the initial treatment for patients with mild to moderate multiple sclerosis who are suffering from bladder complaints.

Incomplete emptying

Bladder emptying is a function that is relatively infrequently performed in health – it is a process that takes only a few minutes, five to seven times over 24 hours. It is therefore unlikely that any medication will be effective in improving a neuronal disruption to this mechanism, and although alpha blockers, which lessen the state of contraction of the bladder neck smooth muscle, have been reported to have some benefit, no medical treatment can restore the normal voiding mechanism. The most effective management is intermittent self-catheterization.

In the 1960s, when Sir Ludwig Guttman introduced intermittent self-catheterization at Stoke Mandeville Hospital, it was regarded as a revolutionary technique. He proposed it as an alternative to permanent catheter drainage in patients following spinal cord injury. Originally the technique was only to be performed using a completely aseptic method, but in the 1970s Lapides *et al.* (1972, 1976) reported 'tremendous improvement' in all abnormal parameters for bladder function, particularly infections, using a clean but non-sterile technique. Intermittent self-catheterization has transformed the management of patients with neurogenic bladder dysfunction, particularly those with MS (Fowler *et al.*, 1992). Those suitable for learning the technique are patients with good bladder capacity and a well-innervated sphincter, who would be able to retain reasonable volumes between catheterizations.

Patients are best taught by an experienced nurse, and ideally a continence advisor working within a multidisciplinary team providing a continence service is a valuable asset. A continence advisor not only teaches patients to catheterize themselves with a disposable catheter two or more times in 24 hours, but also provides access to appropriate diagnostic facilities, follow-up and assistance with the provision of supplies in the community. The plastic catheters that are used are either straight and have a funnel at one end (Neleton catheter) or slightly curved and semi-rigid (Scott catheter). These catheters can be re-used provided they are washed through with clean water and kept dry in a clean bag. Use of antiseptic cleansing solutions is not recommended, since these can cause a chemical urethrocystitis. Disposable catheters should be thrown away after about a week; more frequently if the patient is liable to recurrent infections.

Self-lubricating single-use catheters coated with hydrophilic low-friction materials were first introduced in 1983. The Lofric catheter is covered with polyvinylpyrrolidon (PVP) and sodium chloride, a hydrophilic material with balanced osmolality which, when immersed in water, coats the catheter with a lubricated film, facilitating insertion. Other single-use catheters include the EasiCath and the newly introduced InstantCath, which comes with the lubricant within the plastic sleeve. Clean water is therefore not required to lubricate the catheter prior to use. Ultimately the choice of catheters is determined by patient preference. However, although patients may prefer self-lubricating catheters, they are all considerably more expensive than the plain catheters and the manufacturers recommend they should not be re-used.

Whether or not a patient is able to self-catheterize depends on their physical disability as well as their attitude. Generally, if they have sufficient manual dexterity to be able to write or feed themselves they will be able to manage intermittent self-catheterization. Surprisingly, it is almost impossible to predict a patient's attitude to doing self-catheterization. Most are initially somewhat shocked by the suggestion but if the principle is adequately explained, time taken to demonstrate the technique and best of all if they have the opportunity of speaking to another patient who has benefited from doing it, they will usually agree to learn.

Concern is often expressed about the risk of introducing infection. Although this may be a problem, it is equally the case that having a persistent raised post-micturition residual volume puts the patient at risk of cystitis. Infections are in fact less common than might be expected, provided the technique is carried out cleanly. Furthermore, if patients obtain significant symptomatic benefit from intermittent self-catheterization they are usually willing to manage the occasional episode of urinary tract infection. Long-term antibiotics should be avoided, but a scheme for prompt treatment of the first signs of infection (i.e. change in colour and foul-smelling urine) should be set up so that the patient does not have to wait for the result of culture and sensitivities of the organism before starting a course of antibiotics. The best arrangement is for the patient to be given a specimen bottle, pathology request form and a short course of antibiotics. The patient then sends off a specimen and can start treatment, and by the time the sensitivities are known they will either be better or can change to an appropriate antibiotic.

Self-catheterization is not a method of treatment that suits all patients, and treatment of a patient who has incomplete emptying but is unable or unwilling to have intermittent catheterization is problematic. When incomplete bladder emptying is confirmed there is usually no alternative to learning intermittent self-catheterization, but at the National Hospital for Neurology and Neurosurgery the authors have been looking at the effect of a suprapubic vibrating stimulus. Benefit from this was first described by Peter Nathan in 1977, and a hand-held, battery-operated vibrating device has been found to be effective in improving bladder emptying in up to 80 per cent of patients with MS with a Kurtzke pyramidal function score of 3 or less (DasGupta et al., 1997). The vibrating stimulus may help to initiate micturition, and can improve urinary flow and lessen the post-micturition residual volume. The mechanism of its action is uncertain, although cystometric monitoring during use of the buzzer did show a larger pressure rise compared to 'sham' use of the buzzer (without batteries). However, it is only effective in patients with mild spinal disability who have a residual of less than 400 ml, intact suprapubic sensation and detrusor hyper-reflexia. In some such patients it has obviated the need for self-catheterization.

Treatment of detrusor hyper-reflexia

Effective suppression of hyper-reflexic contractions may sometimes compromise the normal detrusor function. It is therefore important that investigations are carried out to establish satisfactory bladder function (residual urine of less than 100 ml), or that adequate bladder emptying has been achieved, before treatment of detrusor hyper-reflexia is initiated. Considerable advances have been made in the understanding of the muscarinic receptor subtypes in the bladder and, although oxybutynin has been one of the first-line treatments in patients with multiple sclerosis for many years, there is a choice of treatments available. An initial starting dose of 2.5 mg oxybutynin twice a day may be effective, and can be increased to a maximum recommended dose of 5 mg three times a day. The effective dosage is clinically limited by the common side effect of a dry mouth, which in some cases can be significant enough to cause discontinuation of the medication. The impetus for the development of more 'uroselective' anti-muscarinic agents has been driven by the need to avoid the effect on the salivary gland.

Although 70 per cent of the muscarinic receptors in the human bladder are of the M2 subtype, bladder contraction is brought about by activation of the 20 per cent of M3 receptors. Newer anticholinergic drugs such as tolterodine (Detrusitol/Detrol) are more specific for the M3 muscarinic receptor, although this receptor is also present in the detrusor innervation and the innervation of the salivary gland and therefore dry mouth would appear to be inevitable. However, studies comparing tolterodine 2 mg bd with oxybutynin 5 mg tds have shown that for equivalent effects on bladder function, the incidence of dry mouth is reduced by eight times with tolterodine. This apparent anomaly is explained by the differential binding coefficients of these drugs on the entire population of muscarinic receptor subtypes in the bladder and the salivary gland, and also by the fact that a comparatively large dose of oxybutynin was given.

Trospium chloride is an atropine derivative with a quaternary ammonium group, and has also been shown to be more 'urospecific' than oxybutynin. In a study comparing 5 mg oxybutynin tds with 20 mg trospium chloride bd, the incidence of dry mouth was 23 per cent and 4 per cent respectively (Madersbacher *et al.*, 1995). Combination preparations of antimuscarinic agents with calcium channel blockers are being developed, and theoretically potassium channel openers could also be effective in reducing hyper-reflexic contractions. Tolerability is essential for patient compliance, and withdrawal from treatment is much higher with oxybutynin, predominantly due to the dry mouth. A dry mouth is different to a feeling of thirst, and if it is very troublesome artificial saliva can be given or the patient advised to suck pastilles or chew sugar-free gum.

The combination of an anticholinergic and intermittent catheterization is the optimal treatment for patients with bladder symptoms due to MS who have detrusor hyper-reflexia as well as incomplete emptying. However, there are some who use this combination but are still troubled by night-time frequency, and others who are not willing to consider intermittent self-catheterization but, because they are not emptying, cannot be given anticholinergics. It is in these, that it is reasonable to try Desmopressin® (Hilton *et al.*, 1983; Kinn and Larsson, 1990). Desmopressin is a synthetic antidiuretic hormone (DDAVP) that can be administered through a nasal spray. One or two puffs (10 mcg per puff) before retiring has the effect of reducing urine output for 6–8 hours. An anticipated side effect of this medication is hyponatraemia, but fortunately this is rarely symptomatic. However, warning should be given to discontinue the medication if the patient develops a headache or general feeling of malaise. Symptomatic hyponatraemia seems to be more common in the elderly, and extreme caution should be taken when prescribing DDAVP to patients over the age of 65 years. It is not advisable to prescribe this for wheelchair-bound patients with severely limited mobility and dependent oedema; their symptoms of night-time frequency are probably due to re-absorption of oedematous fluid when they are recumbent, and administering DDAVP would put them at risk of water retention.

A number of patients have found that taking DDAVP before a meeting, a journey on public transport or some social occasion may lessen the risk of urinary urgency during that period. This is a reasonable treatment, provided the patient understands that the medication must never be taken more than once in 24 hours.

Intravesical capsaicin

The physiological bladder is under an inhibitory influence from higher brain centres and the pons. Figure 15.4 shows the change in reflex bladder control that occurs following destruction of the pathways conveying afferent innervation from the sacral cord to the periaqueductal grey matter, and then to the pontine micturition centre. In spinal health, afferent impulses from the detrusor muscle are conveyed in the periphery through small myelinated Aδ fibres and then travel to the pontine micturition centre. An interruption in the spinal pathways leads to the emergence of a new reflex at the sacral cord level. The functionally significant afferents of this new emergent reflex are thought to be unmyelinated C-fibres, which, although present in large numbers (about 70 per cent of the afferent innervation in a healthy adult are thought to be C-afferents), are usually quiescent except in conditions of inflammation. It is these unmyelinated C-fibres that are thought to drive the detrusor efferents following disconnection of the sacral cord from the pontine micturition centre. In this way, the normal inhibited state of the detrusor during filling is lost and volume-determined bladder contractions occur instead – i.e. detrusor hyper-reflexia (Figure 15.1).

Capsaicin (8-methyl-N-vannilyl-6-nonenamide) is the pungent ingredient in red-hot chilli peppers, and has been used in the human diet and for medicinal purposes for hundreds of years. C-fibre sensitivity to capsaicin has been documented

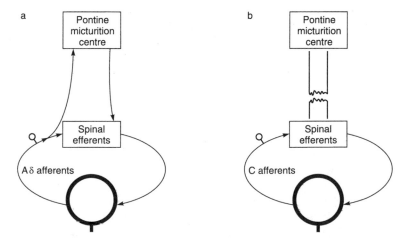

Figure 15.4 Changes in reflex bladder control following spinal injury (see text for details).

in experimental animals (de Groat *et al.*, 1990); indeed, some afferent nerves have been described as capsaicin-sensitive primary afferents (CSPA), based on the effect of capsaicin. Studies in humans suggest that the neurotoxic effect of capsaicin can be an effective treatment for patients with spinal cord involvement due to MS (Fowler *et al.*, 1994). An intravesical instillation of 1 or 2 mmol of capsaicin dissolved in alcohol has been found to lessen detrusor hyper-reflexia, and symptomatic benefit may be derived for nearly 6 months after a single instillation. This prolonged period of effectiveness implies that there has been loss of sensory afferents rather than a functional neuronal block, and a reduction in lamina propria nerve density has been demonstrated 6 weeks following intravesical capsaicin instillation (DasGupta *et al.*, 1998).

Terminal vesicles on sensory nerve axons are thought to contain neuropeptide neurotransmitters such as substance P and calcitonin gene-related peptide. Following capsaicin instillation, ultrastructural studies have shown that there are significant reductions in the numbers of axons containing clear and dense cored vesicles (Hussain *et al.*, 1999). The implication is that degranulation of neuropeptide neurotransmitters from the afferent superficial bladder nerves may also be a possible mechanism of action of intravesical capsaicin. Although it is not always possible to predict which patients will respond favourably, those with severe neurological disability, low compliance bladders and very low bladder capacities are likely to respond less well. The treatment may be repeated, and studies up to 5 years have shown no evidence of pre-malignant change in the detrusor urothelium with repeated applications (DasGupta *et al.*, 1997).

It is likely that the treatment of refractory detrusor hyper-reflexia in multiple sclerosis will eventually make use of ultrapotent capsaicin analogues. The Situs Corporation in the USA is developing innovative drug delivery systems that can be introduced into the bladder during cystoscopy and deliver a known and constant dose of drug for up to a month at a time. These devices may become important in the delivery of newer compounds such as resiniferatoxin (RTX). This is another plant extract (from *Euphorbia resinifera*), and is 1000 times more potent than capsaicin at primary afferent neuronal desensitization (Craft *et al.*, 1995). Caterina *et al.* (1997) used expression cloning to isolate functional cDNA encoding the receptor that binds capsaicin from the dorsal root ganglia cells of rodents, and named it the vanilloid receptor subtype 1 (VR1). The VR1 receptor has also been localized to the spinal cord and visceral organs such as the bladder, urethra and colon (Chancellor and de Groat, 1999). This receptor is an ion channel that can be activated by capsaicin binding, causing calcium and sodium influx and resulting in initial excitation and then desensitization of intravesical C-fibres. Lazzeri *et al.* (1997) reported the use of 10^{-8} mol/l solutions of RTX in 15 humans (six with detrusor hyper-reflexia). They confirmed earlier reports by Cruz *et al.* (1997) that this preparation can cause desensitization without the initial excitation, and therefore avoids the initial deterioration of symptoms and suprapubic discomfort reported during the instillation of capsaicin. The much lower dose of RTX required for therapeutic efficacy is likely to be one cause of the reduced side effect profile. Equally, although both capsaicin and RTX are both vanilloids, they may have different mechanisms of action. RTX is being formally evaluated by means of a randomized, multicentre, placebo-controlled study, and results should become available within the next few years. It is attractive to speculate that a single instillation of a solution of these vanilloid derivatives may render the patient with multiple sclerosis symptom-free from urinary complaints for many months at a time.

Surgery and long-term catheters

Indications for surgical management of the MS bladder remain limited. This is because, unlike traumatic spinal cord injuries, upper tract involvement in multiple sclerosis is relatively uncommon (Sirls et al., 1994; Koldewijn et al., 1995), and hydronephrosis and renal damage seem only to occur in patients who are severely disabled and have long-term in-dwelling catheters (Betts et al., 1993). It is not known why such complications should be infrequent, because patients with MS may develop equally severe spasticity and weakness of the lower limbs to patients who have suffered spinal cord trauma. It may be that the detrusor pressures in multiple sclerosis are lower both in intensity and duration, thus resulting in less damage to the upper tracts. Equally, many of the MS patients who require surgical intervention are those in whom medical management has failed, and they have reached a point in the progression of the disease when they are no longer able to perform intermittent self-catheterization. Understandably, there is a reluctance to submit patients with disabling multiple sclerosis to surgery. Nevertheless, surgical intervention may be carried out to alter urethral resistance, reduce detrusor hyper-reflexia or divert the urine into a conduit in cases of severe and persistent incontinence. Bladder augmentation by means of a clam ileocystoplasty may be a useful means of reducing detrusor hyper-reflexia and increasing bladder capacity, but is complicated by voiding dysfunction in nearly 20 per cent of cases. It is important that patients are assessed to ensure that they can and will perform self-catheterization before such a procedure is considered. A permanent urinary diversion such as an ileal conduit may be indicated when other forms of incontinence management have failed.

Figure 15.5 shows the effect of progression of spinal cord involvement in a patient with MS, their deteriorating mobility and bladder function, and management at each stage. Unfortunately, a point is often reached when medical measures fail and some form of in-dwelling catheter drainage becomes the best option. A long-term urethral catheter is rarely advisable, although as a temporary arrangement it serves to familiarize all concerned with the need to have a continuous drainage bag and has the advantage that it can be easily inserted as an outpatient. However, such a catheter is likely to be extruded and destroy the bladder neck mechanism, and the preferred alternative is a suprapubic catheter. This should be inserted by a urological surgeon, preferably under cystoscopic guidance; this makes it a safer procedure and provides an opportunity to examine the bladder and exclude other pathology such as bladder stones and a tumour. Once inserted it will need to be changed every 6–8 weeks; on the first occasion this will be performed at hospital, but subsequent changes can be done at home. The catheter is left on continual drainage so the bladder is constantly empty, and

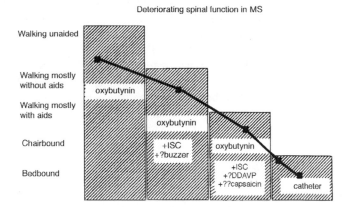

Figure 15.5 The bladder symptoms in MS becoming increasingly difficult to manage with progression of spinal cord disease. This diagram summarizes the various measures that may be effective at each stage.

there is therefore no need for the surgically difficult procedure of urethral closure.

Conclusion

Bladder symptoms in MS are some of the most distressing problems for the patient and their carer, and yet can be effectively managed. In the past there has been an understandable reluctance by neurologists to care for these complaints, since it was considered that imaging of the urinary tract and cystometry were essential in planning management. However, views are changing, and the argument that bladder symptoms should be regarded as a manifestation of neurological dysfunction rather than a symptom of possibly life-threatening urological disease is gaining ground. Essential to management is understanding the extent to which the patient has incomplete bladder emptying whilst complaining predominantly of symptoms of bladder over-activity. The management offered to the patient should suit their current level of disability, and long-term catheterization should only become necessary with advancing neurological disease.

Sexual dysfunction

The problems of sexual function that affect both men and women with MS are now often discussed freely by patients and their medical carers, although this has not always been the case. This is due to a combination of factors, including a shift in opinion concerning public discussion of sexual matters, a better understanding of the organic basis of sexual problems in MS, and the introduction of effective methods of treatment for male erectile dysfunction (ED). Some sexual problems relate to the patient having become disabled and the effect this has both on their own self-image and on their relationship with their partner (Dupont, 1995). However, this section will be confined to discussion of the neurological aspects of patients' sexual dysfunction and how these can be helped. The treatments available for sexual dysfunction in women are still unsatisfactory, but it is apparent that both women and men with MS may welcome the opportunity of discussing their problems with a receptive and sympathetic health-care professional.

Sexual dysfunction in women

The problems for women include loss of libido and loss of ability to achieve orgasm. Lack of vaginal lubrication, impaired or altered sacral sensation, anxiety about incontinence, lower limb spasticity and adductor spasm are all common complaints in women with MS.

Research on female sexual dysfunction in MS is sparse, and was initially carried out only by questionnaire (Lilius *et al.*, 1976; Minderhoud *et al.*, 1984; Valleroy and Kraft, 1984). From these studies, an incidence of about 50 per cent for sexual problems in women with MS was estimated.

In 1981 Lundberg published a study that compared the sexual symptoms of 25 women with mild MS to those of 25 women with migraine, and concluded that problems in MS were mainly of an organic nature (Lundberg, 1981). In these mildly affected patients, transient symptoms were a prominent feature (as illustrated in the two case histories included in the work); however, more than 50 per cent of the group with MS had loss of or decreased libido and/or difficulty in achieving orgasm, whereas sexual problems occurred in only 12 per cent of the migraine patients.

In a more recent study, Hulter and Lundberg (1995) interviewed 47 women with advanced MS. Again, a high proportion of the women reported decreased desire (nearly 60 per cent), diminished orgasmic capacity (nearly 40 per cent) and decreased lubrication (36 per cent). Sensory dysfunction of the genital region was reported by 60 per cent. Perhaps not unexpectedly, symptoms were most marked in those who had other sacral neurological symptoms such as bladder and bowel dysfunction and pelvic floor weakness. Problems with sexual function were reported more by less disabled women. One-third of the group had separated from former sexual partners, and 66 per cent of them said that their MS had been an important factor in their separation.

A finding of particular interest was that the majority of patients said they had never been asked to discuss their sexuality before in connection with their MS, and 83 per cent considered it to have been a positive experience.

In terms of specific treatment, there is little that can currently be done. In the early stages of the disease, reassurance can be given that reported sensory disturbances are likely to be transitory. Effective treatment of incontinence obviously has a positive effect on the situation, as does treatment of spasticity, and possibly advice (which in some situations amounts to 'permission') to explore alternative positions for intercourse. The possible development of a neurotransmitter that may help to induce orgasm in women with spinal cord disease has future therapeutic implications for women with MS, and some years ago vasoactive intestinal peptide was being studied. Today there is considerable interest in the use of the selective phosphodiesterase type-5 inhibitor, sildenafil citrate (Viagra®). Anecdotally its use has been reported in the USA to give improvement in clitoral engorgement and genital lubrication, leading to improved orgasmic capacity. There are no peer-reviewed publications on the use of sildenafil in women, but specific questionnaires for studying sexual dysfunction in women are being developed and validated at present. Until these studies have been carried out and specific pharmacotherapy introduced, discussion between the patient and her health-care contacts (such as physiotherapists, nurses and doctors) about the problems she is facing may be the most helpful factor.

Sexual dysfunction in men

Modern studies have found that 60–65 per cent of males with MS (unselected for their neurological disability) have erectile difficulties (Lilius *et al.*, 1976; Minderhoud *et al.*, 1984; Valleroy and Kraft, 1984), although earlier studies put the figure considerably lower. Miller *et al.* (1965) reviewed the urogenital symptoms of 297 patients with MS and found 62 per cent of males had erectile difficulties but, without any further explanation, stated that in 18 per cent the problem was 'psychological'.

Typically, in the early stages of the disease the chief complaint is of difficulty sustaining an erection for intercourse – i.e. erectile dysfunction (ED). Penile erections occur during the night and on waking in the morning, and normal nocturnal penile tumescence tests have been demonstrated in men with MS complaining of erectile difficulties (Ghezzi *et al.*, 1995). These features may have wrongly contributed in the past to interpretation of the problem as non-organic. With advancing neurological disability, there may be a total failure of erectile function and difficulty with ejaculation.

A few studies have looked at the neurological features associated with this common problem in MS. Of the questionnaire studies, Lilius *et al.* (1976) and Valleroy and Kraft (1984) found an association between lower limb dysfunction and a disturbance of sexual function; Minderhoud *et al.* (1984) did not. Vas (1969) described an association between sensory disturbance and erectile dysfunction, as well as between the distribution of anhydrosis and impotence. Men with complete erectile failure did not sweat below the iliac crests, whereas men with partial ED had a normal pattern of sweating apart from on the lower limbs.

The study by Kirkeby *et al.* (1988) was the first systematically to record the pudendal evoked potential in men with MS, and the finding that it was abnormal in the majority contributed to the changing view that the problem was usually neurologically-based. Betts *et al.* (1994) found that 96 per cent of men with MS attending for treatment of ED had unequivocal bilateral pyramidal signs in their legs, and whereas there was a definite correlation between pyramidal dysfunction and the presence of erectile failure in this group, no other Kurtzke function score was so consistently abnormal. From these clinical data alone it was concluded that spinal cord disease was the major underlying cause of erectile failure, and this was confirmed by neurophysiological studies. Recordings of the tibial and pudendal somatosensory evoked potentials were made in 44 men, and some abnormality was found in 73 per cent. Of particular interest was the finding that the pudendal evoked potential was not abnormal more often than the tibial evoked responses, indicating that the responsible spinal cord disease was suprasacral. A greater sensitivity of the tibial than the pudendal evoked potential in patients with MS and urinary symptoms was reported by Rodi *et al.* (1996). Not only was the pudendal less sensitive than the tibial evoked potential response, but there were also seven men with ED who had normal neurophysiological investigations, four of whom had unequivocal clinical evidence of bilateral pyramidal tract dysfunction in the lower limbs.

Whereas Betts *et al.* (1994) concluded that evoked potential testing was of lesser value than the clinical examination in recognizing relevant spinal cord disease, Ghezzi *et al.* (1995) found neurophysiological abnormalities as commonly in men with MS who did not have ED as in those who did. A correlation was demonstrated between abnormal tibial and pudendal evoked potentials and difficulties with ejaculation (Betts *et al.*, 1994) in that the more severely abnormal the evoked potential, the more likely it was that ejaculation would be difficult or impossible. Miller *et al.* (1965) found that ED was always associated with urinary symptoms, and Betts *et al.* (1993) found that 85 per cent of their group had urodynamically-proven hyper-reflexia; a problem that is also associated with spinal cord involvement in MS.

It has been suggested that a diagnosis of MS should be considered in a man presenting with impotence, but in the absence of clinical spinal cord disease this would seem unlikely. In the series by Betts *et al.* (1994), a single patient had erectile difficulties in association with the first symptoms of MS, but there were no patients who first presented with ED and then developed other neurological features.

Treatment of erectile dysfunction

The aim of ED management is to restore the quality of erection and improve the sexual relationship. Even when MS has been identified as the cause for ED there may be other anxieties contributing to the illness, and although formal psychosexual counselling may not be required, patients often welcome the opportunity to discuss their problem and receive an explanation of their sexual difficulties in relation to their illness. If appropriate, discussions may be conducted with the participation of the patient's partner so that the couple can make an informed choice about management. Although there are numerous management options now available for ED, each has a different profile of efficacy, safety, tolerability and patient satisfaction. The treatment of ED is an area in which pharmaceutical companies are carrying out intensive research, and there are several therapies that have only recently been introduced. Further research is investigating the use of combinations of products and different formulations.

Vacuum constriction devices

These devices consist of a cylinder that is placed over the penis, and when a vacuum is created by pumping air out of the tube the penis can be made to enlarge within the cylinder. After pumping for 5–6 minutes, the increased blood is then maintained in the penis by placing a tourniquet around its base. The resulting penile enlargement is the result of venous rather than arterial engorgement, and the penis is therefore cooler and less stiff, and the base may remain flaccid. Although these devices have been in use for many years, they have not been acceptable to all patients. However, high success rates have been reported in motivated patients who have received enthusiastic instruction. The system has the great advantage of being less invasive than intracorporeal injections.

Intracorporeal pharmacotherapy

Intracorporeal injection of papaverine has been used to treat ED since the early 1980s, although it has now been replaced by prostaglandin E1 (alprostadil), which has been given world-wide licences for self-injection therapy (Porst, 1996). Papaverine has a direct relaxant effect on smooth muscle, and although highly effective, bruising and local discomfort was not uncommon and local fibrosis involving the corpora sometimes occurred. Patients with neurogenic impotence were particularly prone to developing a prolonged erection, which, if it lasted for more than 5 hours, required reversal by aspiration of the corpora or possibly intracorporeal injections of alpha-adrenergic agents such as metaraminol or adrenaline. Prostaglandin E1 is an endogenous substance and is rapidly metabolized, so priapism and local fibrosis are less common. The substance has almost no systemic side effects, and is highly efficacious; the only frequent problem is of penile pain following the injection. A spring-loaded device called a 'peninject' is available to facilitate the injection process in those who are reluctant to self-inject; however, a certain level of manual dexterity is required to set up and use the device.

Transurethral alprostadil

In published series with self-injection therapy, it has been noted that the drop-out rate can be as high as 40–50 per cent (Porst, 1996). A large component of this is attributed to needle phobia, and the introduction of MUSE (medicated urethral system for erection) was the first real alternative to injectables despite remaining an invasive procedure. MUSE is a single-use system for the delivery of a medicated pellet of alprostadil into the urethra, from where it is absorbed into the corpus spongiosum. After micturition a small applicator is inserted into the urethra, a pellet is delivered by depressing the applicator, and erection occurs within 15 minutes. Initial studies during in-clinic testing reported that 65.4 per cent of men were able to achieve erections sufficient for intercourse, although this dropped to 50.4 per cent during home treatment trials. In multicentre cross-over European trials of MUSE, the reported response rates were only 43 per cent with

MUSE compared to 70 per cent after self-injection of alprostadil (and 10 per cent for placebo) (Porst *et al.*, 1996).

The commonest side effect is penile pain, and, surprisingly, a greater proportion of patients are troubled by this during the use of MUSE than with self-injection. Patients should be warned about the need to take great care when inserting the applicator into the urethra, but some may still report urethral trauma and temporary bleeding. It has been suggested that this is unlikely to lead to any long-term sequelae. Priapism is rare, but advice on the need to seek urgent medical attention in the event of a prolonged erection should be given with all forms of therapy for ED. Although the efficacy is lower, many patients prefer MUSE because they are able to avoid self-injection.

Oral medication

A pill for ED is now an effective alternative in most patients with multiple sclerosis. Normal erections are brought about by stimulation of the parasympathetic innervation to the penis with the release of nitric oxide (NO) from the post-synaptic parasympathetic nerve endings. NO has a very short half-life (measured in seconds) and diffuses into the trabecular and arterial smooth muscle cells. By stimulating guanylate cyclase it causes an increase in cGMP, which results in smooth muscle cell relaxation and vasodilatation. Sildenafil citrate (Viagra) is a selective phosphodiesterase-5 inhibitor and, by preventing the breakdown of cGMP, would be expected to restore the natural erectile response to sexual stimulation. The tablets are available in doses of 25 mg, 50 mg and 100 mg, and should be taken as required up to an hour before sexual activity. This drug has now been evaluated in multiple studies in selected groups of patients, including those suffering from multiple sclerosis, diabetes, ED and depression. When efficacy was measured by using the International Index of Erectile Dysfunction (IIEF) questions 3 and 4 (the ability to achieve an erection and to maintain an erection for sexual intercourse), the patients with multiple sclerosis had the best response.

The drug is well tolerated, and although patients may complain of headache, flushing, nasal congestion, dyspepsia and an alteration in blue/green colour appreciation, these are transient side effects and usually resolve within a few hours. However, caution should be exercised in those known to have coronary heart disease. The overall good safety profile has contributed to its popularity since it was approved by the US Food and Drug Administration in March 1998.

Topical creams

Application of a mixture of nitric oxide-releasing vasoactive dilatory creams to the penis (Gomaa *et al.*, 1996) has also been described. In this placebo-controlled cross-over study, 58 per cent of men responded to the active cream while only 8 per cent responded to the placebo.

Prostheses

In contrast to other mammals such as the whale, dog, bear, gibbon and otter, the human male is unusual in not having a penile bone to enforce erections. Some patients may consider having implantation of a penile prosthesis, either rigid or inflatable, if all other treatments fail or are unacceptable (Kirby *et al.*, 1991). However, penile implantation is not recommended in men with MS who may deteriorate neurologically in the future, with worsening bladder control requiring intervention and possible erosion of the prosthesis with increasing sacral sensory loss.

Ejaculation

Yohimbine is a drug that is claimed to improve ejaculatory function and orgasm. It is a reversible alpha-2 adrenoceptor antagonist, and is thought to act both centrally and peripherally. Use of a wide range of doses has been reported in the literature, and both regular and 'as required' therapy have been reported to be effective. For ejaculatory failure, it has been recommended that 5–10 mg should be taken 1–2 hours before intercourse is attempted (Brindley, 1994), but in clinical trials yohimbine has been taken in doses of 15–43 mg per day in divided doses (Eardley, 1998). This variability is a reflection of the difficulty in successfully treating ejaculatory failure.

Bowel dysfunction

Neural control of ano-rectal function

The lower bowel acts to perform two functions; storage and elimination. In neurological disease, these functions may be affected either separately or together. Disorders of elimination cause constipation and difficulty with defecation, and disorders of storage lead to faecal incontinence.

Defecation involves a complex series of neurologically controlled actions, which are initiated in response to the conscious sensation of a full rectum. When this is sensed, and if judged to be appropriate, defecation is initiated by raising the intra-abdominal pressure and straining down, causing descent of the pelvic floor. The outlet of the rectum opens with relaxation of the internal and striated external anal sphincters due to the recto-anal inhibitory reflex.

The role of spinal cord function in controlling the bowel in MS is not clear. If spinal cord disease were a major factor in causing bowel disorders in MS, the prevalence of these symptoms would be expected to be higher in patients with bladder dysfunction than in an unselected population. However, this was found not to be the case, and 32 per cent of patients with clinical evidence of spinal cord disease and significant bladder dysfunction had no complaints of bowel dysfunction (Chia *et al.*, 1995). Nevertheless, patients with MS do often complain of problems with their bowels, and clearly the prevalence of bowel dysfunction is very much higher than in the general population. Sullivan and Ebers (1983) reported that 53 per cent of their patients with MS complained of constipation, and a study of a large number of patients with MS found that 43 per cent had constipation and 53 per cent faecal incontinence (Hinds *et al.*, 1990). Overall, 68 per cent had some form of bowel symptoms (Hinds *et al.*, 1990).

It seems unlikely that there is a single identifiable neurological deficit associated with bowel symptoms, and from the research that has been carried out it appears that there are a number of possible pathophysiological mechanisms for the main symptoms (Table 15.1).

Table 15.1 Symptoms of colo-rectal dysfunction in MS and possible pathophysiological causes (from Fowler and Henry, 1997)

Constipation
• Slow colonic transit
• Abnormal rectal function
• Intussusception

Faecal incontinence
• Absent or decreased sensation of rectal filling
• Poor voluntary contraction of anal sphincter/pelvic floor
• Reduced rectal compliance
• Obstetric injury to the anal sphincters

Constipation

Constipation in MS can vary from being quite minor to being a severe and disabling problem. Abnormalities of colonic activity and a slow transit time have been shown to occur (Glick *et al.*, 1982; Weber *et al.*, 1990; Chia *et al.*, 1995), and in some patients reduced fluid intake, poor mobility and anticholinergic medication may contribute to the problem. Chia *et al.* (1996) speculated that slow transit might be due to an autonomic nervous system deficit such as occurs with a central nervous system lesion rostral to the thoracic cord, but constipation can also occur in patients with little general neurological disability due to MS. An alternative speculative hypothesis is that it is due not to a specific neurological lesion or lesions in the central nervous system, but rather to another mechanism similar to that which causes fatigue in the disease (the cause of which is also unknown).

A complaint that does appear to be associated with a severe paraparesis is difficulty in voluntarily 'switching on' the mechanism of defecation. Spasticity of the pelvic floor is associated with a failure of effacement of the puborectalis during attempts to empty the rectum, and patients may find digitation necessary to assist evacuation. When this is performed during defecating proctography, the index finger is hooked over the puborectalis impression and the muscle pulled downwards until effacement is achieved and rectal emptying can proceed (Gill *et al.*, 1994).

In a study of 11 patients with MS and severe constipation, three were found to have developed an intussusception and in one case this had produced an intrarectal obstruction (Gill *et al.*, 1994). Intussusception is thought to be the result of chronic straining, and such an abnormality should be suspected in patients having severe difficulty in rectal emptying and a continuous sensation of incomplete evacuation. The response to surgical repair of the prolapsed mucosa can be dramatic.

Incontinence

In spinal health, defecation can be delayed when necessary by contraction of the external anal sphincter and pelvic floor. Many patients with MS and faecal incontinence can be shown, either clinically or manometrically, to have poor voluntary squeeze pressures. A study by Nordenbo *et al.* (1996) found a close association between absent or impaired rectal sensation and faecal incontinence. It was suggested that the loss of rectal sensation resulted in the patient being unaware of impending defecation, and because the recto-anal inhibitory reflex has a local intramural pathway (Lubowski *et al.*, 1987) and remains intact in spinal cord disease, relaxation of the internal and external sphincters occurred in response to rectal filling without voluntary input or conscious sensation. The same study also demonstrated a decreased rectal compliance, which further tends to cause the recto-anal inhibitory reflex to be initiated earlier (Nordenbo *et al.*, 1996). A lower motor neurone component of anal sphincter weakness following obstetric injury may be a contributing factor to incontinence in some multiparous women with MS (Swash *et al.*, 1987).

Investigations

Colonic transit times can be estimated by asking the patient to swallow radio-opaque markers and taking serial abdominal X-rays. Defecography is the most valuable investigation in patients complaining of difficulties with defecation. During this investigation, a barium-containing contrast medium is introduced into the rectum and the function of the pelvic floor and sphincters can be studied as the patient attempts to defecate.

In patients whose predominant complaint is incontinence, manometric pressure studies of the rectum and sphincters can be performed. Most studies have shown that faecal incontinence in MS is associated with constipation, and as a general rule a patient with MS who has incontinence without constipation should be investigated for other lower bowel disorders.

Treatment

There are no published studies concerning the effect of medication on bowel symptoms in MS. In general, most patients have tried laxatives and enemas themselves before complaining of their problem to their neurologist, but if constipation is a complaint and lactulose has not been tried, 10 ml daily can be recommended. An enema given in the morning to clear the rectum may reduce the risk of faecal incontinence occurring at some other time during the day.

A study that looked primarily at the value of a vibrating device to assist bladder emptying in patients with MS found that a proportion of the patients also reported this to be of value in assisting effective bowel emptying (DasGupta *et al.*, 1997).

If rectal intussusception is demonstrated, surgical treatment may be highly effective in relieving symptoms.

In general, however, there is little that can be currently offered to help the large number of patients with the distressing symptoms of disturbed bowel function. New approaches and new treatments to this problem are much needed.

References

Betts, C. D., D'Mellow, M. T. and Fowler, C. J. (1993). Urinary symptoms and the neurological features of bladder dysfunction in multiple sclerosis. *J. Neurol. Neurosurg. Psychiatr.*, **56**, 245–50.

Betts, C. D., Jones, S. J., Fowler, C. G. and Fowler, C. J. (1994). Erectile dysfunction in mutiple sclerosis; associated neurological and neurophysiological deficits and treatment of the condition. *Brain*, **117**, 1303–10.

Blok, B., Willemsen, T. and Holstege, G. (1997). A PET study of brain control of micturition in humans. *Brain*, **129**, 111–21.

Brindley, G. (1994). Impotence and ejaculatory failure. In: *The Handbook of Neuro-Urology* (D. N. Rushton, ed.), pp. 331–48. Marcel Dekker.

Caterina, M. J., Schumacher, M. A., Tominaga, M. *et al.* (1997). The capsaicin receptor: a heat-activated ion channel in the pain pathway. *Nature*, **389**, 816–24.

Chancellor, M. and Blaivas, J. (1995). Multiple sclerosis. In: *Practical Neuro-Urology* (M. Chancellor and J. Blaivas, eds), pp. 119–37. Butterworth-Heinemann.

Chancellor, M. B. and de Groat, W. C. (1999). Intravesical capsaicin and resiniferatoxin therapy: spicing up the ways to treat the overactive bladder. *J. Urol.*, **162**, 3–11.

Chia, Y., Fowler, C., Kamm, M. *et al.* (1995). Prevalence of bowel dysfunction in patients with multiple sclerosis and bladder dysfunction. *J. Neurol.*, **242**, 105–8.

Chia, Y., Gill, K., Jameson, J. *et al.* (1996). Paradoxical puborectalis contraction is a feature of constipation in patients with multiple sclerosis. *J. Neurol. Neurosurg. Psychiatr.*, **60**, 31–5.

Craft, R., Cohen, S. and Porreca, F. (1995). Long-lasting desensitization of bladder afferents following intravesical resiniferatoxin and capsaicin in the rat. *Pain*, **61**, 317–23.

Cruz, F., Avelino, A. and Coimbra, A. (1997). Intravesical resiniferatoxin desensitises bladder sensory fibres in a dose-dependent manner. *J. Urol.*, **157**, 79.

DasGupta, P., Haslam, C., Goodwin, R. J. and Fowler, C. J. (1997). Emptying the neurogenic bladder. *Br. J. Urology*, **80**, 234–7.

DasGupta, P., Chandiramani, V. A., Parkinson, M. C. *et al.* (1998). Treating the human bladder with capsaicin: is it safe? *Eur. J. Urol.*, **33**, 28–31.

de Groat, W. C. (1990). Central neural control of the lower urinary tract. In: *Neurobiology of Incontinence* (G. Bock and J. Whelan, eds), pp. 27–56. John Wiley & Sons.

de Groat, W., Kawatani, T. and Hisamitsu, T. (1990). Mechanisms underlying the recovery of urinary bladder function following spinal cord injury. *J. Autonom. Nerv. Sys.*, **30**, S71–8.

Dupont, S. (1995). Multiple sclerosis and sexual functioning – a review. *Clin. Rehabil.*, **9**, 135–41.

Eardley, I. (1998). New oral therapies for the treatment of erectile dysfunction. *Br. J. Urol.*, **81**, 122–7.

Fowler, C. J. (1996). Investigation of the neurogenic bladder. *J. Neurol. Neurosurg. Psychiatr.*, **60**, 6–13.

Fowler, C. J. and Henry, M. M. (1997). Gastrointestinal dysfunction in multiple sclerosis. *Sem. Neurol.*, **16**, 277–9.

Fowler, C. J., van Kerrebroeck, P. E. V., Nordenbo, A. and van Poppel, H. (1992). Treatment of lower urinary tract dysfunction in patients with multiple sclerosis. *J. Neurol. Neurosurg. Psychiatr.*, **55**, 986–9.

Fowler, C. J., Beck, R. O., Gerrard, S. *et al.* (1994). Intravesical capsaicin for treatment of detrusor hyper-reflexia. *J. Neurol. Neurosurg. Psychiatr.*, **57**, 169–73.

Ghezzi, A., Malvestiti, G., Baldini, S. *et al.* (1995). Erectile impotence in multiple sclerosis: a neurophysiological study. *J. Neurol.*, **242**, 123–6.

Gill, K., Chia, Y., Henry, M. and Shorvon, P. (1994). Defecography in multiple sclerosis patients with severe constipation. *Radiology*, **191**, 553–6.

Glick, E., Meshkinpour, H., Haldeman, S. *et al.* (1982). Colonic dysfunction in multiple sclerosis. *Gastroenterology*, **83**, 1002–7.

Gomaa, A., Shalaby, M., Osman, M. *et al.* (1996). Topical treatment of erectile dysfunction: randomised double-blind placebo-controlled trial of cream containing aminophylline isosorbide dinitrate, and co-dergocrine mesylate. *Br. Med. J.*, **312**, 1512–15.

Griffiths, D., Holstege, G., de Wall, H. and Dalm, E. (1990). Control and coordination of bladder and urethral function in the brain stem of the cat. *Neurourol. Urodyn.*, **9**, 63–82.

Hilton, P., Hertogs, K. and Stanton, S. (1983). The use of desmopressin (DDAVP) for nocturia in women with multiple sclerosis. *J. Neurol. Neurosurg. Psychiatr.*, **46**, 854–5.

Hinds, J., Eidelman, B. and Wald, A. (1990). Prevalence of bowel dysfunction in multiple sclerosis. *Gastroenterology*, **98**, 1538–42.

Hulter, B. and Lundberg, P. (1995). Sexual function in women with advanced multiple sclerosis. *J. Neurol. Neurosurg. Psychiatr.*, **59**, 83–6.

Hussain, I. F., Sakakibara, R., DasGupta, P. (1999). Ultrastructural changes in the composition of lamina propria nerves following capsaion therapy, *Br. J. Urol.*, **84**, 145 (abstract).

Kinn, A.-C. and Larsson, P. (1990). Desmopressin: a new principle for symptomatic treatment of urgency and incontinence in patients with multiple sclerosis. *Scand. J. Urol. Nephrol.*, **24**, 109–12.

Kirby, R. S., Carson, C. C. and Webster, G. D. (eds) (1991). *Impotence: Diagnosis and Management of Male Erectile Dysfunction*. Butterworth-Heinemann.

Kirkeby, H. J., Poulsen, E. U., Petersen, T. and Dorup, J. (1988). Erectile dysfunction in multiple sclerosis. *Neurology*, **38**, 1366–71.

Koldewijn, E., Hommes, O., Lemmens, W. *et al*. (1995). Relationship between lower urinary tract abnormalities and disease-related parameters in multiple sclerosis. *J. Urol.*, **154**, 169–73.

Kornhuber, H. and Schulz, A. (1990). Efficient treatment of neurogenic bladder disorders in multiple sclerosis with initial intermittent catheterization and ultrasound-controlled training. *Eur. J. Neurol.*, **30**, 260.

Lapides, J., Diokno, A. C., Silber, S. J. and Lowe, B. S. (1972). Clean, intermittent self-catheterization in the treatment of urinary tract disease. *J. Urol.*, **107**, 458–61.

Lapides, J., Diokno, A. C. and Gould, F. R. (1976). Further observations on self-catheterisation. *J. Urol.*, **116**, 169–71.

Lazzeri, M., Bebeforti, P. and Turini, D. (1997). Urodynamic effects of intravesical resiniferatoxin in humans: preliminary results in stable and unstable detrusor. *J. Urol.*, **158**, 2093–6.

Lilius, H. G., Valtonen, E. J. and Wikstrom, J. (1976). Sexual problems in patients suffering from multiple sclerosis. *J. Chron. Dis.*, **29**, 643–7.

Lubowski, D., Nicholls, R., Swash, M. and Jordan, M. (1987). Neural control of internal sphincter function. *Br. J. Surg.*, **74**, 668–70.

Lundberg, P. O. (1981). Sexual dysfunction in female patients with multiple sclerosis. *Int. Rehabil. Med.*, **3**, 32–4.

Madersbacher, H., Stohrer, M., Richter, R. *et al*. (1995). Trospium chloride versus oxybutinin: a randomised, double-blind, multicentre trial in the treatment of detrusor hyperreflexia. *Br. J. Urol.*, **75**, 452–6.

Miller, H., Simpson, C. A. and Yeates, W. K. (1965). Bladder dysfunction in multiple sclerosis. *Br. Med. J.*, **1**, 1265–9.

Minderhoud, J. M., Leehuis, J. G., Kremer, J. *et al*. (1984). Sexual disturbances arising from multiple sclerosis. *Acta Neurol. Scand.*, **70**, 299–306.

Nordenbo, A., Andersen, J. and Andersen, J. (1996). Disturbances of ano-rectal function in multiple sclerosis. *J. Neurol.*, **243**, 445–51.

Porst, H. (1996). The rationale for prostaglandin E1 in erectile failure: a survey of worldwide experience. *J. Urol.*, **155**, 802–15.

Porst, H. and the European VIVUS–MUSE Study Group (1996). Transurethral alprostadil for the treatment of chronic erectile dysfunction: the European experience. *Int. J. Impot. Res.*, **8**, 131 D35.

Rodi, Z., Vodusek, D. and Denislic, M. (1996). Clinical uro-neurophysiological investigation in multiple sclerosis. *Eur. J. Neurol.*, **3**, 574–80.

Sirls, L., Zimmern, P. and Leach, G. (1994). Role of limited evaluation and aggressive medical management in multiple sclerosis: a review of 113 patients. *J. Urol.*, **151**, 946–50.

Sullivan, S. and Ebers, G. (1983). Gastrointestinal dysfunction in multiple sclerosis. *Gastroenterology*, **84**, 1640–46.

Swash, M., Snooks, S. J. and Chalmers, D. H. K. (1987). Parity as a factor in incontinence in multiple sclerosis. *Arch. Neurol.*, **44**, 504–8.

Valleroy, M. L. and Kraft, G. H. (1984). Sexual dysfunction in multiple sclerosis. *Arch. Phys. Med. Rehabil.*, **65,** 125–8.

Vas, C. J. (1969). Sexual impotence and some autonomic disturbances in men with multiple sclerosis. *Acta Neurol. Scand.*, **45,** 166–82.

Weber, J., Delanger, T., Hannequin, D. *et al*. (1990). Anorectal manometric anomalies in seven patients with frontal lobe brain damage. *Dig. Dis. Sci.*, **35,** 225–30.

16

Neurobehavioural abnormalities

Introduction

There is a wide array of behavioural changes associated with multiple sclerosis (MS). These range from commonly encountered disorders affecting mood, affect and cognition to less frequent manifestations such as psychosis. It is important for the clinician to be able to recognize the signs and symptoms accompanying the various mental state changes, for treatment of many of the disorders, particularly within the realm of mood and affect, is a rewarding area and may significantly enhance the quality of life of MS patients.

This chapter summarizes the essential features that characterize the main neuropsychiatric disorders associated with MS, namely cognitive dysfunction, depression, mania, psychosis, and pathological laughing and crying. It should be stated at the outset that what all these conditions have in common is a paucity of empirically based treatment data. Nevertheless, this chapter combines the results of the few published double-blind, placebo-controlled treatment trials with more numerous anecdotal evidence, thereby providing specific management guidelines for each disorder.

Table 16.1 provides a summary of psychotropic medication in MS patients.

Table 16.1 Psychotropic medication in MS patients

Drug	Indications	Daily dose range	Side effects
Fluoxetine, paroxetine, sertraline, fluvoxamine	Depression	10–40 mg 10–50 mg 25–200 mg 25–200 mg	Anticholinergic effects in 2–10% of patients (dry mouth, blurred vision, constipation, sweating, delayed micturition); CNS effects in 2–15% of patients (drowsiness, sedation, excitement, confusion, headache, fatigue); extra-pyramidal effects > 10% of patients (tremor); cardiovascular problems (orthostatic hypotension > 10%)

Table 16.1 Psychotropic medication in MS patients (*continued*)

Drug	Indications	Daily dose range	Side effects
fluvoxamine (*cont'd*)		25–200 mg	(tachycardia, arrhythmia <2%), gastrointestinal distress in 10–35%; rash in 2%; weight gain in 2%, sexual dysfunction in >30%; seizures in <2%
Lithium carbonate	Depression: adjunct therapy hypomania/mania steroid-induced mania	300–900 mg	Gastrointestinal upset (nausea, vomiting up to 50%; diarrhea up to 20%; (metallic taste, dry mouth are rare); CNS side effects include general weakness and fatigue up to 33%, fine tremor up to 65%, weight gain up to 30%, rarely headache, seizures. Confusion and ataxia are signs of toxicity; CVS side effects include benign ECG changes in 20–30%; renal problems include polyuria and polydipsia in up to 40%, pathological changes in the kidney (e.g. glomerulosclerosis seen in up to 25% of patients after 2 years of treatment); rare dermatological changes include rash, pruritus, acne; long-term risk of hypothyroidism, hyperparathyroidism with hypercalcaemia is very rare
Valproic acid	Hypomania/ mania	250–1000 mg	GIT problems include changes in appetite and weight gain (up to 60%) or weight loss (5%), asymptomatic transaminases elevated (up to 45%), hyperammonaemia (up to 50%); CNS effects are lethargy, tremor (10%), ataxia, dysarthria rare; alopecia (up to 12%); skin rash rare; reversible thrombocytopenia. Oedema, coagulopathies rare; hepatic toxicity rare
Lorazepam, clonazepam, diazepam	Anxiety disorders hypomania/ mania: adjunct therapy	0.5–8 mg 0.25–8 mg 2–20 mg	Sedation, dependency with long-term use, withdrawal symptoms in dependent patients
Haloperidol	Psychosis	0.5–10 mg	High potency antipsychotic drugs like haloperidol carry increased risk of dystonic and extrapyramidal side effects (akathisia, Parkinsonism). Risk of tardive dyskinesia is 40% at 5 years. The less potent antipsychotic drugs have more anticholinergic side effects and less

(*continued*)

Table 16.1 Psychotropic medication in MS patients (*continued*)

Drug	Indications	Daily dose range	Side effects
Haloperidol (*cont.*)	Psychosis	0.5–10 mg	extrapyramidal ones. CNS effects are sedation, impaired memory; CVS problems include hypotension, tachycardia, non-specific ECG changes; GIT symptoms are anorexia, constipation, occasionally diarrhoea; sexual difficulties may include erectile dysfunction, decreased libido, inhibited ejaculation, priapism; raised prolactin
Risperidone, olanzapine, quetiapine, clozapine	Psychosis	0.5–6 mg 2.5–10 mg 25–500 mg 25–600 mg	Less extrapyramidal side effects, but are more strongly anticholinergic. Clozapine associated with prominent sialorrhoea in up to 80% and agranulocytosis in 1–2%

The dosage range and side effect profiles (plus percentages) are derived from patients with mental disorders who do not have MS. The corresponding percentages for MS patients are not known, but are likely to be higher. As such, caution is advocated with respect to drug dosage.

Cognitive dysfunction

Cognitive dysfunction affects approximately 40 per cent of community-based patients with MS (Rao *et al.*, 1991a). Abnormalities of memory (verbal and visual), attention, abstract thinking and executive function have been described (Beatty *et al.*, 1988, 1989; Rao *et al.*, 1991a). Given that MS is primarily a disease of white matter, the pattern of cognitive deficits may be best described as 'subcortical'. In keeping with other prototypical subcortical disorders such as progressive supranuclear palsy and Huntington's disease, patients' speed of information processing is impaired (Albert *et al.*, 1974). The degree of cognitive dysfunction correlates significantly with the total volume of brain lesion load, while more specific cognitive deficits have also been linked to regional brain abnormalities (Rao *et al.*, 1989; Feinstein *et al.*, 1993). The consequences of cognitive decline impinge adversely on many aspects of a patient's daily function, such as the ability to work, manage activities of daily living and maintain relationships (Rao *et al.*, 1991b). Determining the cognitive strengths and weaknesses of a patient is therefore important, and in a young or middle-aged patient struggling to remain in the workforce this becomes imperative.

Treatment

Rehabilitation strategies may be divided into two approaches, namely restorative and compensatory (Sohlberg and Mateer, 1989). The aim of restorative therapy, as the name implies, is to produce an improvement in cognition. An alternative, compensatory approach does not try for recovery in function, but rather emphasizes maximizing those cognitive abilities an individual retains. Rehabilitation for MS patients has largely focused on this approach.

Compensatory strategies

Even before they come to the attention of rehabilitation specialists many MS patients have spontaneously adopted compensatory strategies, the commonest being the use of a memory pad or *aide memoire* (Sullivan *et al.*, 1990). Three principles guide the compensatory approach, namely structuring, scheduling and recording. The aim is to bring structure and stability to the patient's environment, thereby ensuring a degree of predictability. This will in turn produce less demands on planning, organization and memory, areas that are frequently compromised in MS (Sullivan *et al.*, 1989).

As a first step, it is important to know the patient's relative cognitive strengths and weaknesses. Neuropsychological testing is therefore needed, including an index of premorbid IQ. This gives the rehabilitation specialist an indication of what the patient was capable of before the onset of MS, plus a rough guide as to the degree of cognitive decline. Premorbid IQ can be quickly, reliably and accurately obtained via a simple reading test or, alternatively, from the vocabulary subtest on the Wechsler Adult Intelligence Scale.

Having obtained an intellectual baseline, an assessment by an occupational therapist of the patient's environment follows. This provides information on the daily demands confronting the MS patient. Areas of functioning that are most affected by cognitive difficulties are identified and discussed with the patient before a specific plan is implemented. At this stage, enlisting the help of a partner and family members is recommended, because their co-operation may be necessary before changes can take effect.

With the assessment complete, implementation can begin. The use of a day calender to assist impaired memory is often helpful, but it is not enough just to suggest that patients go out and buy the calender; they will also require help in deciding when and what kinds of information need to be recorded (Sullivan *et al.*, 1989). Consistency is the keyword when it comes to structuring the environment, i.e. certain tasks to be performed at the same time each day using items that are always stored in the same place. Depending on a patient's cognitive ability, this structure may be applied to factors ranging from work-related tasks to the more mundane activities of daily living, such as meal preparation, grocery shopping, cleaning, transportation and personal safety issues (Bennett *et al.*, 1991).

Remedial (restorative) strategies

Unlike other neurological disorders, such as head injury (Grafman, 1984), little attention has focused on remedial strategies in MS patients. The reasons probably relate to the nature of cognitive dysfunction in MS. In stroke and head injury, the insult is sudden and followed by a period of expected, albeit variable, recovery. However, MS-related cognitive change follows an altogether different course. The onset may be insidious, and deterioration, if it is to occur over time, is unlikely to be interrupted by periods of cognitive improvement. For this reason, compensation strategies in MS are considered more useful (Minden and Moes, 1990).

Despite a preference for compensatory approaches, remediation has been tried in MS patients. Specific cognitive deficits are identified through detailed neuropsychological testing. Thereafter, interventions are tailored for each deficit. A process of graded practice for improving memory, using computer-run programs, has been implemented in at least one MS rehabilitation setting (LaRocca, 1990). Furthermore, Jonsson *et al.* (1993) reported that 6 months of remediation plus compensation was more effective than non-specific, diffuse mental stimulation in improving some memory functions in a sample of 40 MS patients. Such results, while encouraging, need replication.

Medication to help cognition

As yet, there are no data supporting the use of pharmacotherapy for improving cognition in MS patients. A trial of 4-aminopyridine, a potassium channel blocker which may reduce physical disability in some MS patients (van Diemen *et al.*, 1992), did not result in significant cognitive improvement (Smits *et al.*, 1994). Theoretically, the interferons beta-1b and -1a could produce cognitive improvement by virtue of a reduced brain lesion load. Brief, repeatable neuropsychological batteries are now included in some drug trials, and the results are awaited.

Irrespective of the strategy pursued, attempts at cognitive rehabilitation should not take place in isolation; this should be but one part of a comprehensive treatment strategy that begins at the moment of diagnosis. Such an approach, which focuses primarily on the patient but includes family members when relevant, embraces not only cognitive strategies, but also treatment for neurological symptoms (e.g. the interferon compounds), psychopathology (antidepressant and anxiolytic medication, psychotherapy) and help for psychosocial difficulties.

Depression

The term 'depression' may apply to a symptom or a syndrome, the latter consisting of a constellation of features such as low mood, anhedonia, sleep and appetite disturbances, low energy, poor concentration and suicidal thoughts or intent. This chapter will focus on the syndrome, in particular the diagnostic category 'major depression', which by definition requires a minimum 2-week duration of symptoms. The lifetime prevalence of major depression in patients with multiple sclerosis is approximately 50 per cent (Sadovnik *et al.*, 1996). There is no evidence that MS patients have a premorbid disposition to depression (Minden *et al.*, 1987), nor an increased family history of affective disorder (Joffe *et al.*, 1987). The symptomatology differs from patients with a primary depressive disorder in that feelings of frustration and irritability are prominent, with those of guilt and worthlessness less so (Minden *et al.*, 1987). There is also a higher rate of suicide in MS patients, both in relation to the general population and to sufferers of other neurological disorders (Stenager and Stenager, 1992).

The reasons why so many MS patients develop a disabling depressive illness are unclear. Indirect evidence linking depression to the presence of cerebral plaques comes from two sources. Depression is more likely in MS patients with predominantly cerebral as opposed to spinal cord involvement (Schiffer *et al.*, 1983), and the rates of depression are increased in MS patients compared to those with spinal cord injuries (Rabins *et al.*, 1986). The relationship between the presence of depression and cerebral MRI abnormalities is less clear, with associations for (Honer *et al.*, 1987; Pujol *et al.*, 1997) and against (Reischies *et al.*, 1988; Feinstein *et al.*, 1992a). While the equivocal nature of the MRI results may reflect weaknesses in research methodology, it may also suggest that depression in MS has a heterogenous aetiology (Feinstein, 1995). This must be taken into account when planning treatment.

Treatment

Despite the fact that one in two MS patients will develop a disabling depressive disorder following the onset of demyelination, adding to their morbidity and possibly to mortality as well, there have been few treatment trials, either in the biological or psychological domain.

Antidepressant therapy

In the only published report of a single, double-blind, placebo-controlled study, Schiffer and Wineman (1990) compared the efficacy of desipramine (a tricyclic antidepressant) and individual psychotherapy versus placebo and individual psychotherapy in 14 depressed and 14 non-depressed MS patients. The desipramine group was less depressed at 5-week follow-up when scores on the Hamilton, but not the Beck, Depression rating scales were compared. Patients often reported troubling side effects with desipramine, such as dizziness (postural hypotension), dry mouth and constipation, all attributed to the anticholinergic effect of the tricyclic drug.

Although the authors concluded that desipramine was moderately beneficial in treating MS patients with major depression, the study highlighted a number of salient points. First, MS patients are highly sensitive to the side effects of treatment. Although desipramine is one of the least anticholinergic of all tricyclic compounds, subjects still had difficulty with it. Second, the discrepancy between the Hamilton and Beck Depression scores, indicative of a partial treatment response, was attributed to side effects curtailing adequate dosage. This was confirmed by sub-therapeutic serum desipramine levels.

The late 1980s saw the introduction of a different class of antidepressant drug, the selective serotonin reuptake inhibitors (SSRIs), of which five are now on the market (fluoxetine, paroxetine, sertraline, fluvoxamine and citalopram). Although no more efficacious than their tricyclic predecessors, they have significantly less side effects. There are no double-blind, placebo-controlled studies in MS cohorts, but an open trial of 11 patients involving sertraline 100 mg demonstrated that 10 patients were able to remain on treatment for at least 3 months and showed substantial improvement in mood without troubling side effects (Scott *et al.*, 1995). A retrospective review of pharmacological treatment responses in depressed MS patients supported the greater tolerability of the SSRIs over the tricyclic drugs, and also made the important observation that over 50 per cent of patients relapsed if they discontinued either class of antidepressant therapy prematurely (Scott *et al.*, 1996).

One of the SSRI drugs, fluoxetine (trade name Prozac), has been the subject of some controversy following a report of an exacerbation of MS on beginning treatment (Browning, 1990). However, this was limited to a single case and has not been noted in other studies, and is therefore likely to have been a coincidental occurrence. Fluoxetine reportedly has an 'activating' effect, which makes it a potentially useful treatment in MS-related depression where, in addition to low mood, fatigue often features prominently. An open trial reported mood improvement in all subjects ($n = 20$) without prominent side effects (Flax *et al.*, 1991), while further support comes from a single case report of a patient who did not respond to adequate doses of a tricyclic drug, but on switching to fluoxetine reached an euthymic state (Shafey, 1992).

Although there is no prospective study directly comparing tricyclic and SSRI antidepressant drugs in MS patients, the lower rate of side effects, quicker onset of action, convenient single dosage from day one and their safety in overdose make the SSRIs the drugs of choice in treating the depressed MS patient. A final point to consider when debating the choice of drug is the question of sexual side effects associated with treatment. SSRIs may lower libido and impair sexual performance in at least 20 per cent of physically healthy depressed patients (Walker *et al.*, 1993). MS patients, more than 50 per cent of whom have various degrees of sexual dysfunction, may be particularly susceptible in this regard. A novel antidepressant, buproprion, which works via the dopamine system and reportedly spares sexual difficulties, may be the treatment to consider, but as yet there are no data regarding MS subjects.

Antidepressant medication represents the simplest and most readily available form of therapy for depressed MS patients, but not all patients are willing to take treatment. Reasons may range from an intolerance of side effects to an anti-medication bias. To what extent patients may be helped by a non-pharmacological intervention is unclear, but for those with depression of mild to moderate severity a number of potentially useful options present themselves.

Cognitive–behaviour therapy

The cognitive triad of depression consists of a negative self-perception in which subjects view themselves as inadequate or undesirable, a tendency to experience the world as a negative and self-defeating place, and the expectation of continued hardship and failure. The goal of therapy is to help patients identify and test negative cognitions, develop alternative and more flexible schemas and rehearse new cognitive and behavioural responses (Beck *et al.*, 1979). This therapy is dependent on intact cognition, which may present a problem in many MS patients.

In a study with small sample size, Larcombe and Wilson (1984) demonstrated that cognitive–behaviour therapy (CBT) given weekly over 6 weeks was more effective than no treatment for MS patients with moderately severe depression. Improvement in mood was not only endorsed by the patients, but was also noted on a clinician's rating scale. Unlike medication, there are no adverse side effects of CBT. However, access to a therapist is not readily available in all centres and the treatment is not recommended for cognitively impaired or severely depressed and suicidal patients. A variant of CBT is stress inoculation training (SIT), a short-term, cognitive behavioural approach that targets maladaptive psychological responses to stress, thereby enhancing coping mechanisms. SIT combined with relaxation techniques may also prove beneficial to MS patients and alleviate low mood (Foley *et al.*, 1987).

Psychotherapy

Psychotherapy may be pursued either individually or within a group milieu. An approach to individual therapy has been eloquently outlined by Minden (1992), who stresses the need for flexibility and an absence of dogma on the part of the therapist. She makes the point that MS is a dynamic disease, subject to relapses and remissions, and that consequently a patient's mood or emotional state may also vary. Dalos *et al.* (1983) demonstrated this in a serial study over the course of 1 year. As such, the therapeutic approach to a patient experiencing a disease exacerbation and prey to despondency and hopelessness will differ from the situation when a patient in remission views the future with greater optimism. Similarly, Minden stresses that the psychotherapeutic approach can range from simple support to more insight-oriented therapy, depending on the patient's need and cognitive abilities. This flexibility also extends to the duration of treatment, which may consist of a single session for the patient in crisis to more long-term therapy over months to years for the patient intent on dealing with unresolved and well defended conflicts. The use of pharmacotherapy as an adjunct to the psychotherapeutic process is welcomed. Minden's common-sense approach, although lacking empirical validation, is to be recommended.

Anecdotal evidence supports the use of group psychotherapy with MS patients, the focus varying from the educational (Pavlou *et al.*, 1979) to the psychoanalytical (Barnes *et al.*, 1954) and supportive (Spielberg, 1980). In the single study that attempted to demonstrate experimentally the effectiveness of group therapy, Crawford and McIvor (1985) divided 41 MS patients into three groups, namely insight-oriented psychotherapy, current events discussion, and non-treatment, and found that after 6 months only the first group showed a significant mood improvement.

Interferon beta-1b and depression

The development of depression or the worsening of pre-existing depression has been reported as a side effect of treatment with interferon beta-1b (Neilly *et al.*, 1996). Methodological problems make this study's data hard to interpret, but irrespective of whether the rate of depression is increased or not, treatment of mood change, either with medication or psychotherapy, will improve adherence to interferon beta-1b therapy (Mohr *et al.*, 1997).

Treatment-resistant depression

The percentage of MS patients that fail to respond to antidepressant treatment is unknown. In patients who are physically healthy the figure is approximately

30 per cent; in MS-related depression this is unlikely to be less. Commonly employed strategies include changing from one SSRI to another and, failing that, augmenting the antidepressant with lithium carbonate or T_3 supplements. Electroconvulsive treatment is indicated for the acutely suicidal patient, or when depression is unremitting and debilitating. Treatment is often effective (Gallineck and Kalinowsky, 1958; Krystal and Coffey, 1997), but the number of patients reported on is small. There is also the possibility of ECT precipitating an exacerbation of the MS. The presence of contrast-enhancing lesions on MRI pre-ECT is a putative risk factor (Mattingley *et al.*, 1992).

Herbal remedies

St John's wort (*Hypericum perforatum*) has a weak antidepressant effect in patients who have mild to moderate depression (Linde *et al.*, 1996), but its use in MS has not been assessed. Nevertheless, MS patients with a tendency to self-medicate and with milder forms of depression may find some relief from it.

Bipolar affective disorder

Bipolar affective disorder, also known as manic-depressive psychosis, may manifest as either depression or mania. The depression is indistinguishable from the depressive syndrome described above, and the treatment, in the acute phase, is the same. The 'classic' manic component combines a triad of symptoms; motor overactivity with a decreased need for sleep and racing thoughts, elevated or euphoric mood, and a grandiose thought content. However, in some patients euphoria may be replaced by irritability, and grandiosity by persecutory beliefs.

The prevalence of bipolar affective disorder in MS patients is at least twice that in the general population (Schiffer *et al.*, 1986). Reasons for this increase are unclear, with theories ranging from a shared genetic diathesis for MS and bipolar disorder (Schiffer *et al.*, 1988) to an association with regional cerebral lesion load (Feinstein *et al.*, 1992b; Hutchinson *et al.*, 1993). What is clear, however, is that the increased prevalence cannot be attributed to treatment with steroids.

Treatment

There are no controlled treatment trials of mania in MS. Based on an anecdotal literature, the most frequently prescribed drug is lithium carbonate. Although effective in manic patients with neurological disease (Young *et al.*, 1977), the data pertaining to its use in MS bipolar patients are contradictory, with some (Kemp *et al.*, 1977; Solomon, 1978) finding it effective, but not others (Kellner *et al.*, 1984; Kwentus *et al.*, 1986). An alternative mood stabilizer is valproic acid, which may be equally effective but is better tolerated (Stip and Daoust, 1995). Given that both MS and bipolar disorders may run relapsing–remitting courses, prophylaxis with mood-stabilizing drugs may be required for many years. From a management point of view, three clinical states can be discerned. Although they overlap to varying degrees, the approach to treatment differs in some important ways.

Hypomania

By definition this is a less severe form of mania, with an elevated mood of at least 4 days' duration not severe enough to warrant hospitalization. Treatment may be confined to monotherapy with a mood-stabilizing drug such as lithium.

Mania with psychotic features

Here the manic symptoms are more florid, with an elevated or irritable mood for at least 7 days, accompanied by extreme over-activity, pressured speech and delusional thinking. Neuroleptic treatment needs to be added to the mood-stabilizing drug during the psychotic phase. For additional sedation, benzodiazepines may also be necessary. Admission to hospital is the rule, and often a bed is required on a psychiatric unit as the patient's disruptive behaviour makes containment difficult on a general medical ward. Once the manic psychosis has resolved, maintenance treatment with lithium (or an alternative) is mandatory.

Steroid-induced mania

The mood-altering properties of steroids and ACTH are well known, and mild to moderate degrees of mania may occur in up to one-third of patients (Ling et al., 1981). Risk factors for steroid-induced mania include ACTH as opposed to prednisone, and a premorbid and/or genetic diathesis for psychopathology – particularly depression or alcoholism (Minden et al., 1988). The prophylactic nature of lithium therapy in corticotrophin-induced mania (Falk et al., 1979) means that physicians should not necessarily discontinue treatment if patients become 'high'; rather, the careful monitoring of the mental state on a reduced dose of ACTH, together with the addition of lithium, may allow treatment to continue. Should the manic episode be suggestive of an exacerbation, Peselow et al. (1981) endorse a combination of prednisone plus lithium.

Psychosis

Unlike major depression and bipolar affective disorder, psychosis is uncommon, and does not exceed chance expectation in multiple sclerosis (Davison and Bagley, 1969). A review of case notes in a tertiary referral centre for MS patients unearthed 10 psychotic patients over a 6-year period (Feinstein et al., 1992b). The clinical presentation is characterized by delusional beliefs, usually of a persecutory nature, although the full spectrum of delusional content, ranging from the grandiose and somatic through to the bizarre, may be encountered. Hallucinations may also be present, and are typically of the auditory variety. Feinstein et al. (1992b), in a case–control MRI study, demonstrated that psychotic as opposed to non-psychotic MS patients were more likely to have involvement of the temporal horns bilaterally. However, this finding alone cannot explain the pathogenesis of the psychosis, given that many MS patients have temporal horn involvement and do not become psychotic. The most likely explanation is that lesions in crucial anatomical sites interact with a premorbid diathesis for psychosis to produce the mental state change.

Treatment

Management of psychotic MS patients is fraught with difficulties. By the very nature of their mental illness, psychotic patients lack insight and therefore cannot understand why the physician (and more often their own families) insist on treatment. Should the level of behavioural disturbance be sufficient to prevent patients looking after themselves or to cause considerable distress to family, friends or neighbours, treatment may have to be imposed involuntarily, at least in the acute phase. Once the decision has been made to treat, there are, however, little evidence-based pharmacological data to suggest how it should be done.

Experience has taught that MS patients are frequently sensitive to the side effects of neuroleptic medication. Thus high potency drugs such as the butyrophenones (e.g. haloperidol), which are associated with extra-pyramidal side effects (EPS), may further compromise patients' mobility and balance; at the same time, less potent neuroleptics such as the phenothiazine group (e.g. chlorpromazine) have a higher anticholinergic profile, potentially compounding difficulties with bladder and bowel control and with vision. All neuroleptic medication, irrespective of class, can produce excessive sedation, which may similarly affect already impaired co-ordination and balance.

With these difficulties in mind, neuroleptic dosages should be kept small (i.e. haloperidol in the dose range of 1–4 mg per day). Newer anti-psychotic drugs such as risperidone offer less prominent side effects, and are often well tolerated in the psychotic patient with a co-existing medical illness (Furmaga *et al.*, 1995). Clozapine, which has the advantage of few EPS problems, has a proven efficacy in patients with movement disorders who become psychotic (Chako *et al.*, 1995), and is an alternative to risperidone. Weekly blood checks are required to monitor for the development of agranulocytosis, which affects 1 per cent of patients on treatment. Postural hypotension early in the treatment carries with it the risk of falls in patients who are neurologically impaired, but this difficulty is transient and lessens significantly after a few weeks of treatment. Seizures are another risk factor at higher doses (in excess of 600 mg per day), but such doses are rarely needed. Olanzapine, a thiobenzodiazepine recently introduced to the market, potentially offers the benefits of clozapine without agranulocytosis. Routine blood work is therefore not required, and it also has the advantage of a once-daily dose (recommended range of 2.5–10 mg per day). However, its efficacy in psychotic MS patients has not yet been ascertained.

Should behavioural control still be required despite adequate anti-psychotic dosage, benzodiazepines may be added. Lorazepam is often preferred, because it may be given via either the oral or the intramuscular route.

Feinstein *et al.* (1992b) reported that the median duration of psychosis in their sample of 10 psychotic MS patients was 5 weeks (range 1–72 weeks), and that in

90 per cent of their sample the psychosis resolved. Although there will be patients who are left with a chronic delusional state, they are a minority, and long-term depot neuroleptic medication is not generally indicated (Feinstein and Ron, 1998).

Pathological laughing and crying

Pathological laughing and crying (PLC) refers to a syndrome of emotional dyscontrol whereby patients may spontaneously, or in response to a minimal stimulus, lose control of their emotions. Thus, patients laugh without feeling joy or cry without feeling sadness. This disconnection of the subjective (mood) from the objective (affect) aspect of an emotion often proves embarrassing and disabling. PLC in multiple sclerosis occurs in 10 per cent of patients, and is generally associated with a moderate degree of physical disability and an average disease duration of 10 years (Feinstein *et al.*, 1997).

Treatment

PLC responds well to pharmacotherapy. A double-blind, cross-over treatment trial of low-dose amitriptyline (< 75 mg per day) revealed that two-thirds of patients responded within 48 hours (Schiffer *et al.*, 1985). The improvement in affect was independent of an antidepressant effect, supporting the separation of mood and affect underpinning the syndrome's definition.

However, should patients not respond to amitriptyline, a number of useful alternatives may be tried. An open trial of levodopa (0.6–1.5 g per day) and amantadine (100 mg per day) in patients with PLC of vascular origin demonstrated a 40–50 per cent success rate (Udaka *et al.*, 1984). Once again, a positive response was observed early in the treatment. Finally, fluoxetine may bring about rapid symptom resolution without disabling side effects, although reports in MS and traumatically brain-injured subjects are based on open trials without control groups (Seliger *et al.*, 1992; Sloan *et al.*, 1992).

References

Albert, M. L., Feldman, R. G. and Willis, A. L. (1974). The 'subcortical dementia' of progressive supranuclear palsy. *J. Neurol. Neurosurg. Psychiatr.*, **37**, 121–30.

Barnes, R. H., Busse, E. W. and Dinken, H. (1954). Alleviation of emotional problems in multiple sclerosis by group psychotherapy. *Group Psychother.*, **6**, 193–201.

Beatty, W. W., Goodkin, D. E., Monson, N. *et al.* (1988). Anterograde and retrograde amnesia in patients with chronic–progressive multiple sclerosis. *Arch. Neurol.*, **45**, 611–9.

Beatty, W. W., Goodkin, D. E., Monson, N. and Beatty, P. A. (1989). Cognitive disturbance in patients with relapsing–remitting multiple sclerosis. *Arch. Neurol.*, **46**, 1113–19.

Beck, A. T., Rush, A. J., Shaw, B. F. and Emery, G. (1979). *Cognitive Therapy of Depression*. Guilford.

Bennett, T., Dittmar, C. and Raubach, S. (1991). Multiple sclerosis: cognitive deficits and rehabilitation strategies. *Cog. Rehabil.*, **Sep/Oct,** 18–23.

Browning, W. N. (1990). Exacerbation of symptoms of multiple sclerosis in a patient taking fluoxetine. *Am. J. Psychiatr.*, **147,** 1089.

Chako, R. C., Hurley, R. A., Harper, R. G. *et al.* (1995). Clozapine for acute and maintenance treatment of psychosis in Parkinson's disease. *J. Neuropsychiatr. Clin. Neurosci.*, **7,** 471–5.

Crawford, J. D. and McIvor, G. P. (1985). Group psychotherapy: benefits in multiple sclerosis. *Arch. Phys. Med. Rehabil.*, **66,** 810–13.

Dalos, N. P., Rabins, P. V., Brooks, B. R. and O'Donnell, P. (1983). Disease activity and emotional state in multiple sclerosis. *Ann. Neurol.*, **13,** 573–7.

Davison, K. and Bagley, C. R. (1969). Schizophrenia-like psychoses associated with organic disorders of the central nervous system. A review of the literature. In: *Current Problems in Neuropsychiatry* (R. N. Herrington, ed.), pp. 113–84. Hedley.

Falk, W. E., Mahnke, M. W. and Poskanzer, D. C. (1979). Lithium prophylaxis of corticotrophin-induced psychosis. *J. Am. Med. Assoc.*, **241,** 1011–12.

Feinstein, A. (1995). Multiple sclerosis and depression: an etiological conundrum. *Can. J. Psychiatr.*, **40,** 573–6.

Feinstein, A. and Ron, M. A. (1998). Psychosis due to a general medical (neurological) condition: establishing predictive and construct validity. *J. Neuropsychiatr. Clin. Neurosci.*, **10,** 448–52.

Feinstein, A., Kartsounis, L., Miller, B. *et al.* (1992a). Clinically isolated lesions of the type seen in multiple sclerosis: a cognitive, psychiatric and MRI follow-up study. *J. Neurol. Neurosurg. Psychiatr.*, **55,** 869–76.

Feinstein, A., du Boulay, G. and Ron, M. A. (1992b). Psychotic illness in multiple sclerosis. A clinical and magnetic resonance imaging study. *Br. J. Psychiatr.*, **161,** 680–85.

Feinstein, A., Ron, M. A. and Thompson, A. (1993). A serial study of psychometric and magnetic resonance imaging changes in multiple sclerosis. *Brain*, **116**, 569–602.

Feinstein, A., Feinstein, K. J., Gray, T. and O'Connor, P. (1997). The prevalence and neurobehavioral correlates of pathological laughter and crying in multiple sclerosis. *Arch. Neurol.*, **54,** 1116–21.

Flax, J. W., Gray, J. and Herbert, J. (1991). Effects of fluoxetine on patients with multiple sclerosis. *Am. J. Psychiatr.*, **148,** 1603.

Foley, F. W., Bedell, J. R., LaRocca, N. G. *et al.* (1987). Efficacy of stress inoculation training in coping with multiple sclerosis. *J. Cons. Clin. Psychol.*, **55,** 919–22.

Furmaga, K. M., DeLeon, O., Sinha, S. *et al.* (1995). Risperidone response in refractory psychosis due to a general medical condition (abstract). *J. Neuropsychiatr. Clin. Neurosci.*, **7,** 417.

Gallineck, A. and Kalinowsky, L. B. (1958). Psychiatric aspects of multiple sclerosis. *Dis. Nerv. Sys.*, **19**, 77–80.

Grafman, J. (1984). Memory assessment and remediation. In: *Behavioral Assessment and Rehabilitation of the Traumatically Brain Damaged* (B. A. Edelstein and E. T. Couture, eds), pp. 151–89. Plenum Press.

Honer, W. G., Hurwitz, T., Li, D. K. B. *et al.* (1987). Temporal lobe involvement in multiple sclerosis patients with psychiatric disorders. *Arch. Neurol.*, **44**, 187–90.

Hutchinson, M., Stack, J. and Buckley, P. (1993). Bipolar affective disorder prior to the onset of multiple sclerosis. *Acta Neurol. Scand.*, **88**, 388–93.

Joffe, R. T., Lippert, G. P., Gray, T. A. *et al.* (1987). Personal and family history of affective disorder. *J. Aff. Dis.*, **2**, 63–5.

Jonsson, A., Korfitzen, E. M., Heltberg, A. *et al.* (1993). Effects of neuropsychological treatment in patients with multiple sclerosis. *Acta Neurol. Scand.*, **88**, 394–400.

Kellner, C. H., Davenport, Y., Post, R. M. and Ross, R. J. (1984). Rapid cycling bipolar disorder and multiple sclerosis. *Am. J. Psychiatr.*, **141**, 112–3.

Kemp, K., Lion, J. R. and Magram, G. (1977). Lithium in the case of a manic patient with multiple sclerosis – a case report. *Dis. Nerv. Sys.*, **38**, 210–11.

Krystal, A. D. and Coffey, C. E. (1997). Neuropsychiatric considerations in the use of electroconvulsive therapy. *J. Neuropsychiatr. Clin. Neurosci.*, **9**, 283–92.

Kwentus, J. A., Hart, R. P., Calabrese, V. and Hekmati, A. (1986). Mania as a symptom of multiple sclerosis. *Psychosomatics*, **27**, 729–31.

Larcombe, N. A. and Wilson, P. H. (1984). An evaluation of cognitive–behaviour therapy for depression in patients with multiple sclerosis. *Br. J. Psychiatr.*, **145**, 366–71.

LaRocca, N. (1990). Management of neurobehavioral dysfunction. A rehabilitation perspective. In: *Neurobehavioral Aspects of Multiple Sclerosis* (S. M. Rao, ed.), pp. 215–29. Oxford University Press.

Linde, K., Ramirez, G., Mulrow, C. D. *et al.* (1996). St. John's wort for depression – an overview and meta-analysis of randomised clinical trials. *Br. Med. J.*, **313**, 253–8.

Ling, M. H. M., Perry, P. J. and Tsuang, M. T. (1981). Side effects of corticosteroid therapy. *Arch. Gen. Psychiatr.*, **38**, 471–7.

Mattingley, G., Baker, K., Zorumski, C. F. and Figiel, G. S. (1992). Multiple sclerosis and ECT: Possible value of gadolinium-enhanced magnetic resonance scans for identifying high-risk patients. *J. Neuropsychiatr. Clin. Neurosci.*, **4**, 145–51.

Minden, S. L. (1992). Psychotherapy for people with multiple sclerosis. *J. Neuropsychiatr.*, **4**, 198–213.

Minden, S. and Moes, E. (1990). Management of neurobehavioral dysfunction. A psychiatric perspective. In: *Neurobehavioral Aspects of Multiple Sclerosis* (S. M. Rao, ed.), pp. 230–50. Oxford University Press.

Minden, S. L., Orav, J. and Reich, P. (1987). Depression in multiple sclerosis. *Gen. Hosp. Psychiatr.*, **9**, 426–34.

Minden, S. L., Orav, J. and Schildkraut, J. J. (1988). Hypomanic reactions to ACTH and prednisone treatment for multiple sclerosis. *Neurology*, **38**, 1631–4.

Mohr, D. C., Goodkin, D. E., Likosky, W. *et al.* (1997). Treatment of depression improves adherence to interferon beta-1b therapy for multiple sclerosis. *Arch. Neurol.*, **54**, 531–3.

Neilly, L. K., Goodkin, D. S., Goodkin, D. E. *et al.* (1996). Side effect profile of interferon beta-1b (Betaseron). *Neurology*, **46**, 552–4.

Pavlou, M., Johnson, P., Davis, F. A. and Lefebre, K. (1979). Program of psychologic service delivery in multiple sclerosis centre. *Prof. Psychol.*, **10**, 503–10.

Peselow, E. D., Deutsch, S. I., Fieve, R. R. and Kaufman, M. (1981). Coexistent manic symptoms and multiple sclerosis. *Psychosomatics*, **22**, 824–5.

Pujol, J., Bello, J., Deus, J. *et al.* (1997). Lesions in the left arcuate fasciculus region and depressive symptoms in multiple sclerosis. *Neurology*, **49**, 1105–10.

Rabins, P. V., Brooks, B. R., O'Donnell, P. *et al.* (1986). Structural brain correlates of emotional disorder in multiple sclerosis. *Brain*, **109**, 585–97.

Rao, S. M., Leo, G. J., Haughton, V. M. *et al.* (1989). Correlation of magnetic resonance imaging with neuropsychological testing in multiple sclerosis. *Neurology*, **39**, 161–6.

Rao, S. M., Leo, G. J., Bernardin, L. and Unverzagt, F. (1991a). Cognitive dysfunction in multiple sclerosis. 1. Frequency, patterns, and prediction. *Neurology*, **41**, 685–91.

Rao, S. M., Leo, G. J., Ellington, L. *et al.* (1991b). Cognitive dysfunction in multiple sclerosis. 11. Impact on employment and social functioning. *Neurology*, **41**, 692–6.

Reischies, F. M., Baum, K., Brau, H. *et al.* (1988). Cerebral magnetic resonance imaging findings in multiple sclerosis. Relation to disturbance of affect, drive and cognition. *Arch. Neurol.*, **45**, 1114–16.

Sadovnik, A. D., Remick, R. A., Allen, J. *et al.* (1996). Depression and multiple sclerosis. *Neurology*, **46**, 628–32.

Schiffer, R. B. and Wineman, N. M. (1990). Antidepressant pharmacotherapy of depression associated with multiple sclerosis. *Am. J. Psychiatr.*, **147**, 1493–7.

Schiffer, R. B., Caine, E. D., Bamford, K. A. and Levy, S. (1983). Depressive episodes in patients with multiple sclerosis. *Am. J. Psychiatr.*, **140**, 1498–1500.

Schiffer, R. B., Herndon, R. M. and Rudick, R. A. (1985). Treatment of pathologic laughing and weeping with amitriptyline. *N. Engl. J. Med.*, **312**, 1480–2.

Schiffer, R. B., Wineman, M. and Weitkamp, L. R. (1986). Association between bipolar affective disorder and multiple sclerosis. *Am. J. Psychiatr.*, **143**, 94–5.

Schiffer, R. B., Weitkamp, L. R., Wineman, N. M. and Guttormsen, S. (1988). Multiple sclerosis and affective disorder: family history, sex and HLA-DR antigens. *Arch. Neurol.*, **45**, 1345–8.

Scott, T. F., Nussbaum, P., McConnell, H. and Brill, P. (1995). Measurement of treatment response to sertraline in depressed multiple sclerosis patients using the Carroll scale. *Neurol. Res.*, **17**, 421–2.

Scott, T. F., Allen, D., Price, T. R. P. *et al.* (1996). Characterization of major depression symptoms in multiple sclerosis. *J. Neuropsychiatr. Clin. Neurosci.*, **8**, 318–23.

Seliger, G. M., Hornstein, A., Flax, J. *et al.* (1992). Fluoxetine improves emotional incontinence. *Brain Inj.*, **6**, 267–70.

Shafey, H. (1992). The effect of fluoxetine in depression associated with multiple sclerosis. *Can. J. Psychiatr.*, **37**, 147–8.

Sloan, R. L., Brown, K. W. and Pentland, B. (1992). Fluoxetine as a treatment for emotional lability after brain injury. *Brain Inj.*, **6**, 315–9.

Smits, R. C. F., Emmen, H. H., Bertelsmann, F. W. *et al.* (1994). The effects of 4-aminopyridine on cognitive function in patients with multiple sclerosis: a pilot study. *Neurology*, **44**, 1701–5.

Sohlberg, M. and Mateer, C. (1989). *Introduction to Cognitive Rehabilitation. Theory and Practice*. Guilford.

Solomon, J. G. (1978). Multiple sclerosis masquerading as lithium toxicity. *J. Nerv. Mental Dis.*, **166**, 663–5.

Spielberg, N. (1980). Support group improves quality of life. *Rehabil. Nurse J.*, **5**, 9–11.

Sullivan, M. J. L., Dehoux, E. and Buchanan, D. C. (1989). An approach to cognitive rehabilitation in multiple sclerosis. *Can. J. Rehabil.*, **3**, 77–85.

Sullivan, M. J. L., Edgley, K. and Dehoux, E. (1990). A survey of multiple sclerosis. Part 1: Perceived cognitive problems and compensatory strategy use. *Can. J. Rehabil.*, **4**, 99–105.

Stenager, E. N. and Stenager, E. (1992). Suicide and patients with neurologic diseases. Methodologic problems. *Arch. Neurol.*, **49**, 1296–1303.

Stip, E. and Daoust, L. (1995). Valproate in the treatment of mood disorder due to multiple sclerosis. *Can. J. Psychiatr.*, **40**, 219–20.

Udaka, F., Yamao, S., Nagata, H. *et al.* (1984). Pathologic laughing and crying treated with levodopa. *Arch. Neurol.*, **41**, 1095–6.

van Diemen, H. A. M., Polman, C. H., van Dongen, T. M. M. M. *et al.* (1992). The effect of 4-aminopyridine on clinical signs in multiple sclerosis: a randomised, placebo-controlled, double-blind, cross-over study. *Ann. Neurol.*, **32**, 123–30.

Walker, P. W., Cole, J. O., Gardner, E. A. *et al.* (1993). Improvement in fluoxetine associated sexual dysfunction in patients switched to buproprion. *J. Clin. Psychiatr.*, **54**, 459–65.

Young, L. D., Taylor, I. and Holmstrom, V. (1977). Lithium treatment of patients with affective illness associated with organic brain symptoms. *Am. J. Psychiatr.*, **134**, 1405–7.

17

Multidisciplinary approach

Introduction

The treatment of the multitude of symptoms seen in multiple sclerosis is an integral and fundamental part of the overall management of this chronic, disabling condition (Thompson, 1998) Apart from the sheer number and complexity of symptoms, their management is compounded by the way in which they interact; for example, mobility may be affected by spasticity, weakness, ataxia, visual impairment and sensory disturbance, and it is not unusual for all of these symptoms to be present simultaneously. Therefore, management of one symptom must make allowances for other potential impairments – the use of clean intermittent self-catheterization to manage bladder dysfunction requires reasonable cognitive and upper limb function, and cannot be carried out if there is severe adductor spasticity. Furthermore, drug treatment for one symptom may worsen another; this is well exemplified by the worsening of fatigue with anti-spasticity agents or drugs used to treat tremor. These facts underline the importance of a co-ordinated multidisciplinary approach to the symptomatic management of MS, an approach which is encapsulated within the philosophy of rehabilitation (Thompson, 1996). Rehabilitation provides a co-ordinated multidisciplinary approach to management and, while its role and mechanisms have yet to be adequately defined (Jonsson and Ravnborg, 1998), encouraging results have emerged from a number of recent outcome studies (Aisen, 1999). This chapter provides a broad overview of the principles of rehabilitation, outlines the key aims and elements of successful programmes, and reviews some of the recent advances in evaluation through clinical outcome studies and integrated care pathways.

Rehabilitation

Rehabilitation has been defined as an active process of change by which a person who has become disabled acquires and uses the knowledge and skills necessary for optimal physical, psychological and social functioning (RCP, 1991). The underlying principle is that the affected person and his or her family are central to planning and participating in the programme. To achieve this, they require an understanding of the condition and the strategies that will help in coping with it and managing it (Hatch, 1997). Education is hence a key factor in the rehabilitation process.

In essence, rehabilitation aims to assist people in achieving the best possible quality of life within the limits of their disease (Kesselring, 1999) by:

1. Providing a comprehensive assessment of their physical, social and psychological needs
2. Promoting physical, psychological and social adaptation to disability and handicap
3. Facilitating independence in daily activities
4. Maximizing life satisfaction for both patient and carers
5. Empowering the person
6. Preventing secondary complications such as contractures, pressure areas and pain.

Impact of MS on the individual

Multiple sclerosis has a major, widespread and long-term impact on many aspects of life for the affected individual, their family and friends. The first symptoms of MS tend to occur in young adults, generally between 20 and 50 years of age, at a stage in their lives when they are establishing their careers, setting up home and having a family. The variable and unpredictable nature of the disease course means that people with MS not only face the prospect and reality of increasing disability, but also the uncertainty of not knowing when new relapses will occur or established disability set in (Campion, 1996). These problems are lifelong, evolving over decades; the lifespan of people with MS is only marginally reduced (Koch-Henriksen and Bronnum-Hansen, 1999).

Because all parts of the central nervous system (CNS) can be affected, a wide range of diverse symptoms may occur which interact in a complex, disabling way. They may interfere with mobility, upper limb function, bladder, bowel and sexual function, speech and swallowing, and vision and cognition; they may result in severe fatigue, temperature lability, and both acute and chronic pain. In relation to mobility, it is estimated that 50 per cent of patients require a walking aid or use of a wheelchair 15 years after diagnosis (Weinshenker, 1994). The impact on full-time employment is dramatic. Unemployment rates range from 53 per cent (Rodriguez *et al.*, 1994) to as high as 75–80 per cent (Harvey, 1995), with many of those leaving work within the first 5 years of diagnosis. Perhaps not surprisingly, MS is associated with high divorce rates and high incidences of depression and suicide (Sadovnick *et al.*, 1996).

Rehabilitation in multiple sclerosis

The process of rehabilitation in MS has been described by a number of authors (Scheinberg *et al.*, 1981; Schapiro, 1990; LaRocca and Kalb, 1992; Johnson and

Thompson, 1996). While no two centres deliver care in an identical way, the literature demonstrates that there is a shared conceptual and practical framework to its practice. Some of the key elements have been identified as:

1. A multidisciplinary approach
2. Assessment and selection
3. An individually tailored, patient-centred, goal-setting approach
4. Collaboration with health, social and voluntary service sectors.

A multidisciplinary team approach

To be effective, rehabilitation must be carried out by co-ordinated input from a range of professionals (European Federation of Neurological Societies Task Force, 1997). While the precise composition of this team varies, a number of services have been identified that are considered central to comprehensive rehabilitation (Table 17.1). Additional team members usually include psychologists, social workers and dieticians.

Table 17.1 Services central to a rehabilitation service

Physical, occupational and speech therapy
Medical and nursing staff
Continence service
Orthotics service
Pressure sore policy and service
Wheelchair service
Environmental control and communication aids service
Counselling service

Assessment and selection

Accurate, comprehensive and detailed assessment enables appropriate targeting of resources, and is the first and most crucial step in the rehabilitation process. Given the wide variety of interacting physical, psychosocial and cognitive problems that exist in MS, this can be an extremely challenging and difficult process. It must therefore be carried out on a basis of knowledge, experience and expertise. This is achieved most effectively by a multidisciplinary team, each of whom utilizes information from their own disciplines, and who work together to identify areas of potential improvement (Johnson and Thompson, 1996).

An individually tailored, patient-centred, goal-setting approach

The initial assessment should allow the team to identify the extent of change possible (a long-term goal) and the length of time required to achieve it. This is a difficult process, and one that should be tailored to meet the needs of the individual at a specific point in time. It must take into account factors such as fatigue, temperature lability and cognitive problems, which are common in MS. The programme focuses on achieving this long-term goal through a series of small, measurable steps (short-term goals), which are designed to be easily identified and appreciated by the person with MS, the carer and all members of the rehabilitation team. By focusing on different elements of the problem in a co-ordinated fashion, the overall goals of intervention can be achieved – for example, mobility can be improved by strengthening muscles, teaching new techniques for transferring, providing information about tone and fatigue management, improving access to the home, etc. Crucial to its success is the fact that the goals must be important to the person with MS; if not, there is a high likelihood that goals will not be achieved or, if they are, will not be maintained on return to the home environment.

Collaboration with health, social and voluntary service sectors

Rehabilitation is only one part of the comprehensive model of care for persons with MS, and should not be viewed in isolation (Thompson *et al.*, 1997). It should not be considered as a separate phase of care, but as an integral part of the long-term management process. Communication and co-operation between the rehabilitation setting and other health-care, social service and voluntary sectors is essential to meet the needs of the person in an effective and timely manner.

Measuring the effectiveness of rehabilitation intervention

Rehabilitation is labour-intensive and costly (Bourdette *et al.*, 1993). The need for evaluating its effectiveness is well recognized as being fundamental in enabling evidence-based clinical decision making and ensuring continued improvements in patient management (Rosenberg and Donald, 1995). To be credible, effectiveness needs to be established in a scientifically sound and clinically relevant manner. The difficulties in achieving this have been well documented both in the fields of MS (Whitaker *et al.*, 1995; Thompson, 1999) and rehabilitation (Pollock *et al.*, 1993). It is thus extremely challenging, containing a number of difficult methodological issues.

Measuring outcome

It is widely accepted that measuring the results of an intervention (its outcome) is an important means of determining its effectiveness (Sackett *et al.*, 1931). In evaluating rehabilitation, it is necessary to select relevant outcomes and identify appropriate instruments with which to measure them. This requires a thorough knowledge of the problems of MS, the broad aims of rehabilitation, and what can be expected to change as a result of the intervention. Furthermore, it involves

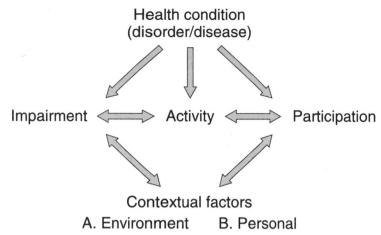

Figure 17.1 New WHO classification.

choosing instruments that measure the anticipated change and are both scientifically sound and clinically useful.

Over the past decade, many clinical trials have used the International Classification of Impairments, Disabilities and Handicaps (ICIDH) (Figure 17.1; World Health Organization, 1980) as a framework for choosing which outcomes to measure. These concepts are well defined (Table 17.2), but do not include the patient's perspective – as is incorporated in quality of life measures. This classification is currently being extensively reviewed to play down the inherent implication that there is a linear relationship between impairment, disability and handicap, and to underline the importance of personal and environmental factors. The new system, termed the International Classification of Impairments, Activities and Participation (ICIDH 2; World Health Organization, 1997), is undergoing systematic field trials, the results of which will be published in the near future.

Although this framework provides a valuable structure for measurement, it does not capture other important aims of rehabilitation such as goal achievement, self-efficacy, and the patients' perception of their capacity to cope. Some of these aspects may be measured by the use of Integrated Care Pathways (ICPs), which have the additional benefit of being an excellent audit tool for monitoring many aspects of the rehabilitation process (Campbell *et al.*, 1998).

Integrated Care Pathways

An ICP is a document that details the expected interventions occurring during a given episode of care, including aspects of service delivery and patient management, (such as number and timing of assessments and treatments, goal achievement etc.). It records when and why variations have occurred from the expected procedure of the rehabilitation process. These departures from the pathway, termed variances, are documented, coded and analysed to provide information directly related to the rehabilitation process and to the individual's progress in

Table 17.2 Levels of measurement and examples of generic and MS-specific measures

Term	Definition	Outcome measures	
		Generic	MS-specific
Impairment	Clinical signs/symptoms resulting from nervous system damage		Functional systems of EDSS Composite measure (US Task Force)
Disability	Limitations on activities of daily living from neurological impairment	Barthel Index (BI), Functional Independence Measure (FIM), Functional Independence Measure/ Functional Assessment Measure (FIM/FAM)	Guy's Neurological Disability Scale (GNDS), Incapacity Status Scale
Handicap	Social and environmental consequences from impairment and disability	London Handicap Scale (LHS)	Environmental Status Scale (ESS)
Health-related quality of life (QOL)	The satisfaction that a person has with health-related dimensions of life, as judged by him or herself	Short Form 36 (SF-36) Nottingham Health Profile Sickness Impact Profile	MS QOL 54 Functional Assessment of MS QOL Instrument (FAMS) MS QOL Inventory (MAQLI)

Reprinted from Thompson (1999), by permission of Thieme Medical Publications.

terms of goal achievement. Group analysis of this information enables the identification of difficulties or inadequacies within the rehabilitation process, and highlights the reasons behind the failure to achieve specified goals. This, in turn, enables informed changes to be made regarding the delivery of care.

This process is well illustrated by a recent study that compared three sequential cohorts of inpatient rehabilitation patients with MS (Rossiter *et al.*, 1998). The three groups ($n = 37$, 50 and 38, respectively) were all of similar age (39–43 years) and severity of disease (median EDSS 7.0). In terms of goal achievement, the results of the first cohort indicated that the key factors preventing success were an underestimation of cognitive dysfunction, inadequate management of fatigue, and neurological deterioration. As a consequence, clinicians were encouraged to increase the number of goals pertaining to cognitive function and fatigue management. Analysis of the latter two cohorts demonstrated an increase in the number of goals achieved from 79–87 per cent. In terms of the rehabilitation process, the ICP highlighted difficulties including inadequate carer involvement, poor secretarial support and badly timed admissions. Once these issues were addressed, the mean length of stay decreased from 28 days to 18 days, carer involvement increased from 66 per cent to 75 per cent, and the achievement of standards relating to documentation were improved. Thus the ICP is useful as a tool to improve both process and outcome.

Outcome measures

The quality of outcome data is determined in part by the quality of the instruments used to produce it. Consequently, considerable care is required in choosing appropriate measurement instruments. It is essential that the instruments have been carefully evaluated in terms of both clinical usefulness and scientific properties (Hobart *et al.* 1996). Clinical usefulness refers to aspects such as whether the instrument is user friendly, practical to administer and inexpensive. Scientific soundness refers to whether the instrument is reliable, valid and recognizes to clinically relevant change. Knowledge about these properties in relation to the clinical setting under study is essential to enable accurate interpretation of the information gained (Streiner and Norman, 1989).

An increasing range of instruments, measuring many aspects of health status, is now available for use in the evaluation of rehabilitation (Table 17.2). These may be divided into generic measures such as the Barthel Index (Mahoney and Barthel, 1965), Functional Independence Measure (Granger *et al.*, 1990) or London Handicap Scale (Harwood and Ebrahim, 1995), which allow comparison across disease groups, and disease-specific measures such as the Expanded Disability Status Scale (Kurtzke, 1983) or Environmental Status Scale (Stewart *et al.*, 1995), which in theory may be more sensitive to changes in the disease under study. Measures may also focus on specific functions involving the upper limb, e.g. the nine-hole peg test (Goodkin *et al.*, 1988), mobility, e.g. the 10 m timed walk and the Rivermead Mobility Scale (Vaney *et al.*, 1996), and cognition, e.g. the Rao battery (Rao, 1990) and the VESPAR (Langdon and Warrington, 1995). In general these instruments are rated by health professionals (although self-report measures of impairment and disability are being developed; Schwartz *et al.*, 1999) and, although patient-oriented in their focus, rarely take into account the patient's perception of disease impact. This perspective is addressed by health-related quality of life (QoL) measures which, by definition, are patient rated. Examples of such measures include: the 36-item Short Form Health Survey Questionnaire (SF-36; Ware *et al.*, 1993) and the MS QoL 54 (Vickrey *et al.*, 1995). It is important to emphasize that, although these QoL instruments assess many important areas addressed by rehabilitation (such as emotional status, pain and fatigue), they may not be sufficiently detailed to pick up the small but clinically relevant changes that might be captured by instruments measuring more specific constructs (Krupp, 1997).

It is recognized that there are areas which are not addressed by the instruments described, but which may well be influenced by the educational philosophy of rehabilitation. These include development of coping skills, increased understanding of the condition, improved self-management and self-efficacy. Instruments addressing some of these areas are currently being developed (Schwartz *et al.*, 1996).

Clinical trials evaluating rehabilitation

Different approaches exist in evaluating the outcome of rehabilitation intervention; measuring each component of the rehabilitation process ('the parts'), or measuring the culmination of multidisciplinary inputs (the 'package' of care). Each approach is valid, providing different but complementary information.

Trials evaluating the component parts

Recently three randomized controlled studies that have investigated the effectiveness of specific aspects of intervention have been published (Petajan *et al.*, 1996; Fuller *et al.*, 1996; Vahtera *et al.*, 1997). The study by Petajan and colleagues (Petajan *et al.*, 1996) evaluated the effectiveness of a 15-week aerobic training programme on fitness and quality of life in 54 MS patients. Their results demonstrated significant improvements in a range of physiological benefits at the end of 15 weeks, and transient psychological benefits between weeks 5 and 10 of the study period. The study by Fuller and colleagues (1996) evaluated the effectiveness of a single inpatient admission for physiotherapy on mobility and related activities of daily living. Forty-five patients with MS were randomized to either treatment or delayed treatment groups, and were assessed at baseline and 9 weeks. At the 9-week assessment, the only statistically significant difference found between the two groups was a reduction in the treatment group of mobility-related distress as measured on a visual analogue scale. Finally, the study by Vahtera and colleagues (1997) evaluated the role of pelvic floor exercises together with electric stimulation in the management of urinary symptoms, and demonstrated a significant benefit – particularly in male patients.

Trials evaluating the package of care

Over the past decade, a number of clinical trials have investigated the outcome of the package of comprehensive multidisciplinary rehabilitation (Table 17.3;

Feigenson *et al.*, 1981; Greenspun *et al.*, 1987; Reding and LaRocca, 1987; Carey *et al.*, 1988; Francabandera *et al.*, 1988; Kidd *et al.*, 1995; Aisen *et al.*, 1996; Kidd and Thompson, 1997; Freeman *et al.*, 1997). In recent months two further trials have been published (Freeman *et al.*, 1999; Solari *et al.*, 1999), which have been described as moving the justification of neurorehabilitation a few steps forward (Aisen, 1999). The results of the earlier trials suggest that rehabilitation in MS has a beneficial effect on disability, which is more marked in the relapsing–remitting group when compared to those in the progressive phase (Carey *et al.*, 1988; Kidd *et al.*, 1995; Aisen *et al.*, 1996; Kidd and Thompson, 1997). The few studies that have addressed handicap (Kidd *et al.*, 1995; Kidd and Thompson, 1997; Freeman *et al.*, 1999) and quality of life (Jonsson *et al.*, 1998; Di Fabio *et al.*, 1997; Freeman *et al.*, 1999) suggest that positive benefits also occur in these areas. Unfortunately, the interpretation of many of these studies is limited by their design; most are uncontrolled single-group studies with small sample sizes, and in the main assessments are limited to those undertaken on admission and discharge, with relatively little attention made to the duration of benefit. Despite these limitations, valuable information has been gathered. Importantly, improvements in methodology have been made. The results of a stratified randomized wait-list controlled study involving 66 patients with progressive MS has recently been published (Freeman *et al.*, 1997). The treatment group underwent a short period (25 days) of multidisciplinary inpatient rehabilitation. All patients were assessed at zero and 6 weeks with a range of measures including disease severity (EDSS and Functional Systems), disability (the Functional Independence Measure) and handicap (the London Handicap Scale). At the end of the 6 weeks, although the neurological status in both groups remained the same, the treatment group showed significantly improved levels of disability ($P < 0.001$) and handicap ($P < 0.01$) compared to the control group.

Another more recent trial compared 3 weeks of inpatient rehabilitation with a home exercise programme in 50 ambulatory patients in a randomized, single-blind, controlled trial (Solari *et al.*, 1999). Patients were evaluated at 3, 9 and 15 weeks with the EDSS, FIM and SF-36. Although no effect was seen in the EDSS in either group, significant benefit was seen in the study group in the FIM ($P = 0.004$), particularly at 3 weeks. The study group also improved in overall health-related quality of life profile compared with controls, although this was only significant for the mental composite score at 3 ($P = 0.008$) and 9 weeks ($P = 0.001$).

These studies did not, however, address the key issue of the longer-term maintenance of change once the patient has returned home, and only a few uncontrolled studies have addressed this question to date (Francabandera *et al.*, 1988; Aisen *et al.*, 1996; Kidd and Thompson, 1997; Freeman *et al.*, 1999). These studies suggest that benefit may be maintained (at least in part) following discharge in a variety of dimensions, including disability (Francabandera *et al.*, 1988; Kidd and Thompson, 1997; Freeman *et al.*, 1999), handicap (Kidd and Thompson, 1997; Freeman *et al.*, 1999), emotional wellbeing and quality of life (Freeman *et al.*, 1999). The most recent of the studies measured these dimensions at 3-monthly intervals for 1 year following rehabilitation (Freeman *et al.*, 1999), and showed that improvements in disability and handicap were maintained for an

Table 17.3 Summary of outcome studies of comprehensive inpatient rehabilitation in people with MS

Reference	Trial method	Sample (*n*)	Main outcomes/instruments	Timing of assessments
Feigenson *et al.* (1981)	Prospective, single group, pre- and post-study design	20	Impairment, disability and handicap: MS Functional Profile (a modified version of BUSTOP), Costs of intervention	Admission and discharge Costs were also measured at 12 months (by telephone interview)
Greenspun *et al.* (1987)	Retrospective, single group, pre- and post-study design	28	Disability: CRDS	Admission, discharge, and 3-month review (by telephone if necessary)
Reding and LaRocca (1987)	Retrospective study, using case-matched analysis	20 pairs	Disability: ISS Hospital re-admission rate Cost of intervention The need for home help assistance	Review at 16 months (by telephone)
Carey *et al.* (1988)	Retrospective multicentre study assessing a range of conditions Single group, pre- and post-study design	6194, of whom 196 had MS	Disability: LORS-II	Admission and discharge
Francabandera *et al.* (1988)	Prospective, stratified randomized study	84	Disability: ISS Need for home assistance (hours)	Admission, and at 3-monthly intervals for 2 years (3-month results reported in this publication)
Kidd *et al.* (1995)	Prospective, single group, pre- and post-study design	79	Impairment: DSS Disability: Barthel Index Handicap: ESS	Admission and discharge
Aisen *et al.* (1996)	Retrospective, single group, pre- and post-study design	37	Impairment: FS and EDSS Disability: FIM	Admission, discharge and telephone follow-up (from between 6 and 36 months post-discharge)

Study	Study design	n	Measures	Timing
Kidd and Thompson (1997)	Prospective, single group, pre- and post-study design	47	Impairment: EDSS Disability: FIM Handicap: LHS	Admission, discharge and 3-month follow-up
Freeman et al. (1997)	Stratified, randomized, wait-list controlled study design	66 (all in the progressive stage)	Impairment: FS and EDSS Disability: FIM Handicap: ESS	Baseline and 6 weeks
Freeman et al. (1999)	Prospective, single group, longitudinal study design	50 (all in the progressive stage)	Impairment: FS and EDSS Disability: FIM Handicap: LHS Quality of life: SF-36 Emotional wellbeing: GHQ-28	Admission, discharge and at 3 monthly intervals for 1 year
Solari et al. (1999)	Prospective, randomized, single-blind, controlled study	50 ambulatory patients	Impairment: EDSS Disability: FIM Quality of Life	Baseline, 3, 6, 9 and 15 weeks

BUSTOP, Burke Stroke Time-oriented Profile; CRDS, Computerised Rehabilitation and Data System; DSS, Disability Status Scale; EDSS, Expanded Disability Status Scale; ESS, Environmental Status Scale; FIM, Functional Independence Measure; LORS-II, Revised Level of Rehabilitation Scale; FS, Functional Systems; ISS, Incapacity Status Scale; LHS, London Handicap Scale; SF-36, Short Form 36 Health Survey Questionnaire; GHQ-28, 28-item General Health Questionnaire. Reprinted from Freeman, J. A. and Thompson, A. J. *International MS Journal* (1998); 5: 16-23, by permission of Cambridge Medical Publications.

Time series plots of the group's scores for each outcome measure

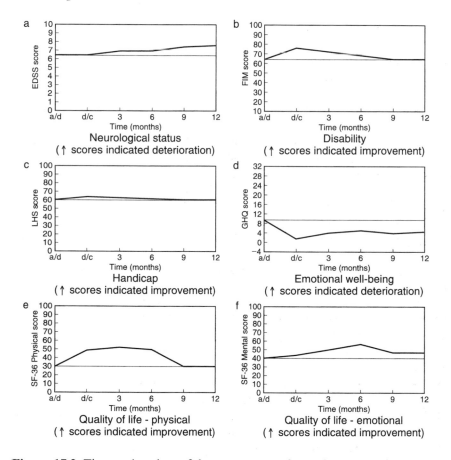

Figure 17.2 Time series plots of the group scores for each outcome measure.
a. Neurological status. Expanded Disability Status Scale (EDSS);↑ scores indicate deterioration.
b. Disability. Functional Independence Measure (FIM);↑ scores indicate improvement.
c. Handicap. London Handicap Scale;↑ scores indicate improvement.
d. Emotional wellbeing. General Health Questionnaire (GHQ);↑ scores indicate deterioration.
e. and f. Health-related quality of life, physical (e) and mental (f). Thirty-six-item Short Form Health Survey Questionnaire (SF-36) ;↑ scores indicate improvement.

average of 6 months and quality of life for an average of 10 months, despite a deterioration in the group's neurological status (29 per cent of patients' EDSS scores had increased ≥ 1.0 point by the 12-month assessment; Figure 17.2). Interestingly, two studies (Kidd and Thompson, 1997; Freeman et al., 1999) demonstrated that handicap continued to improve following discharge form rehabilitation, peaking at between 3–6 months.

The more difficult area of outpatient multidisciplinary rehabilitation has also been evaluated recently (Di Fabio et al., 1998). Forty-six patients with progressive MS were randomly assigned to a group receiving treatment for 1 year ($n = 20$) and a waiting list ($n = 26$). Treatment consisted of 5 hours 1 day a week for 1 year. Receiving treatment was a significant predictor of reduced symptom frequency, and fatigue was significantly reduced in the treatment group. There was also less loss of functional status in the treatment group, although this did not reach statistical significance.

The results of these studies emphasize the need to use a range of scientifically sound outcome measures to detect changes and evaluate the impact of rehabilitation. They also emphasize the importance of continuity of care between the rehabilitation environment and the community and social service sectors if the needs of the person with MS are to be met effectively in the longer term (Hatch et al., 1999). There is a need to continue evaluating rehabilitation input, both to identify the crucial components contained within it and to compare different models of service delivery.

References

Aisen, M. L., Sevilla, D. and Fox, N. (1996). Inpatient rehabilitation for multiple sclerosis. J. Neurol. Rehabil., 10, 43–6.

Aisen, M. L. (1999). Justifying neurorehabilitation: a few steps forward. Neurology, 52, 8–10.

Bourdette, D. N., Prochazka, A. V., Mitchell, W. et al. (1993). Health care costs of veterans with multiple sclerosis: implications for the rehabilitation of MS. VA Multiple Sclerosis Rehabilitation Study Group. Arch. Phys. Med. Rehabil., 74, 26–31.

Campbell, H., Hotchkiss, R., Bradshaw, N. and Porteous, M. (1998). Integrated care pathways. Br. Med. J., 316, 133–7.

Campion, A. (1996). Meeting multiple needs. Nursing Times, 92, 28–30.

Carey, R. G., Seibert, J. H. and Posavac, E. J. (1988). Who makes the most progress in inpatient rehabilitation? An analysis of functional gain. Arch. Phys. Med. Rehabil., 69, 337–43.

Di Fabio, R. P., Choi, T., Soderberg, J. and Hansen, C. R. (1997). Health-related quality of life for patients with progressive multiple sclerosis: Influence of rehabilitation. Phys Ther, 77/12, 1716.

Di Fabio, R. P., Soderberg, J., Choi, T. et al. (1998). Extended outpatient rehabilitation: its influence on symptom frequency, fatigue, and functional status for persons with progressive multiple sclerosis. *Arch. Phys. Med. Rehabil.*, **79**, 141–6.

Disability Committee of the Royal College of Physicians (1991). *National Concept of Rehabilitation*. Royal College of Physicians Publications.

European Federation of Neurological Societies Task Force (1997). Standards in neurological rehabilitation. *Eur. J. Neurol.*, **4**, 325–31.

Feigensen, J. S., Scheinberg, L., Catalano, M. *et al.* (1981). The cost-effectiveness of multiple sclerosis rehabilitation: a model. *Neurology*, **31**, 1316–22.

Francabandera, F. L., Holland, N. J., Wiesel-Levison, P. and Scheinberg, L. C. (1988). Multiple sclerosis rehabilitation: inpatient vs outpatient. *Rehabil. Nursing*, **13**, 251–3.

Freeman, J. A., Langdon, D. W., Hobart, J. C. and Thompson, A. J. (1997). The impact of inpatient rehabilitation on progressive multiple sclerosis. *Ann. Neurol.*, **42**, 236–44.

Freeman, J. A., Langdon, D. W., Hobart, J. C. and Thompson, A. J. (1999). Inpatient rehabilitation in multiple sclerosis: do the benefits carry over into the community? *Neurology*, **52**, 50–56.

Fuller, K. J., Dawson, K. and Wiles, C. M. (1996). Physiotherapy in chronic multiple sclerosis: a controlled trial. *Clin. Rehabil.*, **10**, 91–7.

Goodkin, D. E., Hertsgaard, D. and Seminary, J. (1988). Upper extremity function in multiple sclerosis: improving assessment sensitivity with box-and-block and nine-hole peg tests. *Arch. Phys. Med. Rehabil.*, **69**, 850–54.

Granger, C. V., Cotter, A. C., Hamilton, B. B. *et al.* (1990). Functional assessment scales: a study of persons with multiple sclerosis. *Arch. Phys. Med. Rehabil.*, **71**, 870–75.

Greenspun, B., Stineman, M. and Agri, R. (1987). Multiple sclerosis and rehabilitation outcome. *Arch. Phys. Med. Rehabil.*, **68**, 434–7.

Harvey, C. (1995). Economic costs of multiple sclerosis: How much and who pays? *National Multiple Sclerosis Society Health Research Reports*, Document ER-6005, 2–48.

Harwood, R. H. and Ebrahim, S. (1995). *Manual of the London Handicap Scale*. University of Nottingham, Department of Health Care of the Elderly.

Hatch, J. (1997). Building partnerships. In: *Multiple Sclerosis: Clinical Challenges and Controversies* (A. J. Thompson, C. H. Polman and R. Hohlfeld, eds), pp. 345–51. Martin Dunitz.

Hatch, J., Johnson, J. and Thompson, A. J. (1999). Standards of health care for people with MS. *MS Management*, **5**, 16–25.

Hobart, J. C., Lamping, D. L. and Thompson, A. J. (1996). Evaluating neurological outcome measures: the bare essentials (editorial). *J. Neurol. Neurosurg. Psychiatr.*, **60**, 127–30.

Johnson, J. and Thompson, A. J. (1996). Rehabilitation in a neurosciences centre: the role of expert assessment and selection. *Br. J. Ther. Rehabil.*, **3**, 303–8.

Jonsson, A., Dock, J. and Ravnborg, M. H. (1996). Quality of life as a measure of rehabilitation outcome in patients with multiple sclerosis. *Acta Neurol. Scand.*, **93**, 229–35.

Jonsson, A. and Ravnborg, M. H. (1998). Rehabilitation in multiple sclerosis. *Phys. Rehabil. Med.*, **10**, 75–100.

Kesselring, J. (1999). Long-term rehabilitation in multiple sclerosis. In: *Frontiers of Multiple Sclerosis* (A. Siva, J. Kesselring and A. J. Thompson, eds), pp. 243–52. Martin Dunitz.

Kidd, D., Howard, R. S., Losseff, N. A. and Thompson, A. J. (1995). The benefit of inpatient neurorehabilitation in multiple sclerosis. *Clin. Rehabil.*, **9**, 198–203.

Kidd, D. and Thompson, A. J. (1997). Prospective study of neurorehabilitation in multiple sclerosis. *J. Neurol. Neurosurg. Psychiatr.*, **62**, 423–4.

Koch-Henriksen, N. and Bronnum-Hansen, H. (1999). Survival in multiple sclerosis. In: *Frontiers of Multiple Sclerosis II* (A. Siva, J. Kesselring and A. J. Thompson, eds), pp. 75–84. Martin Dunitz.

Krupp, L. B. (1997). Mechanisms, measurement, and management of fatigue in multiple sclerosis. In: *Multiple Sclerosis: Clinical Challenges and Controversies* (A. J. Thompson, C. H. Polman and R. Hohlfeld, eds), pp. 283–94. Martin Dunitz.

Kurtzke, J. F. (1983). Rating neurologic impairment in multiple sclerosis: an expanded disability status scale (EDSS). *Neurology*, **33**, 1444–52.

Langdon, D. W. and Warrington, E. K. (1995). VESPAR: A Verbal and Spatial Reasoning Test. Lawrence Erlbaum.

LaRocca, N. C. and Kalb, R. C. (1992). Efficacy of rehabilitation in multiple sclerosis. *J. Neurorehabil.*, **6**, 147–55.

Mahoney, F. I. and Barthel, D. W. (1965). Functional evaluation: the Barthel Index (BI). *Maryland State Med. J.*, **14**, 61–5.

Petajan, J. H., Gappmaier, E., White, A. T. *et al.* (1996). Impact of aerobic training on fitness and quality of life in multiple sclerosis. *Ann. Neurol.*, **39**, 432–41.

Pollock, C., Freemantle, N., Sheldon, S. *et al.* (1993). Methodological difficulties in rehabilitation research. *Clin. Rehabil.*, **7**, 63–72.

Rao, S. M. (1990). *A Manual for the Brief Repeatable Battery of Neuro-psychological Tests in Multiple Sclerosis*. National Multiple Sclerosis Society.

Reding, M. J. and LaRocca, N. G. (1987). Acute hospital care versus rehabilitation hospitalisation for management of non-emergent complications in multiple sclerosis. *J. Neurol. Rehabil.*, **1**, 13–17.

Rodriguez, M., Siva, A., Ward, J. *et al.* (1994). Impairment, disability and handicap in multiple sclerosis: a population based study in Olmsted County, Minnesota. *Neurology*, **44**, 28–33.

Rosenberg, W. and Donald, A. (1995). Evidence-based medicine: an approach to clinical problem solving. *Br. Med. J.*, **310**, 1122–6.

Rossiter, D. A., Edmondson, A., Al-Shahi, R. and Thompson, A. J. (1998). Integrated care pathways in multiple sclerosis: completing the audit cycle. *Multiple Sclerosis*, **4**, 85–9.

Sackett, D. L., Rosenberg, W. M. C., Gray, J. A. M. *et al.* (1931). Evidence-based medicine: what it is and what it isn't. It's about integrating individual clinical expertise and the best external evidence. *Br. Med. J.*, 72.

Sadovnick, A. D., Remick, R. A., Allen, J. *et al.* (1996). Depression and multiple sclerosis. *Neurology*, **46**, 628–32.

Schapiro, R. T. (1990). The rehabilitation of multiple sclerosis. *J. Neurol. Rehabil.*, **4**, 215–17.

Scheinberg, L., Holland, N. J., Kirschenbaum, M. *et al.* (1981). Comprehensive long-term care of patients with multiple sclerosis. *Neurology*, **31**, 1121–3.

Schwartz, C. E., Coulthard-Morris, L., Zeng, Q. and Retzlaff, P. (1996). Measuring self-efficacy in people with multiple sclerosis: a validation study. *Arch. Phys. Med. Rehabil.*, **77**, 394–9.

Schwartz, C. E., Vollmer, T., Lee, H. and The North American Research Consortium on Multiple Sclerosis (1999). Reliability and validity of two self-report measures of impairment and disability for MS. *Neurology*, **52**, 63–70.

Solari, A., Filippini, G., Gasco, P. *et al.* (1999). Physical rehabilitation has a positive effect on disability in multiple sclerosis patients. *Neurology*, **52**, 57–62.

Stewart, G., Kidd, D. and Thompson, A. J. (1995). The assessment of handicap: an evaluation of the Environmental Status Scale. *Disabil. Rehabil.*, **17**, 312–16.

Streiner, D. L. and Norman, G. R. (1989). *Health Measurement Scales: A Practical Guide to the Development and Use.* Oxford University Press.

Thompson, A. J. (1996). Rehabilitation of progressive neurological disorders: a worthwhile challenge. *Curr. Opin. Neurol.*, **9**, 437–40.

Thompson, A. J., Johnston, S., Harrison, J. *et al.* (1997). Service delivery in multiple sclerosis: the need for co-ordinated community care. *MS Management*, **4**, 11–18.

Thompson, A. J. (1998). Symptomatic treatment in multiple sclerosis. *Curr. Opin. Neurol.*, **11**, 305–9.

Thompson, A. J. (1999). Multiple sclerosis: rehabilitation measures. *Sem. Neurol.*, **18**, 397–403.

Vahtera, T. Haaranen, M., Viramo-Koskela, A. L. and Ruutiainen, J. (1997). Pelvic floor rehabilitation is effective in patients with multiple sclerosis. *Clin. Rehabil.*, **11**, 211–19.

Vaney, C., Blaurock, H., Gattlen, B. and Meisels, C. (1996). Assessing mobility in multiple sclerosis using the Rivermead Mobility Index and gait speed. *Clin. Rehabil.*, **10**, 216–26.

Vickrey, B. G., Hays, R. D., Harooni, R. *et al.* (1995). A health-related quality of life measure for multiple sclerosis. *Quality Life Res.*, **4**, 187–206.

Ware, J. E., Snow, K. K., Kosinski, M. and Gandek, B. (1993). *SF-36 Health Survey: Manual and Interpretation Guide.* The Health Institute.

Weinshenker, B. G. (1994). Natural history of multiple sclerosis. *Ann. Neurol.*, **36(Suppl.),** S6–11.

Whitaker, J. N., McFarland, H. R., Rudge, P. and Reingold, S. C. (1995). Outcomes assessment in multiple sclerosis clinical trials: a critical analysis. *Multiple Sclerosis*, **1**, 37–47.

World Health Organization (1980). *International Classification of Impairments, Disabilities and Handicaps.* World Health Organization.

World Health Organization (1997). *ICIDH-2: International Classification of Impairments, Activities, and Participation. A Manual of Dimensions of Disablement and Functioning*. World Health Organization.

Drug synonyms

Drug name	Synonym
Alprostadil	Caverject, Muse, Prostaglandin E1, Prostin VR, Viridal
Amantadine	Symmetrel
Aminopyridine	4AP
Amitriptyline	Domical, Elavil, Lentizol, Tryptizol
Azathioprine	Berkaprine, Imuran
Baclofen	Lioresal
Botulinum toxin	Botox, Dysport
Carbamazepine	Tegretol, Teril CR, Timonil retard
Chlorpromazine	Largactil, Thorazine
Cladribine	2CDA, 2-chlorodeoxyadenosine, Leustat, Leustatin
Clonazepam	Klonopin, Rivotril
Clonidine	Catapres, Dixarit
Clozapine	Clozaril
Cyclophosphamide	Cytoxan, Endoxana
Cytosine arabinoside	Alexan, Cytarabine, Cytosar
Dantrolene sodium	Dantrium
Desmopressin	DDAVP, Desmotabs, Desmospray
Diazepam	Dialar, Diazemuls, Rimapam, Stesolid, Tensium, Valclair, Valium
Etoposide	Etopophos, Vepesid
Fluoxetine	Prozac
Fluvoxamine	Faverin, Luvox
Gabapentin	Neurontin
Glatiramer acetate	Copaxone, Cop-1, Copolymer-1, Copolymer, Co-polymer, Glatiramer, Glatiramate
Haloperidol	Dozic, Fortunan, Haldol, Serenace
Imipramine	Tofranil
Immunoglobulin	Alphaglobin, Gammagard, Octagam, Sandoglobulin, Vigam
Interferon alpha-2a	Roferon-A
Interferon beta-1a (Ares-Serono)	Rebif
Interferon beta-1a (Biogen)	Avonex

Interferon beta-1b	Betaferon, Betaseron
Isoniazid	Rifamate, Rimifon
Lactulose	Duphalac, Kristalose, Lactugal, Laxose, Osmolax, Regulose
Lithium carbonate/citrate	Camcolit, Eskalith, Eskalith CR, Liskonum, Litarex, Li-Liquid, Phasal, Priadel
Lorazepam	Almazine, Ativan
Melphelan	Alkeran
Metaraminol	Aramine
Methotrexate	Maxtrex
Methylprednisolone	Depo-medrone, Medrone, Solu-Medrol, Solu-medrone
Mitoxantrone	Mitozantrone, Novantrone
Nortriptyline	Allegron, Pamelor
Olanzapine	Zyprexa
Ondansetron	Zofran
Orphenadrine	Biorphen, Disipal, Norflex, Norgesic
Oxybutynin	Cystrin, Ditropan, Ditropan XL
Paroxetine	Paxil, Seroxat
Pemoline	Cylert, Volital
Pentoxifylline	Oxpentifylline, Trental
Piracetam	Nootropil
Prednisolone	Deltacortril, Precortisyl, Prednesol
Propranolol	Angilol, Apsolol, Berkolol, Beta-Prograne, Cardinol, Inderal, Propanix
Quetiapine	Seroquel
Risperidone	Risperdal
Sertraline	Lustral, Zoloft
Sildenafil citrate	Viagra
Sodium valproate	Convulex, Depacon, Depakene, Epilim, Valproate, Valproic acid
Tizanidine	Zanaflex
Tolterodine	Detrol, Detrusitol

Index

Activity modification, 248
Adhesion molecules, inhibition of, 169–70
Adrenocorticotrophic hormone (ACTH)
    treatment, 15–16
    steroid-induced mania, 291
Adverse drug effects, *See* Side effects
Aetiology, 2–3
Allergic skin reactions, azathioprine
    therapy and, 123
Alprostadil, erectile dysfunction
    management, 273–4
    intracorporeal, 273
    transurethral, 273–4
Altered peptide ligands (APLs), 165
Amantadine, fatigue treatment, 248–9
    relative efficacy, 249–50
American multicentre study, glatiramer
    acetate therapy, 77–82
Aminopyridines, fatigue treatment, 250
    basis of pharmacological effect, 250–1
Amitriptyline, pathological laughing and
    crying management, 293
Ano-rectal function, neural control of,
    275–6
    See also Bowel dysfunction
Anti-idiotypes, 98
Anti-inflammatory agents, 170
Anti-spastic agents, *See* Spasticity
Antidepressant therapy, 287–8
Ataxia, 228–37
    basis of, 229
    classification of, 228–9
    management:
        cannabinoids, 233–4
        occupational therapy, 237
        orthoses, 236–7
        physiotherapy, 237
        tetrahydrocannabinol, 233–4
Austrian Immunoglobulin in MS (AIMS)
    study, 101
Autoantibodies, to interferon beta-1a, 51
Autoantigens, oral tolerance to, 168

Avonex®, 39–40
    Multiple Sclerosis Collaborative
        Research Group Trial (MSCRG),
        44–5
    See also Interferon beta-1a therapy
Axonal loss, 6–7, 171–2
    prevention of, 171–2
Azathioprine therapy, 114–27
    combination therapy, 126–7
    effect on disability, 119–21
        mean change in EDSS score, 120–1
        probability of disability progression,
        119–20
    future trials, 127
    magnetic resonance imaging, 115
    mechanism of action, 114–15
        pharmacokinetics, 115
        pharmacology, 114–15
    patient selection, 126
    regime, 124–6
        dosage, 124–5
        monitoring blood tests, 125–6
    relapses and, 116–19
        odds ratio of remaining relapse free,
        117
        relapse rate, 117–19
    side effects, 121–4
        allergic skin reactions, 123
        cancer risk, 123–4
        gastro-intestinal (GI) disturbance,
        122–3
        haematological effects, 122
        hepatic effects, 122
        infections, 122
        teratogenicity, 123

B cells, immunoglobulin effects on, 98–9
Baclofen, spasticity treatment, 189–91
    clinical efficacy, 189–90
    dosage, 190
    intrathecal usage, 195
    mechanism of action, 189

pharmacology, 189
side effects, 190
Benzodiazepines:
    psychosis treatment, 292
    spasticity treatment, 189
    See also Diazepam
Bipolar affective disorder, 290–1
    hypomania, 291
    mania with psychotic features, 291
    steroid-induced mania, 291
Bladder dysfunction, 258, 259–69
    detrusor hyper-reflexia, 259–61
        treatment of, 264–6
    management, 261–9
        detrusor hyper-reflexia, 264–6
        incomplete emptying, 262–4
        intermittent self-catheterization,
            263–4, 265–6
        intravesicle capsaicin, 266–8
        surgery and long-term catheters,
            268–9
    neural control of the bladder, 59
    symptoms, 259–61
Blood–brain barrier, 168–9
    breakdown of, 3–4
        steroid effects, 15
    inhibition of adhesion and
        inflammatory cell migration,
        168–70
Bone marrow depression, mitoxantrone
    therapy and, 139
Bone marrow transplantation (BMT),
    167–8
Botulinum toxin, spasticity management,
    201–23
    commercial preparation of toxin, 207–8
    contraindications, 212
    effectiveness, 212–13
        cost-effectiveness, 213–14
    history of botulinum toxin, 202–3
    injection technique, 217–22
        flexed wrist/clawed hand, 219
        hip flexor/thigh adductor spasticity,
            219
        post-injection care, 222–3
        spastic upper arm/shoulder, 218
        talipes equino-varus foot, 222
    mechanism of action, 203–7
    non-response, 209–11
    toxicity, 208–9
    treatment rationale, 214–17
        aim of treatment, 214
        patient assessment, 214–17
Botulism, 202
Bowel dysfunction, 258, 275–8

constipation, 276–7
incontinence, 277
investigations, 277
neural control of ano-rectal function,
    275–6
treatment, 277–8
British and Dutch Multiple Sclerosis
    Azathioprine Trial Group, 117

Cancer risk, azathioprine therapy, 123–4
Cannabinoids:
    ataxia and tremor management, 233–4
    spasticity treatment, 194–5
Capsaicin, bladder dysfunction
    management, 266–8
Carbamazepine, tremor management, 233
Cardiotoxicity, mitoxantrone therapy,
    139–40, 143
Catheterization:
    intermittent self-catheterization, 263–4,
        265–6
    long-term catheters, 268–9
2-Chlorodeoxyadenosine, progressive
    disease treatment, 155–6
Cladribine®, progressive disease
    treatment, 155–6
Clonidine, spasticity treatment, 192–4
    clinical efficacy, 193
    dosage, 193
    mechanism of action, 192
    pharmacology, 192–3
    side effects, 193
Clozapine, psychosis treatment, 292
Cognitive dysfunction, 284–6
    compensatory strategies, 285
    medication to help cognition, 286
    remedial strategies, 285–6
Cognitive–behaviour therapy (CBT),
    288–9
Combination therapy, 126–7
Complement, immunoglobulin effects on,
    98
Congestive heart failure, mitoxantrone
    therapy and, 140
Constipation, 276–7
Copaxone®, See Glatiramer acetate
    therapy
Crying, pathological, 293
Cyclophosphamide, progressive disease
    treatment, 155
Cytokines:
    cytokine based treatments, 166–7
    immunoglobulin effects on, 100
Cytoxan®, progressive disease treatment,
    155

Dantrolene sodium, spasticity treatment,
191–2
clinical efficacy, 191
dosage, 191–2
mechanism of action, 191
pharmacology, 191
side effects, 192
Deconditioning, 247–8
Demyelination, 3, 4–5
See also Remyelination
Depression, 286–90
interferon beta-1b and, 289
treatment, 287–90
antidepressant therapy, 287–8
cognitive–behaviour therapy, 288–9
herbal remedies, 290
psychotherapy, 289
treatment-resistant depression,
289–90
Desipramine, depression treatment, 287
Desmopressin (DDAVP), detrusor hyper-
reflexia treatment, 265–6
Detrusor hyper-reflexia, 259–61
treatment of, 264–8
intravesicle capsaicin, 266–8
3-4 Diaminopyridine, fatigue treatment,
250
Diazepam, spasticity treatment, 187–9
clinical efficacy, 188
dosage, 188
mechanism of action, 187
pharmacology, 188
side effects, 188
Disability:
azathioprine therapy effect on, 119–21
fatigue relationship, 244–5, 246–7
interferon beta-1a therapy relevance,
62–3
progression of, 6–7

Ejaculatory failure management, 275
Environmental factors, 3
Erectile dysfunction, 258, 271–2
treatment of, 272–5
ejaculatory function, 275
intracorporeal pharmacotherapy, 273
oral medication, 274
prostheses, 274–5
topical creams, 274
transurethral alprostadil, 273–4
vacuum constriction devices, 273
European Secondary Progressive MS
(EUSP MS) trial, 149–51
European–Canadian Study, glatiramer
acetate therapy, 82–6

EUROQOLs, 116
Exercise therapy, 247–8
Experimental allergic encephalomyelitis
(EAE), 3, 71, 164–5

Faecal incontinence, 277
Fatigue, 237–51
definition of MS fatigue, 238
distinction from fatigue in chronic
illness/disability, 244–5
distinction from fatigue in healthy
adults, 238–9
management approach, 246–8
activity modification/lifestyle
change, 248
deconditioning, 247–8
disability and, 246–7
medication, 246
sleep disturbance, 246
measurement of, 240–4
Fatigue Assessment Instrument,
242–3
Fatigue Impact Scale, 240–1
Fatigue Severity Scale, 243–4
MS-specific Fatigue Scale, 244
use of scales in clinical trials,
244
multifactorial causation, 245–6
pharmacological treatments, 248–51
amantadine, 248–50
aminopyridines, 250–1
pemoline, 249–50
physiological basis of, 239–40
Fc receptor, immunoglobulin effects on,
99
Fertility problems, mitoxantrone therapy
and, 140–1
Fluoxetine, depression treatment, 288
French and British multicentre controlled
trial, mitoxantrone, 133–6

GABA agonists, spasticity treatment, 194
Gastro-intestinal (GI) disturbance,
azathioprine therapy and, 122–3
Genetic factors, 2–3
Glatiramer acetate therapy, 71–90
biochemistry, 71–2
future prospects, 89–90
mechanisms of action, 72–5
progressive disease, 86–8
relapsing disease, 75–86
American multicentre study, 77 82
European–Canadian Study, 82–6
first double–blind, placebo-controlled
trial, 76–7

side effects, 88–9
Glucocorticoids, *See* Steroid treatment
Glutethimide, tremor management, 232–3
Gonadal function, mitoxantrone therapy
 and, 140–1

Haematological effects:
 azathioprine therapy, 122, 125–6
 mitoxantrone therapy, 139
Haloperidol, psychosis treatment, 292
Hepatic effects of azathioprine therapy,
 122
Herbal remedies, depression, 290
Hypericum perforatum (St John's wort),
 depression treatment, 290
Hypomania, 291

Immunoglobulins, 95–6
 See also Intravenous immunoglobulin
  (IVIg) therapy
Immunological factors, 3
Impotence, *See* Erectile dysfunction
Incontinence, *See* Bladder dysfunction;
 Bowel dysfunction
Infections, azathioprine therapy and, 122
Inflammation, 4, 7
 anti-inflammatory agents, 170
Integrated Care Pathways (ICPs), 303–5
Integrins, inhibition of, 169–70
Interferon beta, 24, 38–9
 actions of, 38–9
Interferon beta-1a therapy, 38–64
 adverse effects, 49–50
 autoantibodies, 51
 clinical issues, 52–63
  clinical relevance for long-term
   disability, 62–3
  dose–response effects, 54–62
  heterogeneity, 52–4
 clinical trials, 41–9
  Multiple Sclerosis Collaborative
   Research Group Trial (MSCRG),
   44–5
  new clinical trials, 63–4
  Once-Weekly Interferon for MS Trial
   (OWIMS), 45–6
 Prevention of Relapses and Disability by
  Interferon beta-1a
 Subcutaneously in Multiple Sclerosis
  (PRISMS) trial, 46–9
 neutralizing antibodies, 51–2
 pharmacokinetics, 40
 pilot studies, 41
 safety, 49–50
Interferon beta-1b therapy, 24–34

adverse effects, 30
clinical usage, 33–4
depression and, 289
effect in secondary progressive disease,
 31–2, 148–51
history of, 24
mechanism of action, 25
molecular structure, 24–5
neutralizing antibodies, 30–1
pilot trial, 25–6
pivotal trial, 26–30
 first publication, 26–9
 MRI results, 29
 primary endpoints, 28
 second publication, 29–30
 secondary endpoints, 28–9
Interferon gamma, 25
International Classification of
 Impairments, Activities and
 Participation (ICIDH), 303
Intravenous immunoglobulin (IVIg)
 therapy, 95–106
 current role of in MS treatment, 105–6
 immunoglobulin properties, 95–6
 interval treatment of
  relapsing–remitting MS, 101–4
 mechanisms of action, 96–100
  effects on immune system
   components, 98–100
  effects on remyelination, 100, 171
  reduction of fixed deficit, 104
 side effects, 104–5
Intravenous methylprednisolone (IVMP)
 treatment, 16, 18–19
 cyclical pulses for progressive disease
  management, 153–4
 practical guidelines, 19–20
 See also Steroid treatment
Isoniazid, tremor management, 230–2
 mechanism of action, 232
Italian multicentre controlled trial,
 mitoxantrone, 136–7

Laughing, pathological, 293
Left ventricular ejection fraction (LVEF),
 mitoxantrone therapy and, 140
Lifestyle changes, 248
Lithium carbonate, bipolar affective
 disorder treatment, 290
Lorazepam, psychosis treatment, 292

Magnetic resonance imaging (MRI), 4–5
 American multicentre study, 81–2
 azathioprine effects, 115
 European–Canadian Study, 82–6

mitoxantrone studies, 133–5, 137
Major histocompatibility class II antigens (MHC), 72–3
Manic-depressive psychosis, *See* Bipolar affective disorder
Matrix metalloproteinases (MMPs), 170, 172
Medicated urethral system for erection (MUSE), 273–4
Metalloproteinases, 170
Methotrexate therapy (MTX), 151–3
Methylprednisolone treatment, *See* Intravenous methylprednisolone (IVMP) treatment
Mitoxantrone (Mx) therapy, 131–44
  animal model studies, 132
  clinical trials:
    controlled phase III MIMS trial, 137–8
    French and British multicentre controlled trial, 133–6
    Gd-DTPA enhanced MRI, 133
    Italian multicentre controlled trial, 136–7
    single-arm open-label trials, 132–3
  mechanism of action, 131, 143
  pharmacology, 131
  role in progressive disease, 142, 156–7
  role in very active disease, 142
  sequential treatment, 144
  short- versus long-term clinical efficacy, 142–3
  toxicity profile, 138–41
    bone marrow depression, 139
    cardiotoxicity, 139–40, 143
    effects on usage, 143
    gonadal function, 140–1
    treatment after mitoxantrone therapy, 143–4
Monoclonal antibody therapy, 166
MS-Specific Fatigue Scale, 244
Multiple sclerosis:
  aetiology, 2–3
  definition of, 2
  disease process, 3
  impact on the individual, 300
  progression of disability, 6–7
  types of, 5–6
Multiple Sclerosis Collaborative Research Group (MSCRG), interferon beta-1a clinical trial, 44–5
MUSE (medicated urethral system for erection), 273–4
Myelin basic protein (MBP), 71, 72–5, 164–5

Myelin oligodendrocyte glycoprotein (MOG), 73

N-acetyl aspartate (NAA), 171–2
Neuroleptic medications, 292–3
Neurotoxins, 202–3
  See also Botulinum toxin
Neutralizing antibodies:
  botulinum toxin, 209–11
  interferon beta-1a, 51–2
  interferon beta-1b, 30–1
Non-Hodgkin's lymphoma, azathioprine therapy and, 124
North American secondary progressive MS (NASPMS) trial, 149–51
Novantrone®, *See* Mitoxantrone

Occupational therapy, ataxia management, 237
Olanzapine, psychosis treatment, 292
Once-Weekly Interferon for MS Trial (OWIMS), 45–6
Ondansetron, tremor management, 233
Optic neuritis, 16–17, 19, 104
Orphrenadrine, spasticity treatment, 194
Orthoses, ataxia and tremor management, 236–7
Outcome measures, 305–6
  spasticity treatment, 186
Oxybutynin, detrusor hyper-reflexia treatment, 264–5

Papaverine, erectile dysfunction management, 273
Pathological laughing and crying (PLC), 293
Pemoline, fatigue treatment, 249
  relative efficacy, 249–50
Phenol, intrathecal, spasticity treatment, 195
Physiotherapy, ataxia management, 237
Prednisolone treatment, 17–18, 19
  guidelines, 20
Prevention of Relapses and Disability by Interferon beta-1a Subcutaneously in Multiple Sclerosis (PRISMS) trial, 46–9
Primary progressive disease (PP), *See* Progressive disease
Progressive disease:
  primary progressive disease (PP), 5–6
  secondary progressive disease (SP), 5–6, 148, 181–2
  treatments for, 148–58
    2-chlorodeoxyadenosine, 155–6

choice of therapy, 157–8
cyclical pulses of intravenous
    methylprednisolone, 153–4
cyclophosphamide, 155
glatiramer acetate therapy, 86–8
interferon beta-1a therapy, 63–4
interferon beta-1b therapy, 31–2,
    142, 148–51
methotrexate therapy (MTX), 151–3
mitoxantrone, 142, 156–7
steroid therapy, 17–18
treatment strategies, 181–2
trial results, 155–7
Propranolol, tremor management, 233
Prostaglandin E1, See Alprostadil
Prostheses, erectile dysfunction
    management, 274–5
Proteolipid protein (PLP), 73
Psychosis, 291–3
    treatment, 292–3
Psychotherapy, 289
Psychotropic medication, 282–4
    See also Specific drugs

QALYs, 116

Rebif®, 39–40
    Once-Weekly Interferon for MS Trial
        (OWIMS), 45–6
Prevention of Relapses and Disability by
    Interferon beta-1a
        Subcutaneously in Multiple
    Sclerosis (PRISMS) trial,
    46–9
    See also Interferon beta-1a therapy
Rehabilitation, 299–311
    assessment and selection, 301
    clinical trials, 306–11
        evaluating the component parts, 306
        evaluating the package of care,
        306–11
    collaboration with health, social and
        voluntary
        service sectors, 302
    individually tailored approach, 301–2
    measuring the effectiveness of, 302–6
        Integrated Care Pathways (ICPs),
        303–5
        measuring outcome, 302–3
        outcome measures, 305–6
    multidisciplinary team approach, 301
Relapsing–remitting disease, 118
    azathioprine therapy, 116–19
        odds ratio of remaining relapse free,
        117

relapse rate, 117–19
glatiramer acetate therapy, 75–86
    American multicentre study, 77–82
    European–Canadian Study, 82–6
    first double-blind, placebo-controlled
        trial, 76–7
interferon beta-1a therapy, 44–63
interferon beta-1b therapy, 25–30
interval immunoglobulin treatment,
    101–4
mitoxantrone, 133–38
steroid use, 18–19
    clinical efficacy, 15–17
    practical guidelines, 19–20
treatment strategies, 178–80
    current practice amongst
        neurologists, 18–19
    with moderate cumulative disability,
        179–80
    with no/minor cumulative disability,
        178–9
Remyelination:
    immunoglobulin effects on, 100, 171
    promotion of, 171
Resiniferatoxin (RTX), bladder
        dysfunction management,
        267–8
Rheumatoid arthritis (RA), 151–2
Risperidone, psychosis treatment, 293

St John's wort, depression treatment, 290
Secondary progressive disease (SP), See
        Progressive disease
Selective serotonin reuptake inhibitors
        (SSRIs), depression
    treatment, 287–8
Self-catheterization, 263–4, 265–6
Sequential treatment, 144
Sexual dysfunction, 258, 269–72
    in men, 271–2
        ejaculatory failure, 275
        See also Erectile dysfunction
    in women, 270–1
Side effects:
    azathioprine, 121–4
    baclofen, 190
    clonidine, 193
    diazepam, 188
    glatiramer acetate, 88–9
    interferon beta-1a, 49–50
    interferon beta-1b, 30
    intravenous immunoglobulin (IVIg),
        104–5
    mitoxantrone, 138–41
    tizanidine, 193

Sildenafil citrate (Viagra), erectile
dysfunction
management, 274
Sleep disturbance, 246
Spasticity, 184–5, 201
botulinum toxin treatment, *See*
Botulinum toxin
non-pharmacological treatment, 186–7
pharmacological treatment, 187–95
baclofen, 189–91, 195
cannabis, 194–5
clonidine, 192–4
dantrolene sodium, 191–2
diazepam, 187–9
GABA agonists, 194
general points, 187
intrathecal usage, 195
orphrenadrine, 194
phenol, 195
L-threonine, 194
tizanidine, 192–4
treatment goals, 185
treatment outcome measures, 186
Staphylococcal B antigen, 72
Stereotactic thalamotomy, tremor
management, 234–6
Steroid treatment:
possible modes of action, 14–15
stabilization of blood–brain barrier,
15
progressive disease, 17–18, 153–4
relapses, 15–17, 18–19
practical guidelines, 19–20
steroid-induced mania, 291
See also Intravenous
methylprednisolone (IVMP)
treatment
Steroid-dependency, 17
Systemic lupus erythematosus (SLE), 244

T-cell receptor (TCR) immunotherapy,
164–5
T-cells:
immunoglobulin effects on, 98
neutralization of activation markers,
166–8
bone marrow transplantation, 167–8
chimeric and humanized monoclonal
antibodies, 166
cytokine based treatments, 166–7
Talipes equino-varus foot, botulinum toxin
injection, 222

Teratogenicity, azathioprine, 123
Tetrahydrocannabinol, ataxia and tremor
management, 233–4
Thalamic stimulation, tremor
management, 236
L-Threonine, spasticity treatment, 194
Tissue inhibitors of matrix
metalloproteinases (TIMP), 170
Tizanidine, spasticity treatment, 192–4
clinical efficacy, 193
dosage, 193
mechanism of action, 192
pharmacology, 192–3
side effects, 193
Tolterodine, detrusor hyper-reflexia
treatment, 265
Toxicity, *See* Side effects
Transforming growth factor beta (TGFβ),
25
Tremor, 228–37
basis of, 229
classification of, 228–9
management, 230–7
cannabinoids, 233–4
carbamazepine, 233
glutethimide, 232–3
isoniazid, 230–2
ondansetron, 233
orthoses, 236–7
propranolol, 233
stereotactic thalamotomy, 234–6
tetrahydrocannabinol, 233–4
thalamic stimulation, 236
Tricyclic antidepressants, 287, 288
Trospium chloride, detrusor hyper-reflexia
treatment, 265
Tumor necrosis factor (TNF) antagonists,
167

Upper motor neurone (UMN) syndrome,
184–5

Vacuum constriction devices, erectile
dysfunction
management, 273
Valproic acid, bipolar affective disorder
treatment, 290
Viagra, erectile dysfunction management,
274

Yohimbine, ejaculatory failure
management, 275